The DOCTOR *in History*

The DOCTOR *in History*

By

HOWARD W. HAGGARD

ASSOCIATE PROFESSOR OF APPLIED PHYSIOLOGY
IN YALE UNIVERSITY

DORSET PRESS
New York

THIS BOOK

IS HOPEFULLY DEDICATED TO

HOWARD JR., WILLIAM II, AND MARJORIE MARIE

This edition published by Dorset Press
a division of Marboro Books Corporation
by arrangement with The Estate of Howard Haggard
1989 Dorset Press
ISBN 0-88029-437-X
Printed in the United States of America
M 9 8 7 6 5 4 3 2 1

Preface

DAUDET, presumably with a view to their moral sophistication, wrote *Sapho* for his children to read when they were twenty-one. Chesterfield wrote his letters in the interest of his son's social elegance. I know nothing of the effect on Daudet's children; Chesterfield's son did not appear to benefit. Nevertheless, hopeful, as parents will be, I have followed the example and written this book for my children. Not, let me hasten to say, for their morals or their manners. Perhaps it is a reflection of changing times, or possibly merely of my own interests, that I am frankly concerned less with these matters than I am with some other aspects of their education and their health—especially their health.

What I have tried to write for them is a history of health. I have little doubt that their generation will live to see this new kind of history come much to the front—the movement is rapid in that direction. History as the older of us knew it in school was almost wholly the story of man's struggle against man and against geographical barriers. We saw the pageant of human affairs through the eyes of the explorer, the warrior, the politician, the economist, the priest, even the refugee and the slave, but we did not see it with the doctor or the humanitarian. And that in spite of the fact that man's greatest and longest struggle has been to survive against disease.

Before us today an epoch in medicine is beginning. The physician is regaining a social leadership lost 2300 years ago when medicine was separated from religion. Medicine is rapidly ceasing to be a private matter of the bedchamber; it is becoming a guiding influence in everyday life. Now—and it will be even more obvious in the future—for the sake of health, medical matters must be known, must be interpreted correctly by the layman.

This educational aspect was once called hygiene—but hygiene of the kind we knew in school is a failure. I have taught for many years what is generally called hygiene and I have gained from the experience a thorough conviction of the inadequacy of the so-called rules of health. I should prefer my children to think logically and soundly on the social matters of medicine in these years of faddism, quackery, and commercially exploited "health appeal," than to be able to recite glibly the hygienic dicta of today, many of which will surely become the absurdities of tomorrow. On the other hand, the history of health is the clue to the logic of modern medicine; if people know the past they will be able to interpret the present.

That is what I had in mind when I wrote these pages. But having written them, I doubt my complete sincerity. I wonder, too, if Daudet and Chesterfield were wholly honest in their purpose. Was it entirely guidance they sought to give? Or were they led on by the hope, the parent's longing so often doomed to disappointment, that sons and daughters will feel a kindred enthusiasm for scenes and deeds that stirred the parent?

The scenes and deeds of medicine are not to be comprehended in the sentimental story of the "good fight" for the sake of humanity. They are part, rather, of the grim tale of man's ignorance and hope, his life and death. I want my children to see the reeking, sweating, savage medicine man struggling with the spirits of disease—the savage who gave us the principle of nearly everything we have in medicine today and much besides that we have tried to get rid of. I want them to join the temple throngs and pay their respects to Imhotep and Æsculapius; stand for a moment beside the philosophers who rescued medicine from religion and beside the physicians who rescued it from the philosophers. I want them to meet Galen, admire his intellect and condone his egotism. I want them to see the jigsaw puzzle of medieval scholasticism, hear the vulgar words of Paracelsus, and follow Paré through court intrigue and battle. I want them to recognize the primitive medicine man disguised as King of England, the mountebank of the street corner, and the quasi-scientist of today. I want them to witness the rise of mental contagions, and see civilizations crumble before disease and rise again with the aid of medical discovery. . . . I want them to follow the Doctor in History.

I wish to express here my thanks for the valuable suggestions and criticisms of my friends Professor Samuel Harvey and Professor Erwin Goodenough who read the manuscript in preparation. To Miss Ella Holliday of the Yale University Press I extend my gratitude for her tireless effort in checking dates and quotations.

HOWARD W. HAGGARD

Contents

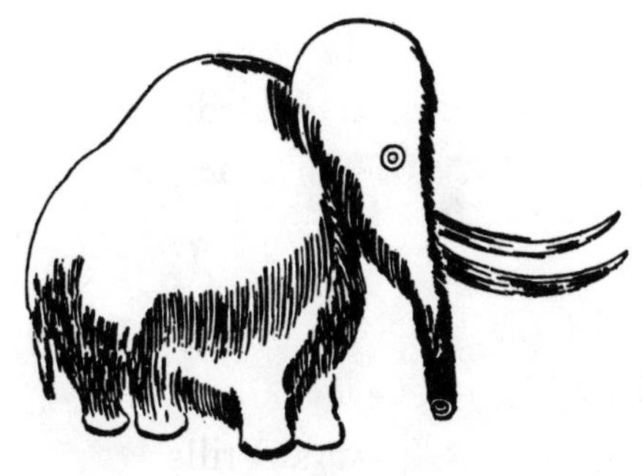

Part One

AN UNKNOWN HERO OF MEDICINE

SPIRITS, DEMONS, GHOSTS, AND WITCHES

THEORIES AND FACTS

THE DOCTOR IN HISTORY

CHAPTER I

An Unknown Hero of Medicine

DISEASE is older than man.

There were no men in the Age of Reptiles, in those days before the surface of the land was for the last time covered with a blanket of ice. But there were diseases.

The story of disease is written in records of rock and soil. We find in the fossil remains of gigantic dinosaurs the signs of injuries. There are broken bones, the only record of some mighty struggle to the death enacted perhaps a hundred million years ago. There are traces to show that broken bones had healed in some great beast that once limped across a world man never saw.

Such injuries were to be expected; what is more important is that there are signs of infection. Dinosaurs, cave bears, and saber-toothed tigers had toothache; their fossil teeth show cavities and decay. In prehistoric bones there are roughened spongy places, traces left by a sort of rheumatism of the joints. In one skeleton of a horned dinosaur that has been uncovered there are marks of an abscess of the leg that once held nearly half a gallon of pus.

We know today that all infections are caused by living parasites that grow upon the flesh, parasites such as bacteria.

There were disease bacteria before there were men.

Many hundreds of centuries ago the forces were being marshaled, the scene set, for the great struggle which was in time to confront the human race—disease against man and man against disease.

Then like a curtain separating the acts in a play, the glacial period descended upon the Continent of Europe. For centuries the ice lay upon lands barren of life. Gradually it began to melt. A new scene opened, another era began, and a new actor appeared upon the stage—man.

Thirty or forty thousand years ago the glacier was slowly moving back toward the mountains. Streams from the melting ice were cutting wide valleys in the land. The level of the ocean was rising, but still it had not yet covered the strip of land that connected England with the continent. There was no English Channel. The Baltic Sea was a great fresh-water lake. The weather was still cold, but the air was becoming drier, and dust storms swept across the land. Along the seacoast forests were springing up; inland there were wind-swept prairies sparsely grown with grass, widening each year as the ice receded.

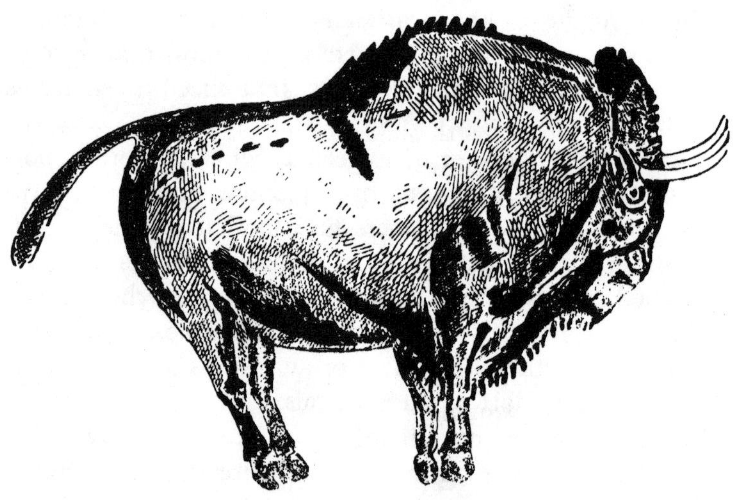

A bison painted on the wall of a cave by a prehistoric artist.

It was the grass, always the grass, that drew the animals to the new-found prairies. Slowly, over centuries, they came, first the warm fur animals; then, as the climate changed, the thin-coated grazing animals.

Their story, like that of the great reptiles before them, is written in records of rock and soil. From fossil bones we can identify the woolly rhinoceros, the mammoth with enormous tusks, the musk-ox, the bison, the reindeer, and the wild horse. The horses came in droves, queer little ponies with tufted beards like goats.

In the wake of the grass-eaters followed the animals of prey; the bear, the fox, the cave hyena—and man. He came across North Africa, following the slow migration into the new lands of a changing world. These men who followed the reindeer and horses into France were not the first to live there. But they were the first men of whom we have record who looked like modern men. The earlier inhabitants were not handsome by our standards nor were they, we should judge, intelligent. They were short and stocky, with bowed legs, overhanging brows, receding chins. They were probably more savage, more primitive and beastlike than any people living today, even in the most remote jungle.

Our story concerns the reindeer men and they, at least in appearance, do not suffer by comparison with modern men, for they were giant fellows, well over six feet tall, straight bodied, strong limbed, large headed. We call them Cro-Magnon men because it was in the Cro-Magnon caves at Dordogne, France, that the remains they left were first discovered.

The reason why these people have an especial interest for our story is that among them we find the first record of a doctor.

Twenty thousand years ago the struggle between man and disease was already under way. A leader had been chosen to direct the forces that men employed to fight for health and life.

We have no records to tell us what sort of a struggle the earliest men, those bowlegged squat fellows of fifty thousand years ago, made against disease. But we can guess and guess closely. Certainly they had no doctors. Probably they had no tribes or tribal organization, but lived in scattered families made up of a leader followed by a few women with their babies. Their life was hard and cruel and short. Men, women, and children suffered from accidents and diseases. But they knew, we are sure, little more about how to cure or prevent disease or treat the injuries from accidents than do brute beasts.

An animal struggles alone against disease or injury; none of its kind helps it. The crippled beast hides from others, lest it be torn to pieces; it licks its sores in solitude; sick, it crawls into a dark corner to die unattended. No doubt the earliest men behaved in the same way when confronted with accident and disease. The hale man killed the injured man and took for himself his skins and weapons; the sick savage died neglected, shunned by his companions. Such primitive men did not even bury their dead.

Sympathy, the willingness to aid the injured and the ill, to enlist in their defense against disease, was the first forward step in man's struggle against disease. No man can fight sickness alone, and least of all the man to whom disease has come.

This sympathy in some measure at least had developed among the Cro-Magnon people twenty thousand years and more ago, for, as we have said, their tribes had leaders in the struggle against disease—medicine men. We must not think of these primitive doctors as being like modern doctors. Their medical practice was as primitive as were their weapons and their homes. But they deserve a place in our story because as far as we know they were the first among men to join together in the struggle against disease. They gave us the first principle of medicine, a very important one: that there shall be men whose duty it is to devote themselves to the care of the sick and injured, to use their efforts to save their companions from disease. These primitive tribesmen originated the doctor.

Hundreds of centuries before the Christian Era, the Cro-Magnon people vanished; they either died off entirely or were absorbed into other tribes of men that came later. The climate of the lands where they lived changed, forests grew up, the animals they had hunted disappeared. Forest tribesmen far more civilized than they came into their lands. In

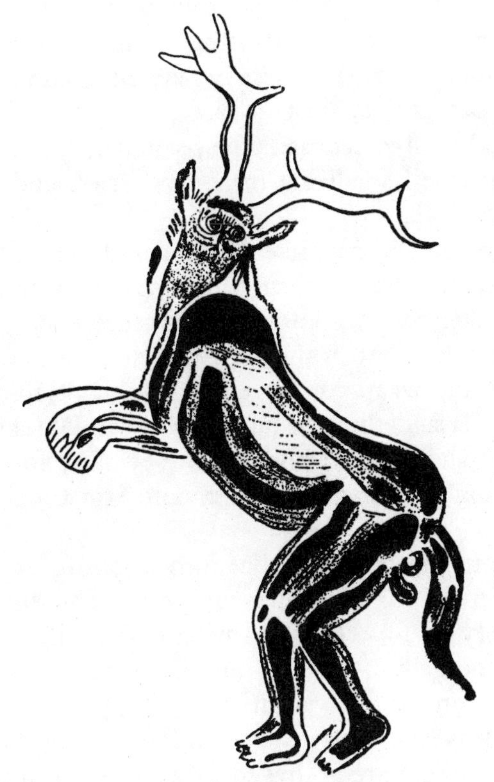

The Cro-Magnon medicine man dressed in his ceremonial costume.

time from the East there arrived men in steel helmets—the Romans—advancing civilization, driving back the barbarians. Then in turn the barbarians drove back the Roman legions, but civilization lingered. Castles arose and feudal lords reigned, then kings. Wars were fought over the lands where the Cro-Magnon men once chased wild horses. Cities grew, fields and orchards spread across the land. Factories were built, railroads spanned the countryside, automobiles sped over paved roads, perhaps carrying the modern doctor to his patient, and steamboats churned their way through rivers where the Cro-Magnon man had once speared fish. The panorama of recorded history unfolded over the land where he had lived and where he had enlisted in man's first organized struggle against disease.

For two hundred centuries the records of the Cro-Magnon people and their medicine men lay buried undisturbed in caves in the hills.

These people did not, like the savages before them, desert their dead; they buried them with ornaments and weapons. From the skeletons we know their stature and build. From the remains they left in the caves which were their homes—stone tools and weapons, carved bones and perforated skulls—we can tell something of how they lived. We can tell even more: how they looked and what they saw, for they have left amazing paintings on the smooth stone walls of deep caverns.

It was only in our time that men began to explore these caves, deserted for thousands of years. The entrances are often merely narrow clefts at the base of a hill, perhaps partially submerged in streams and now nearly sealed with stalactites formed by centuries of dripping water. From them the way leads into upper galleries, long, high-walled caves where there are hollowed rocks into which grease was once poured to form crude lamps. There are pictures on the walls of these chambers—bison in red and black, half-finished sketches of reindeer, and drawings of wild horses.

The paintings are mostly of animals—flat-looking one-sided pictures, lacking the foreshortening that gives perspective and a sense of depth. They are, in fact, much like the paintings made by the early American Indians.

You would hardly believe that these paintings could have

survived for twenty thousand years, but they have, and for a peculiar reason. The Cro-Magnon artists used grease paint, and the grease has preserved the colors against moist air and trickling water. The grease was the fat from some animal, tallow mixed with colored dirt and pushed inside a piece of broken bone—not a bad sort of paint tube for a primitive artist.

There is one cave in particular at Ariège, France, that holds our attention. It was discovered by the three sons of Count Begouën and is called in their honor *Trois Frères*—the three brothers. It contains one of the few prehistoric pictures of a man—a Cro-Magnon medicine man. This is the first known representation of a doctor.

He is shown dressed fantastically in the skin of an animal. On his head he wears the antlers of a reindeer; his ears look like those of a bear; on his hands are mittens with claws; a long flowing beard and the tail of a horse complete his costume.

He is half crouching as if in the step of a ceremonial dance, and he presides over the painted animals as he did in life, when through his magic he brought game to the hunters of his tribe and kept his people free from disease. He is the Cro-Magnon sorcerer—and doctor.

The Cro-Magnon people had no written or picture language. Such things came much later. We do not know, and never shall, the name of this primitive doctor. We shall never know what feats of magic he performed, what wonderful cures he effected. But we do know that his companions turned to him for aid in illness. He was the early leader in man's struggle against disease.

To him and his kind we today owe the principle of medicine: that there shall be doctors to lead men in a united warfare against disease.

CHAPTER II

Spirits, Demons, Ghosts, and Witches

WE owe to primitive man the origin of the doctor and the beginning of medicine. But such a queer creature is man that, having pointed the direction and taken the first steps toward the control of disease, he lost his way and wandered into a maze of bypaths that led him not to science but to magic and mystery and superstition. In consequence for hundreds of centuries he fought a sham battle with disease in a region where disease does not exist.

The thing that led him astray was a belief, a false belief which held back the progress of medicine for thousands of years. Until it was discarded, all the meager advances resulted from accident and chance.

Primitive man believed that disease came not from natural causes but from supernatural ones; that it arose from the action of unfriendly spirits, ghosts, and demons, or from witchcraft. It was accordingly to be prevented and treated by magic directed against supernatural forces.

The greatest single advance ever made in controlling disease was not the acquiring of something new but the giving up of something that was old—the discarding of a false belief. The great difference between the futile efforts of the Cro-Magnon medicine man and the success of the modern doctor in treating and preventing disease is not so much in their relative skills as in their opposing beliefs. The Cro-Magnon medicine man, because of his beliefs, attempted to treat disease by dealing with spirits and ghosts; the modern doctor attempts to deal with the facts of nature. The one fought a sham battle; the other meets the enemy in reality.

We have spoken here as if we knew what the beliefs of the Cro-Magnon medicine man were. The only record we have of him is his picture. But in spite of that we do know what he believed about disease as well as if we had lived with him and spoken his language. His costume gives us the clue to his beliefs. It was the ceremonial dress he wore to frighten away the evil spirits that tormented his tribesmen with disease. We know his beliefs because of another reason—a curious one: All the medicine men of all primitive peoples in all times of which we have any record have held, and still hold the same beliefs about disease, and used the same measures to contend against it.

You could go as an explorer to some little-known tropical island where there are primitive people and learn the beliefs of the medicine man. You would find that he thought that disease was caused by spirits and demons and ghosts, and that his tribesmen believed that illness could be cured only by magic and witchcraft. Or you could land thousands of miles away in Africa and trek far into the interior to a people who had never heard of the Islanders, who spoke a different language, were a different race, and you would find that they too believed that disease was caused by spirits and demons and ghosts. Explore wherever you wish, among primitive peoples, and you will always discover beliefs similar to those held by the Cro-Magnon medicine man.

Turn to the records of our Indians. They once thought that spirits were the cause of disease. On page 12 is a picture of a medicine man of the Blackfoot tribe, dressed in his professional costume. He wears the hide of the uncommon yellow bear; strung to it are skins of snakes, frogs, and mice, the feathers of birds, and the hoofs of the deer and goat. In one hand he holds a decorated wand and in the other a rattle. When called to treat a sick man, he brandished the wand and shook the rattle, hopped and jumped about his patient, gave wild Indian yells, growled like a bear, and ordered the demon of disease to depart.

We find these same beliefs among the Druids of ancient Britain, among the barbarians who once roamed the forests of Germany, and in the ancient records of Egypt, Babylon, Greece, and Rome. As we go on with our story we shall dis-

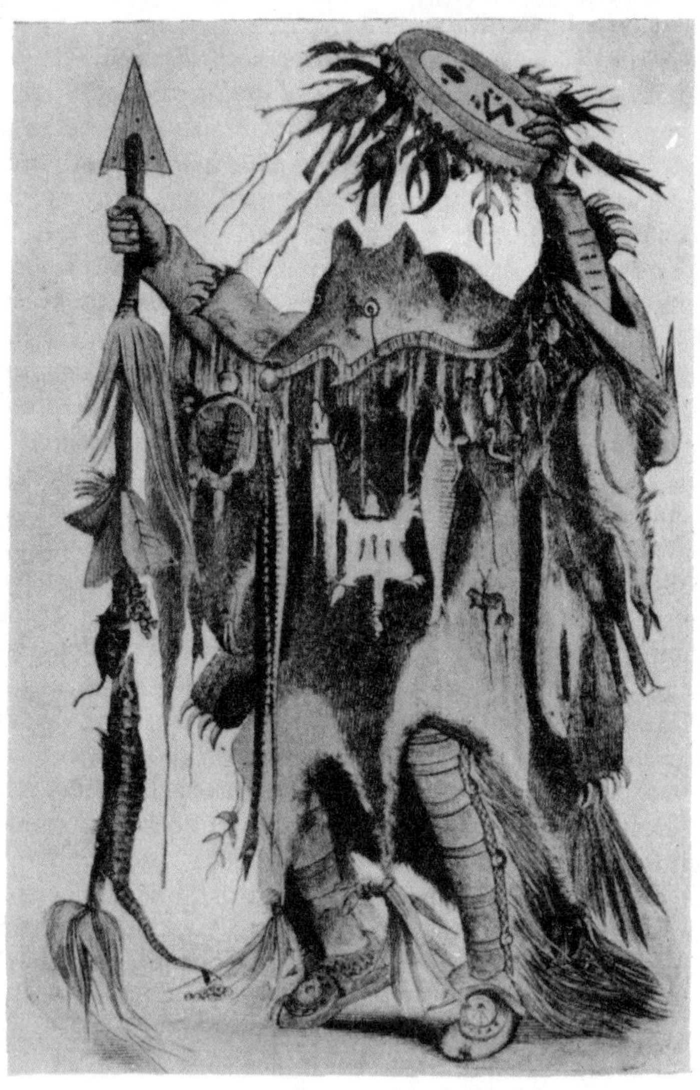

Medicine man of the Blackfoot Indians dressed in his professional costume.

cover that the idea of the supernatural origin of disease has persisted in civilization and exists in our own time.

You perhaps may wonder—great scientists certainly have—how it happened that all primitive peoples, although they lived widely separated, shared this common belief concerning disease. Some scientists think that the idea was carried from a common center during ancient migrations of people or was spread by travel in days when there was more land above the water than there is now and tribes were not cut off and isolated. The Cro-Magnon men when they came out of North Africa brought their beliefs with them, as did the Lake Dwellers who migrated into Europe after them. The American Indians, the Eskimos, the Islanders, the Africans migrated centuries ago to the lands where they are now. We do not know where they came from. Did the basic idea concerning disease spring from one common meeting place and so spread everywhere? It is possible. Also it is true that once primitive peoples adopt a belief they do not readily change it, but keep it unaltered for centuries; they are the victims of tradition even more than are civilized men.

The theory of migration does not, however, explain at all where or why belief in spirits as a cause of disease arose, but merely tells how it may have spread.

Other scientists do not consider migration necessary to account for this uniform belief. They think that there may have been no common source, but that the idea arose many times quite independently and would occur naturally among any untutored men living the life of savages.

Men are very much alike everywhere. They differ, of course, in strength and size and color and certainly in intelligence, but always their natural tendency is to reason about the dangers of life in a certain way. This peculiarly human way of reasoning accounts for the ideas that made spirits the cause of disease.

By extensive education the natural faults of reasoning can be corrected. Native people were, of course, educated, but not to this extent. They were trained in the folkways of their people and in tribal tradition. Beyond these things their education did not go. The child educated in civilized surroundings is, for the first ten or twelve years of his schooling, trained in precisely the same things—the folkways and traditions of his people. During the centuries of civilization many facts have been accumulated; folkways and traditions have changed. The school child of today has knowledge of many things unknown to the savages and, if he continues with his education, he may go beyond the stage of the mere acquiring of knowledge; he may learn to correct his faults of reasoning and to think independently. That is an ideal of education held only by civilized peoples.

Unfortunately, education is not hereditary; we are born ignorant and untrained. If a child of civilized and educated parents were placed among savages and raised by them, he would grow up to think and believe as they do. This has happened, and the child—unlike the heroes of some jungle tales—did not become superior in education to the natives, or teach himself to read and write, or learn to think logically. He remained an ignorant savage with the savage's beliefs and fears.

Primitive man is like a child not yet educated to think independently, but a child without parents to protect him. In spite of his ignorance he must take all responsibilities himself. He is a man; and he is confronted by the most serious things that can occur to men—disease, injury, and death. From these things he wants to escape, to protect himself. But his thoughts on the problems of health and disease, life and death, are guided only by the peculiar and natural qualities that are always in the human mind, that we are born with.

Curiosity is one of these qualities; no education is required for its attainment. Conceit or egotism is another. Egotism makes us believe that what we accomplish successfully is due to our own fine qualities, and that what we do poorly is owing to no fault of our own but to some outside influence. Like the savage, we all wish to take credit for our success and to blame our failures on someone else.

Native peoples confronted by disease blamed their misfortunes on something other than their own ignorance, on something outside themselves. Because they were curious they sought the influences that brought their misfortunes. They found them in spirits.

Men from the very beginning have seen their companions killed or injured by falling trees, gored or trampled by animals, knocked down or murdered by other men. In each case there was a cause for the misfortune. The tree that fell, the animal that turned, the man that struck, were the visible agents of misfortune. But men also saw their companions fall ill, suffer, and die when nothing visible had injured them. Since, so reasoned the savage, the effects were there—the pain and death—there must be an agent. It was invisible but still it must exist—a malicious, vindictive "something."

Invisible forces then could bring misfortune. But where were they? What were they?

Dreams and motion supplied the material for the solution of the problem. In his dreams primitive man saw men he knew were far away or dead. He saw animals that threatened him. He awoke in fear, but the bodies of the men or animals were no longer there.

Men and animals, so reasoned the savage, have then something—let us call it a spirit—which can separate from them and travel long distances, which persists even after death.

He reasoned further: Men and animals have spirits; men and animals are alive; things that are alive move; movement means life. The water in the rivers moves, the clouds in the skies move, the branches of the trees move, the sun and moon and stars seem to move; the wind moves. These things must be alive; being alive they must have spirits.

Like a small child, the savage made no clear distinction

between living and nonliving things. When he stepped on a bent stick and the end flew up and struck him, he turned and kicked the stick to get even with it. When he slipped and fell in a mud puddle, he might throw a rock into the water for vengeance, because it had been unkind to him.

Primitive men think of everything about them as having the qualities of men. The trees can talk, the thunder is the voice of a great spirit, the sun eats up the moon each day, the rocks that men stumble over have deliberately crawled into the path. Such things sound much like fairy tales. And so they are. When the small child of today reads and prattles of whispering brooks and animals that talk, of good fairies and roaring giants, he is living over in play the things that were serious to savage men.

It was not in play that primitive man peopled the world with spirits. Spirits were the invisible agents of misfortune. A spirit could attack a man, hurt him, kill him.

Sometimes a man's own spirit left him for a time. Then the man fell down as if dead, but when his spirit returned, he came to life again. We should say he had fainted or was unconscious.

Occasionally a wandering spirit found its way into a man's body, crawled into it, and overcame the man's true spirit. Such a man might speak with a queer voice and behave in most peculiar ways. His body was possessed by a strange spirit, said the savage; we should say that he was insane.

Again a man thus possessed might throw himself on the ground and writhe and squirm and beat his arms and legs against the earth. Surely, reasoned the savage, no spirit would so abuse the body to which it rightfully belonged. Here, said he, is proof that an alien spirit has entered the body; we should say the man had a fit.

The belief in spirits offered an explanation for every misfortune that could happen to men. And what is more, it satisfied curiosity as to the cause of misfortune and it pleased conceit. Misfortunes could be blamed on the spirits. It was a very satisfying belief indeed.

You would call these beliefs of the savage superstitions. And so they are if people hold them today. Among primitive peoples they were not superstitions. A superstition is a belief derived logically, but from ideas that are not consistent with generally prevailing knowledge. When a savage, seeing his image in a mirror, believed that it was his spirit looking at him, he was following the ideas thought to be true by all of his people. If he broke a mirror, he believed that bad luck would come to him, for he had injured his spirit. His reasoning was logical. He was not truly superstitious; he was ignorant. When, on the other hand, men learned the principles of optics and knew the image to be merely a reflection of light, then the belief that it was a spirit became a false idea, one no longer consistent with generally prevailing knowledge. To believe that a broken mirror brought bad luck thus became merely a superstition.

Nearly every superstition that exists today is a survival of the beliefs that primitive men developed to account for their misfortunes. You have seen superstitious people do something, such as tapping wood, to prevent the bad luck they expect. This is to drive away the evil spirits and the ghosts and demons that may be lingering about. A childish idea, of course, but a serious matter to ignorant peoples. Ideas like this guided primitive man in his struggle against disease.

For him there were literally thousands of things that he must or must not do to keep away the spirits that brought illness. Of course the details of these acts varied among different tribes, but they existed everywhere. Food must be eaten in a certain way, caves or tents entered in a special manner, spears stacked in a peculiar position, charms carried as lucky pieces, like a rabbit's foot, or like a horse-chestnut to prevent rheumatism, and so on through the range of every conceivable act. Today we sometimes think we are trammeled and cramped by the conventions of social etiquette, but we are free compared with primitive man who imposed upon himself prohibitions for every act of life.

When, in spite of constant "wood tapping and salt throwing," so to speak, bad luck came to the savage, as it often did, it was the business of the medicine man to set matters right. He was the one who was nearest to the spirits, who knew where they lived and how to frighten or bribe them away. He had developed many methods of controlling them. Some spirits disliked noises, others feared water, some dashed away when smoke was about, and many disappeared into thin air when certain magic words were spoken.

The medicine man built his treatment into a ceremony. He came to the patient and "made medicine." His efforts were always intended to remove the evil spirits that he imagined caused the illness. He dressed to impress the spirits and carried charms to make them obey him; he danced, he shouted, he shook his rattle, and made a frightful din about the sick man to frighten the demons away. Sometimes he threw water over the invalid or even dipped him in a stream. He filled the tent with smoke. He gave the man vile tasting medicines to make his body unpleasant for the spirits. And finally he mumbled curious words that no one except the medicine man and the spirit could understand, and produced weird and rare things to convince the spirits of his powers—a deformed frog, a snake with legs, or, in modern times, as a result of contact with civilized people, a broken dollar watch, or a collar button.

The antics of the medicine man had no influence upon the nonexistent spirits, but they did make a deep impression on those who watched him. The medicine man did everything possible to increase the awe in which he was held. He lived apart from other men, he behaved differently, he dressed differently. He never missed an opportunity to impress upon people that he was different from other men; he controlled the spirits. It was this belief held by his companions that gave him his main influence upon disease.

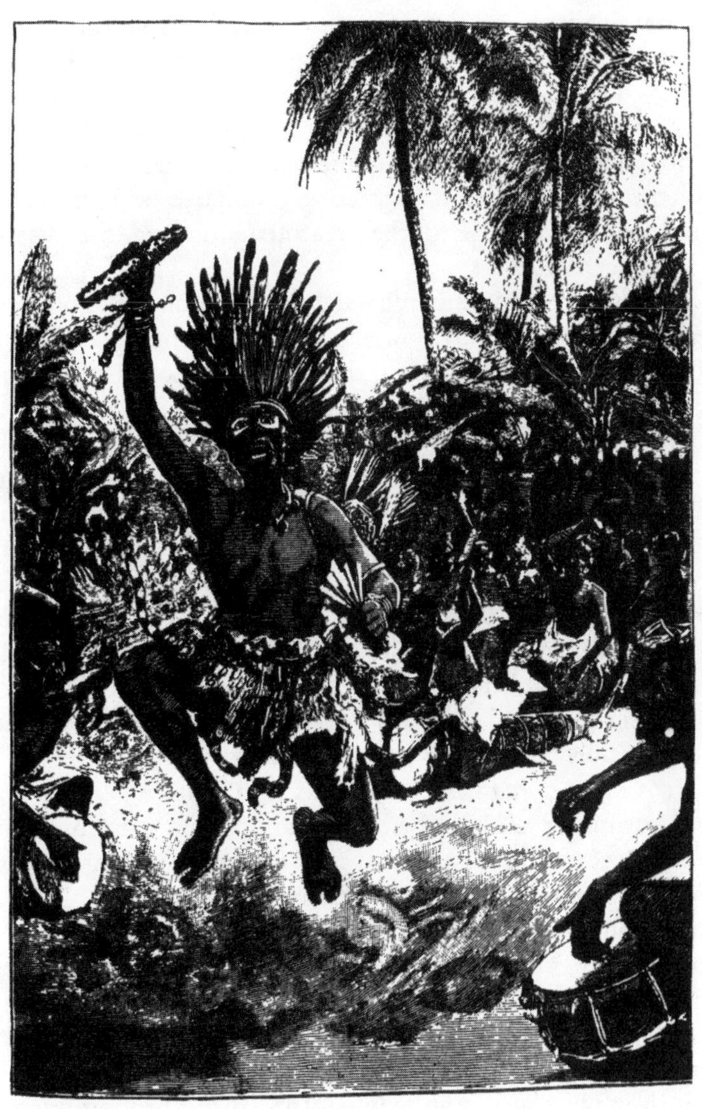

A medicine man of an African tribe driving away evil spirits.

He did have some effect on the illness of those he treated. In disease there is always an element that is purely mental; often it is the most unpleasant part of illness. The fears and discouragements of the sick man make his sufferings more severe. The medicine man encouraged him, comforted him, removed his fears; he took over responsibility for the disease and so relieved the patient's mind of responsibility. In consequence the sick man might feel better, and suffer less, become more confident of recovery because he believed in the medicine man. But the treatment affected the disease itself very little.

Almost everyone has played "medicine man." You have seen a small child fall down and bump his head. What did you do? First you picked up the child and looked to see how severely he was hurt. Then when you found his injury was slight, did you not use the medicine of the savage—make faces, try to stand on your head perhaps, shout to drown out his wails, and swing your watch in front of him to catch his attention, and make him "forget the pain"? After the tears stopped, perhaps you gave him a piece of candy to keep him from thinking of the hurt. The candy was like the savage's amulet, a charm to keep away disease. This kind of treatment for the child—or for the savage—while it may stop pain and fear and anxiety, does not heal a wound or cure an infection, nor does it prevent disease.

It seems never to have occurred to primitive peoples that wounds might heal of themselves and that a man might recover from disease without any treatment. Many people today do not realize the enormous recuperative ability of the human body. There are many diseases the modern doctor cannot cure, but he does help the sick man recover by aiding in every way the healing powers of the body.

Primitive peoples, however, as they always attributed the cause of disease to some outside force also attributed recovery to it. The medicine man controlled the healing agency.

He received full credit for curing every man who lived through an illness.

Some of his patients died, but such failures were quickly forgotten; only successes were remembered and talked about. People were pitifully eager to believe in the powers of the medicine man. Doubt and uncertainty are unpleasant. Confidence brings hope and peace of mind even when it is misplaced confidence.

Then, too, the medicine man always had ready an explanation for his failures. The most effective one was that some enemy of the sick man, in his tribe or perhaps in another tribe far away, had put a curse upon him, sent a spirit to torment him. The spirit of course could not be driven away until the enemy was found. Often the patient died before the search was finished.

This explanation for his failures brings up an unpleasant side of the medicine man, one on which we have not touched—that of black magic. When the medicine man tried to heal the sick by driving away evil spirits, he was practicing what is called white magic. But he was expected to aid his tribe not only by preventing their misfortunes but also by bringing misfortunes on their enemies. He then called on the spirits to cause disease. Such a practice is black magic.

It is doubtful whether the medicine man's efforts at black magic influenced the members of a tribe at a distance, but they did affect the people about him. They were in constant fear of offending him and so bringing down upon themselves his black magic. So strong was this belief that when the medicine man worked his magic on a member of his own tribe, the man might actually become ill and even die from fear.

In terror of this black magic or witchcraft, primitive peoples often carefully buried the parings of their finger nails, bits of loose hair, a tooth, or anything that had been a part of their bodies; they thought that if a sorcerer found such things he could use them to work a magic spell and so send an evil spirit to torment them. Some peoples even believed that their names were as much a part of them as their eyes, or teeth, or arms. Consequently they were very cautious about telling their true names, often giving fictitious ones to strangers.

Such beliefs did not stop with primitive or barbarian peoples. They were carried on far into civilization. We shall meet black magic again under the names of sorcery and witchcraft. We shall find men making little wax images of their enemies, sticking pins in them, and melting them in order to cause disease. We shall find judges in courts of law in civilized countries, only a century or two ago, maintaining that men who were mentally ill were possessed by demons. We shall find epidemics of disease attributed to the wrath of the gods; men hanged in the belief that they have caused death by black magic; and poor, harmless old women burned as witches.

And yet amid the welter of false beliefs of early man there were hidden great principles of medicine, the very foundations of modern medicine. We saw in the first chapter how the tribesmen gave us the principle of the doctor—a man who devoted himself to the care of the sick and to the prevention of disease. In the next chapter we shall find that, in spite of their false beliefs, these same tribesmen laid the crude foundations of hygiene, the use of medicaments, of surgery, and even of medical education.

CHAPTER III

Theories and Facts

CENTURIES before the rise of civilization, primitive peoples developed what may be called a theory of disease. A theory affords an explanation for known facts. The theory concerning spirits served to explain every fact that primitive people knew about disease.

Theories, when correct, are very useful indeed, for they serve as guides in the search for new facts. But when incorrect, they obscure the truth.

In the early nineteenth century, as we shall see, most physicians held the theory that infectious diseases resulted from evil smells and peculiar conditions of the air. Their theory was wrong, and when they attempted to prevent disease by following it, they failed. Later in the century scientists advanced the theory that infection was caused by bacteria. They found that by preventing the spread of bacteria they could prevent the spread of disease, and so the theory was proved to be a fact. But without the theory the fact perhaps would not have been discovered.

Occasionally, even in following out a false theory, important facts may be stumbled upon by accident. Some primitive peoples believed that the sun was born each morning and was eaten up each night at dusk; the ancient Greeks believed that the sun was a glowing chariot driven across the sky by Apollo. Both theories were wrong; but that did not prevent men from discovering that they could tell the passage of time from the position of the sun. False theories do not alter facts.

Likewise even though primitive people followed an incorrect theory of the cause of illness, they nevertheless occasionally stumbled upon important facts about disease. The knowledge that we have gained since their time shows that the explanation they gave for the facts was wrong, but the facts themselves remain unaltered.

Early man had stomach aches, just as we do, from eating indigestible things such as unripe fruit, but he had no one to tell him that indigestible material irritates and inflames

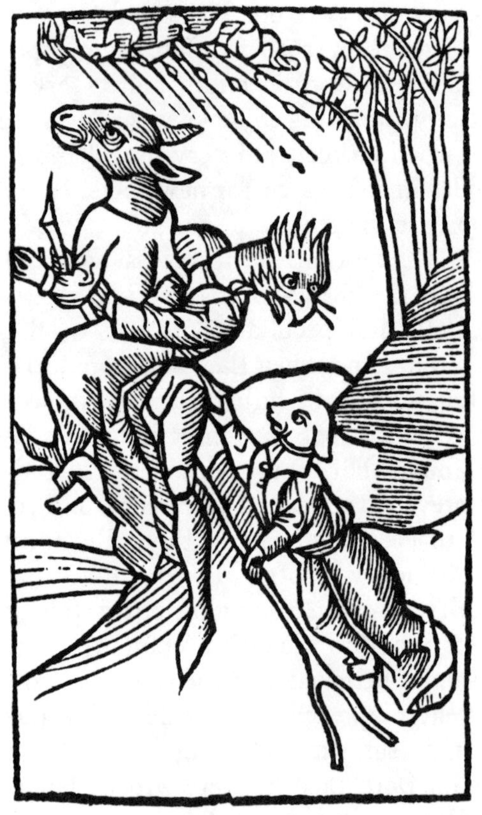

Humans changed to beasts by black magic.

the interior of the stomach and so causes pain. He did not even know he had a stomach. All that he was aware of was the pain. He explained it by saying that a spirit tormented him. That was his theory.

However, after many stomach aches from eating unripe fruit, the idea gradually dawned upon him that there was some connection between the fruit and the pain. The fruit, so he reasoned, following his theory, was the abode of an evil spirit. Evil spirits were to be shunned, and so he avoided the fruit.

Gradually in the same way he learned many facts concerning what we should call hygiene. He found that certain berries had in them spirits that killed men. He discovered that fish which had rotted in the sun acquired a particularly violent spirit that brought great pain to men: fish were to be eaten fresh and thrown away when stale. He found that when the leaves of certain trees, such as the swamp oak, or of certain vines, such as poison ivy, touched him, a spirit crept under his skin and made it raw and sore. Such plants were to be let alone.

He discovered that there were whole tracts of land, the home of buzzing flies which rose from the bushes to bite men and animals; in such places lived spirits that gave men a sleeping illness. There were marshes where spirits dwelt that caused men to shake in chills and burn with fever. These places were to be avoided.

Step by step from sad experience man gained practical knowledge of hygiene. This knowledge he handed on to his children.

In matters of hygiene, early man was not always either a careful or a critical observer. His fears and his false theories made him too ready to believe that harm lay where there was none. He often made mistakes in picking out the places where evil spirits were to be found, and so prohibitions grew up about many things and many acts which were not harmful. His life was burdened with the host of things that he must or must not do to prevent misfortune.

Just as efforts to avoid evil spirits led to the first attempts at hygiene, so attempts to drive away the spirits after disease had occurred led to the first use of medicaments. Primitive man in thinking of the spirits always imagined that their likes and dislikes were much the same as his own. He reasoned that bitter herbs, vile tasting messes, since they were unpleasant to man, should make his body unpleasant for the spirits and thus hasten their departure. Following this theory, he concocted medicaments from berries, barks, roots, dirt, the flesh of animals, anything in fact that seemed likely to rout the spirits. The vast majority of these concoctions had no real effect upon disease, but some made the sick man vomit, some were physics, and a very few were real remedies against disease or its symptoms.

Hemp and mistletoe and the juice of the poppy drove away the evil spirits of pain. The bark of the willow and the black birch relieved the aches of rheumatism. The fresh buds of hemlock cured the scurvy. A toad boiled in water, made into a mess like the witch's caldron of Macbeth and given to a man swollen with dropsy, seemed to benefit him. Pure fancy? That is what scientists thought until a few years ago when they discovered that the toad has in its skin a drug called bufonin that may actually be helpful in treating dropsy.

From ancient China came the belief that eating bits of dragons' bones drove away the evil spirit that caused babies to have fits. Foolish as this sounds, dragons' bones were really those of dinosaurs buried in the sands of the Gobi Desert. Today for a certain kind of convulsion that babies may have the doctor prescribes calcium, and the dinosaur bones, like all others, contain calcium!

Would you believe that the ashes from a burnt sponge could help relieve a swelling in the neck? Ashes were used, and they drove away the spirit that caused the swelling—according to the ancient theory. Modern science has shown that a swelling of the neck called a goiter may occur when there is too little iodine in the food and drinking water, as is the case in some parts of our country. Small amounts of iodine are given to prevent goiter. The ashes of sponge contain iodine.

From what has been said about these few remedies you must not think that all the medicaments used by primitive peoples were beneficial. We use very few of them today.

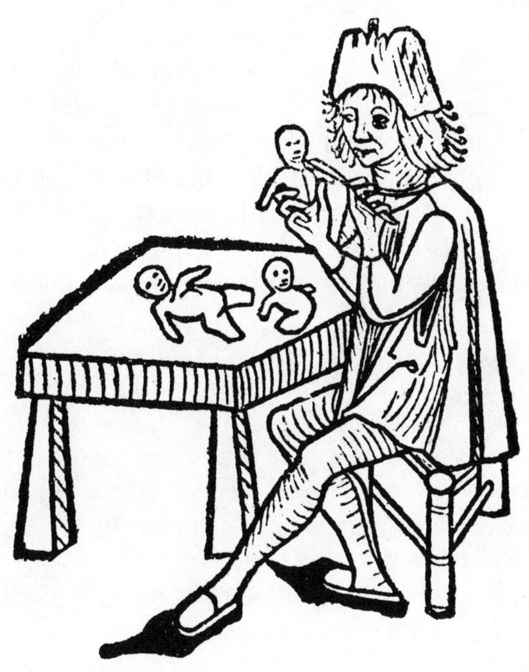

Black magic with wax images.

The vast majority were utterly worthless—weird concoctions and nasty messes. It was only the exceptional one or two out of many thousands that had any real healing virtue. Our debt to primitive man is not that he found a few things that were useful, but that, following his wrong theory, he developed the broad principle of using medicaments.

The general principle of treating disease by taking medicaments was carried over into civilization and so also were many of the horrible mixtures the savages had concocted. The great Roman writer on natural history, Pliny, recommended that a mouse be eaten once a month to prevent toothache; the doctors of the sixteenth century used ground-up mummy and horn supposed to come from the fabled unicorn, spices, bezoar stones, powdered jewels, and even fly specks. In the seventeenth century when Robert Boyle, "the father of modern chemistry," revised the list of useful remedies—the pharmacopœia—he included the ground-up sole of a well-worn shoe for the treatment of stomach ache. There were more unpleasant remedies in use than these.

If scientists of the seventeenth century could not tell that shoe leather was useless in the treatment of disease, the ignorant savage can hardly be blamed for his choice of medicines.

The savage on the one hand and most men of the seventeenth century on the other had something more in common than a poor choice of medicines. They had a peculiar way of thinking in such matters that convinced them that the useless medicines they employed were valuable remedies. This is an error of logic that is very common in the thinking of all people who are untrained in science.

It explains why many people even today believe in cures that the physician knows are useless.

This error of reasoning lies in the confusion of cause and effect. Just because one thing happens *after* another does not mean that the second happened *because* of the first. A man is sick; he takes some medicine; he gets well. He got well after he took the medicine but not necessarily because he took it. He might have recovered as quickly without it. Spring flowers bloom after the winter but not because of it. There are five Latin words that express the essence of this, the commonest of all faults of reasoning: *Post hoc: ergo propter hoc* (after it; therefore because of it)—a sentence that everyone would do well to remember and apply as a test to his way of thinking.

Through this type of reasoning the medicine man of primitive peoples received credit for curing everyone who got well under his treatment. And because of it many worthless substances were used as medicaments long after belief in spirits as a cause of illness was given up.

When a man became sick, he was given medicine or treated in some way. If he recovered from his illness, it was, so it is always natural to believe, the medicine or the treatment which cured him. It is only in modern times that science has raised the questions: "Might not the man have recovered from his illness if he had taken no medicine, or some other medicine, or used some other treatment? Did the treatment cure him, or did he get well in spite of it?" Questions of this kind led to studies by "statistics" and control experiments. We shall have much more to say of these things when we have gone further in our story and reached the time when the useless medicaments of the savage were finally discarded. The remedies used by the modern physician have been proved to be beneficial by scientific tests. Science with means of experimental proof came late in civilization; it has altered many of our ways of thinking but it has not altered the fact that it was the savage who gave us the great principle of using medicines. Nor was this the only form of treatment we owe to him.

It was he who originated what is called physical treatment, or physiotherapy. Physiotherapy makes use of exercises, massage, baths, the application of heat and cold. It seems a far cry from belief in spirits as the cause of disease to using massage. But the savage originated massage when he tried to pound the spirits out of the flesh. He sometimes placed his patient on the ground and prodded and poked and pounded him in a manner that would make the massage of an athletic trainer seem gentle stroking. Often under this treatment the evil spirits in stiff joints and sore muscles seemed actually put to flight. The joints became more limber and the soreness left the muscles.

Physical therapy is a useful form of treatment as applied by the modern doctor, but it was harmful as well as useful in the hands of the medicine man. Very definite harm may come from following the wrong theory in treating disease. The savage might use massage for any kind of illness, because he believed that all disease was due to a common cause. Today we know that rough massage may be harmful in certain diseases, especially infections, just as the wrong medicine may be harmful. The modern doctor must choose his treatment carefully to suit the disease.

Physiotherapy and medicaments by no means exhausted the list of treatments that the savage used and that we have adopted. As we have already said, he used suggestion. His magic and ceremony, his beating on the tom-tom and shouting did not impress the spirits, but they did impress the sick man and make him believe that he was getting well and that his pain was disappearing. Suggestion, the influence of the mind on the body, may be beneficial, or useless, or harmful. Primitive man made no distinctions, nor, as we shall see, did the healing priests of early civilization. The modern doctor has adopted the principle of suggestion which the savage originated, but again he must decide carefully when to apply this treatment.

Physiotherapy, medicaments, and psychotherapy (the medical term for mental treatment) were originated in crude form by native peoples, and so also was surgery.

Today surgery is looked upon as a method of repairing injured parts of the body, removing diseased flesh, and correcting abnormalities. The savage no doubt tried some of these things in a rough sort of way when he straightened out broken legs, but his interest even in surgery centered about the spirits. He mutilated the body rather than repaired it. Thus he might cut off the tip of a finger to provide a means of exit for a troublesome spirit, or bore a hole through the skull so that the spirit which caused headaches might escape. Explorers find in the ancient burial places skulls upon which this operation has been performed not only once but many times.

Present-day surgery is always associated in our minds with antiseptics, substances to destroy bacteria and hence to prevent infection. But antiseptics as we know them did not come into use until late in the nineteenth century. Nevertheless primitive man did have an antiseptic of a kind. It was fire. Fire was itself a spirit, one that could be used to frighten away other spirits. Burning embers or a red-hot stone held for a moment in a wound drove off evil spirits of disease, so the savage thought; and incidentally they did kill the bacteria of infection, of which he knew nothing.

A traveler to Russia some forty years ago relates how he saw fire thus applied by a native boy of the Yakuts. The boy had an infected finger. He and his friends had come to the conclusion that a spirit had established itself in the finger. To drive the spirit out, the boy took a burning coal and began to touch it to the place, while blowing upon it. When the burned flesh blistered and finally burst with a little crackle, the curious group which had crowded around to watch him jumped back with cries of terror, and the wounded boy with a smile of satisfaction said: "You saw how he jumped out."

Among civilized people fire continued in use as an antiseptic until the sixteenth century, not always because of belief in spirits, but because it was thought that some wounds were poisoned, and that fire destroyed the poison. We shall tell later how the great French war surgeon of the sixteenth century, Ambroise Paré, was the first to discourage the torture of wounded men with fire and boiling oil. But fire is used occasionally even today when nothing else is available and an especially strong antiseptic action is needed, as in the case of bites from mad dogs; now we call its use cauterizing.

Still another practice of primitive peoples which, like the use of fire, was carried over into civilization and then largely discarded, was bleeding. If you have read of Dr. Sangrado in the story of *Gil Blas* you know what is meant by that—the actual opening of a vein and letting out blood, with the idea that health is thus improved and disease prevented or cured. The method is now rarely resorted to, but even in the eighteenth century it was one of the commonest practices in medicine. It has been said that George Washington was bled to death by his physician, Dr. Craik, who treated him in his last illness; he was certainly bled, but since he had a severe throat infection, possibly diphtheria, the bleeding alone probably was not responsible for his death.

The practice of bleeding was originated by primitive peoples as a sort of peace offering to the ghosts and spirits. A man gave some of his blood to flatter them into favoring him. It was in miniature a duplication of the practice of human sacrifice to appease the gods, a practice that held so gruesome a place in the religions of savages and even, long ago, in those of civilized men.

Physicians in the time of Washington did not, of course, "bleed" for that reason; by that time the old belief had changed and been replaced by the theory that blood-letting removed impurities from the body—let out what some people still absurdly call "bad blood."

It is a long way from the hygiene, the medicines, the physiotherapy of primitive man to these same things in the hands of the modern doctor. The difference is as great as that between a rude straw hut and a skyscraper. Yet in that hut may be found all the principles of the skyscraper—the principle of the roof, the floor, the walls, the rooms, the windows, the doors, and even the stairs. We have simply elaborated, refined, extended the structure.

Today we have great medical schools where young men are trained to become physicians, and rigorous examinations given by the State before the doctor can treat the sick. Primi-

les, too, had these things in a crude form. We owe -, then, still another principle.

In earliest times the medicine man was probably simply the chosen leader, the strongest and the most intelligent man of the tribe. Later, as tribal organization grew more complex and there were both chiefs and medicine men, the choice was sometimes made for other reasons. A man might be selected

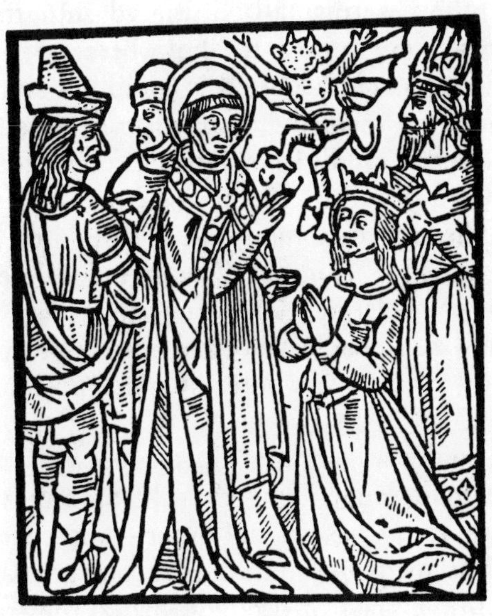

A saint delivering a princess from a demon.

because of something in his appearance—physical disfigurement by a birthmark perhaps, or crossed eyes, or even blindness. Even today some superstitious people talk of the "evil eye" and fear one-eyed people, for as Dickens says, "Popular prejudice is in favor of two."

The way that one tribe of African natives chose a medicine man is related by an explorer: One of the natives climbed a tree and chopped off the limb on which he was seated. He fell to the ground, but although he fell a long way, he landed on his feet unhurt. Obviously the spirits must have protected him and kept him from harm. He was therefore a friend of spirits and hence a medicine man.

Rarely, however, was the test so easy. These primitive physicians guarded their order jealously. They accumulated a great fund of beliefs and customs and methods which they handed on to young men, and sometimes young women as well, who studied with them as apprentices. And these pupils, before they were finally initiated into the order of medicine men, were forced to show before the assembled tribe the skill they had acquired in handling spirits.

To the accepted medicine man a life of ease and importance was assured. He did not labor in the fields; his food, his shelter were provided for him; he was respected, even venerated. The medicine man had leisure, and fortunately he sometimes used it profitably; he served as the artist and the historian of the tribe. These functions passed on to the priests of civilized people who, not so many centuries ago, were the only men in a whole kingdom able to read and write.

With the many advantages that went with the position of medicine man, one might think that any young man would choose to join such an order—but there was one drawback. The medicine man had to be successful. When disease or famine, flood or drought visited the tribe, he was responsible. Unless fortune favored him or he could explain away his failure, he might find himself in an uncomfortable position. Natives may be gullible, but they may also be violent. The medicine man who failed too often paid for his failures with his head.

What we have attempted in this chapter is to marshal many things both good and bad that find their places again and again in the story of medicine.

Long before the days of recorded history great principles of medicine were shaped by rude medicine men living in caves and jungles; but these men also originated false theories of disease. The modern doctor has accepted and used many of the beneficial principles, but discarded the false beliefs. These two, the savage medicine man and the modern doctor, lie at the extremes of a hundred, perhaps two hundred, centuries of medical progress. Our story covers the years between, and in these intervening years we shall recognize the old beliefs recurring in changing forms but, knowing their origin, we shall know their meaning.

We shall find belief in the supernatural origin of disease, in evil spirits, in demons, and in sorcery, magic, witchcraft, kept alive in civilization, in Egypt, Greece, Rome, and in Christian Europe.

The primitive medicine man with all his fears and his false reasoning stalks on for centuries in the midst of civilization. Finally the doctors outdistance him, acquiring fresh theories and knowledge, and using new and effective weapons in the age-long struggle of man against disease.

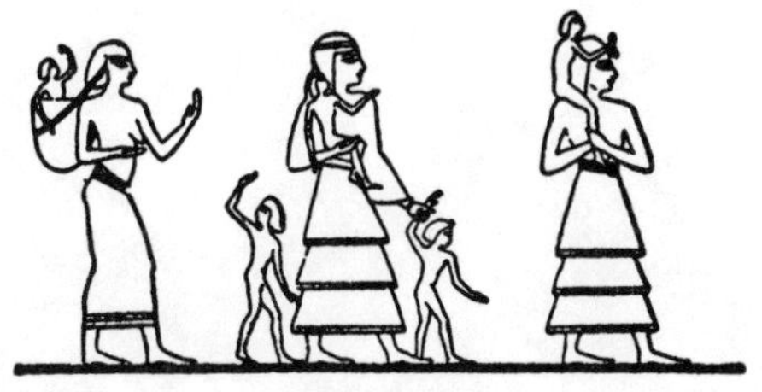

Part Two

IMHOTEP, THE GOD
ÆSCULAPIUS, THE MYTH
HIPPOCRATES, THE NAME

CHAPTER IV

Imhotep, the God

THOUSANDS of years ago man first put his foot to the endless ladder of civilization and began his stumbling progress from the lowest savagery. We today still climb onward, rising from the steps reached by men before us. As we look down from our elevation far above the savage, far above the men of early civilization, we can see the steps they took. The savage climbed one rung when he first used fire, another when he chipped crude weapons and tools from stone. Then, each step a rung higher, the family group gave way to the tribe with a chief, animals were domesticated, crops were raised, rough dwellings built. Centuries went by while men worked out the barest rudiments of government and acquired the simplest elements of culture.

Civilization had its greatest growth when men built towns and cities. Wandering tribesmen had scant time to devote to art, or science; their ways of living remained crude and primitive as they are today among the Bedouins of the desert, or among the Eskimos. When men settled in cities, some of them had leisure to devote to what we call "culture," and in settled communities improvements could be made that were impossible among migrating tribes.

The settlements flourished best where the climate was warm and water abundant, and where there was natural protection against the men of the tribes that still wandered about. The valley watered by the river Nile, and protected by a desert on one side and by a sea on the other, afforded a place particularly suited to the growth of cities. Civilization flourished there at an early period.

In the more peaceful settled life of towns men progressed far beyond the culture of the wandering tribesmen and of the cave dwellers before them. But this advance consisted less in finding new things than in improving and refining the old. The tribal chief became a king. The cave or rude hut became a house of stone or brick. The pictures daubed on the walls of caverns grew into writing.

Writing—the use of symbols to record the thoughts, the knowledge, and the deeds of men—marks perhaps the greatest of all steps in man's progress. It is the one thing beyond all others that marks him as civilized.

It is also the step that has given us history. History in contrast to legend has its beginning in written records. When knowledge was handed from generation to generation only by the spoken word, the stories told grew and changed in the telling, as happens today with gossip. But with the invention of writing the original facts could be found out as long as the writing was preserved.

In moist climates paper decays unless it is carefully preserved; inscriptions cut in stone or scratched on clay soon weather away. But in the dry climate of sandy Egypt, Assyria, and Babylon, buildings and writing too have been preserved through the centuries. We can decipher many of the inscriptions. We know from them what men of ancient Egypt did and thought and believed from actual records written by their hands.

Egypt is the burial ground of early civilization. Still hidden in the sands, or already uncovered by explorers, is the record of man's rise from the primitive state to one of high culture and art. There are the beginnings of masonry, and also, from much later periods, magnificently designed buildings, with water pipes and even sewers. There are rough attempts at carpentry and metal working buried almost side by side with exquisite furniture, tapestries, and wonderfully designed jewelry. Such seemingly modern devices as candles, razors, steam baths, manicure sets, and lip-sticks were known to ancient Egyptians.

The same dry climate and sandy soil that have preserved

the records of Egypt have also helped preserve some of the men themselves; men who lay buried for centuries with the things they wore and used when they were alive.

The art of preparing mummies grew out of the belief that after death the spirit of a man survived and would live on in another world. It would have need of a body and of food.

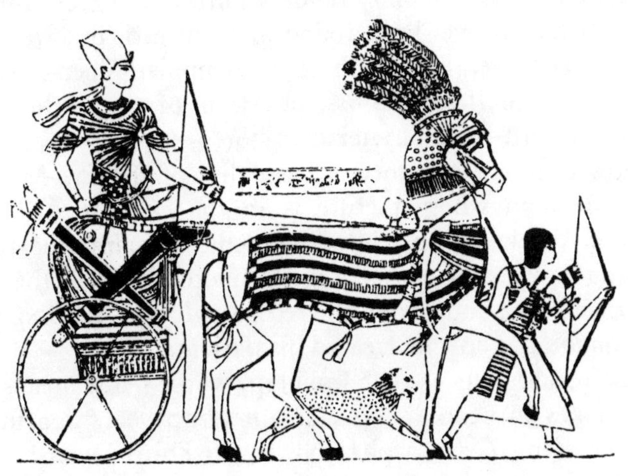

Rameses II and his chariot.

In preparing for the after-life the Egyptian learned by heart the *Book of the Dead*, a guide to the other world. And then at death his body was preserved, made into a mummy, and buried in a tomb with food and clothes and weapons. The earliest mummies were crudely prepared, but as time went on the art was perfected and became an elaborate ritual. First the brain was removed, the organs of the abdomen taken out, the space filled with spices, and the wound sewn up. Then the body was soaked for more than two months in a solution of salt or sodium bicarbonate. Next it was wrapped in bandages smeared with gum and resin and placed in a coffin shaped to resemble a man. This coffin, together with four jars containing the organs removed from the abdomen, was then put carefully into the tomb.

From study of mummies we know something of the diseases from which the Egyptians suffered. There are signs of broken bones, infections, appendicitis, rheumatism, decayed teeth, and many other diseases that we have today.

One particular mummy holds additional interest for our story. It has not yet been found or identified, but we know that it lies buried in a tomb near Memphis. When it is discovered, we shall see the first physician of whom there is a written record—the physician Imhotep.

How different his story is from that of the Cro-Magnon medicine man whose picture is in the cave at Ariège in France! We know only how the medicine man appeared—nothing of what he actually did. Imhotep lived in the days of writing. We know from the records what he did and what he thought and how he treated his patients.

The records tell us that Imhotep, whose name means "he who comes in peace," lived about 5,000 years ago in the reign of King Zoser, a pharaoh of the Third Dynasty. His father was an architect. When Imhotep reached manhood, such were his abilities and learning that he became Grand Vizier to the Pharaoh. If you wonder what his duties were, these titles which he held may give the answer: "chief judge, overseer of the King's records, bearer of the royal seal, chief of all the works of the King, supervisor of that which Heaven brings, the Earth creates, and the Nile brings, and supervisor of everything in this entire land."

One might gather that, though the pharaoh held the higher position, the vizier did most of the work. Indeed, in the old kingdom of Egypt at least, the vizier seems to have been chosen because he was the wisest man in the land. And of all of the viziers Imhotep was the wisest.

It was probably he who designed the great Step Pyramid which still stands near Memphis, the earliest large stone structure known to history. Imhotep also helped design the first temple of Edfu, one that preceded the temple standing there today.

It may have been in this ancient temple that Imhotep held

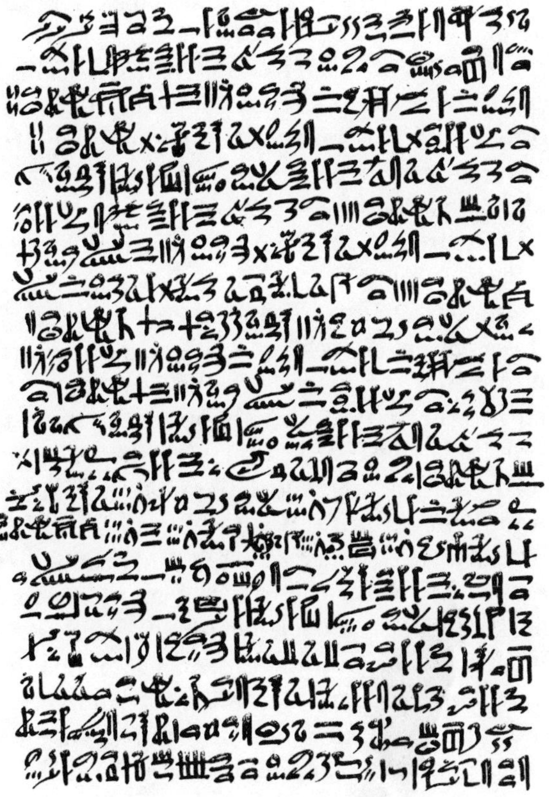

Facsimile of a portion of the Ebers papyrus

office as the high priest and magician, for Imhotep was a physician, and even in the civilization of Egypt, as among the Cro-Magnon people, the magician, the sorcerer, was the physician.

The physician was also the priest. It was his duty to deal

with the gods and spirits that caused disease, for the Egyptians, like primitive peoples, still believed disease to be of supernatural origin. But the spirit world of the Egyptians was more highly organized than that of the savage. Just as the society of men in becoming civilized had become more complex, so the spirit world had become more and more complicated.

The spirits were no longer crude creatures living in trees and rivers, in beasts and stones; they were denizens of another world, of various ranks, like soldiers in an army. And like soldiers, the spirits of lesser rank were led by powerful commanders, gods. Each village had its own patron god or goddess represented in the temple by an idol often wearing the head of some animal.

Just as soldiers change in rank, the gods of Egypt might gain or lose power. A local god might gain in reputation from the tales told by his priests and come to be feared or worshiped in other cities. So it happened in time that Ra, the Sun God, was worshiped throughout the whole of Egypt.

The enemy of Ra was Apop, the God of Darkness, who each morning fought with Ra to prevent the rising of the sun and was always defeated. These family squabbles among the gods were indirectly the cause of many misfortunes to man. The god Osiris quarreled with his brother Seth, the god of Upper Egypt, who in consequence of his defeat became a constant evildoer. He and his friends created evil and spread disease. Their tears, dropped upon the ground, made plants poisonous; and their sweat turned into scorpions and deadly snakes. At every chance these evil demons sought to inflict harm upon men, and could be kept away only by magic which brought protection from the gods friendly to man.

The gods of Egypt, like men, might suffer from disease. Ra occasionally had a disease of the eye, so that there was darkness for a time—an eclipse we should call it. He nearly died when stung in the heel by a scorpion. Horus, the son of

Isis, had headaches, and, like Ra, nearly lost his life from a scorpion's sting.

When a god was stricken with disease he turned for aid to his friends among the gods. That was precisely what men did. They turned to the gods. The sick went to the temples for aid.

The priests knew the mystery of the gods and the magic formulæ to drive away evil spirits. The priests of Egypt were medicine men. Their principles, for all their greater knowledge, were the same as those of the medicine man of primitive peoples. Only, the wild and grotesque behavior of the primitive medicine man had under the restraint of civilization given place to mystery and magic and charms.

The greatest of the priests of ancient Egypt, the man who best controlled the evil spirits of disease and brought the friendly gods to the aid of his fellow men, was Imhotep.

He not only treated the sick, but he wrote in proverbs the things he had learned of men and of life. So deeply were his countrymen impressed by his great learning that his words became a national tradition.

When he died, he was buried with the highest honors; and his reputation lived on. A man so kindly, so wise in life, so successful in healing, would surely continue to aid men in spirit from the other world. So people prayed to Imhotep. They called to him for help in illness. Statues of him were built, and these statues had healing powers. With each century after his death his reputation grew. Men placed him near the gods—he was a demigod. Finally 2500 years ago, when Egypt was conquered by the Persians under Cambyses, Imhotep had become a god—the Egyptian God of Healing and of Medicine. Temples were erected in his honor. These temples where he was worshiped were in a way hospitals; they were schools of medicine and of magic. The sick came to them, and the lame and the maimed, to pray to Imhotep, the beloved god. Upon these people the priests of Imhotep worked their healing magic and prescribed such remedies as they knew.

The priests wrote on papyrus descriptions of the diseases they saw and the treatment they gave. One of these papyri, discovered by the archæologist Edwin Smith, is fifteen feet in length and describes forty-eight injuries, wounds, and broken bones, together with the treatment given and the magic formulæ used. These temple papyri were the first written records of medicine—the first medical books.

CHAPTER V

Æsculapius, the Myth

IN time civilizations grow old just as men do. As we grow older our interest turns back to the past, to scenes of earlier and more vigorous days. The old man talks of his childhood; the old civilization adheres to its earlier customs and makes them into formal traditions. In each case progress ceases.

Three thousand years ago the civilization of Egypt had reached its peak and was declining, dying. Stiff with age, its art, its architecture, its literature, had become formal, unchanging. But this country of tombs and mummies became with the passage of centuries a vast storehouse of wisdom from which other and younger civilizations, more progressive, were to learn something of the mysteries of life and death, of health and disease.

Such a civilization was rising to the north and west. There a poet, a story-teller, blinded, so legend says, to keep him from leaving the tribe he entertained, was singing of a new civilization. Homer, as he was called, told tales of warlike, sturdy barbarians, who in their wanderings had come upon an ancient civilization on the shores of the Mediterranean Sea and had conquered its cities. The barbarians had taken over the civilization of their predecessors. They had settled in towns. Homer's tale was only an incident in the age-long conflict between the settler and the nomad.

New cities—Athens, Sparta, Thebes, and Corinth—grew up where old ones had been. Although the people spoke a common language, their cities were not united, but each was ruled as a little state.

These men, the Hellenes, or as we should call them, the Greeks, were a free and independent people who knew no binding traditions. They were acquisitive, not only of lands and riches, but of knowledge and beliefs as well. Their civilization was young.

They believed in gods and had gods of their own, but unlike the Egyptians they obeyed no rigid rule of the temple.

The Greeks were willing to respect the gods of all people, but they gave to no god a profound reverence. They were free-minded and open-minded. When at length their sailors and merchants came to Egypt, they saw in Imhotep not a rival deity but their own god under a different name. They called him Imuthes and linked his name with their own God of Healing, Æsculapius.

The Greeks, like their nomadic ancestors and like the Egyptians, believed in the supernatural origin of disease. They turned to their gods for aid in misfortune, for the cure and prevention of disease. Gods were supreme, powerful beings with enormous magic powers, but with all the bad habits and weaknesses of men. They could walk on earth, mingle with men, and enjoy men's pleasures. They were likable gods to whom one could speak as man to man.

In early times all the cities and villages had their own favorite gods and goddesses, but they respected each other's deities just as they did Imhotep. Gradually some of the gods grew in reputation and rose to supremacy. The legends that were built about them have come down to us—the legends of Zeus, and Apollo, and Artemis, and all the rest of the great galaxy that mirrored the adventurous and nature-loving spirit of the Greeks.

Apollo, the averter of ills, was chief god of healing. His arrows visited plagues and pestilence upon men, but he could, if he desired, recall them and free men from disease. He was physician, so Homer tells us, to the gods on Mount Olympus, and treated their wounds with the root of the peony. Some men believe that the name "Sons of Pæan," which is sometimes applied to physicians, comes from that story.

Apollo, so legend records, communicated all his knowledge of healing to the son of Cronus, the centaur Chiron, half horse, half man. Chiron, who was versed in history and music as well as medicine, was intrusted with the education of the heroes Jason, Hercules, Achilles, and, particularly, Æsculapius, who was destined in time to become the great healing god of Greece, greater even than Apollo.

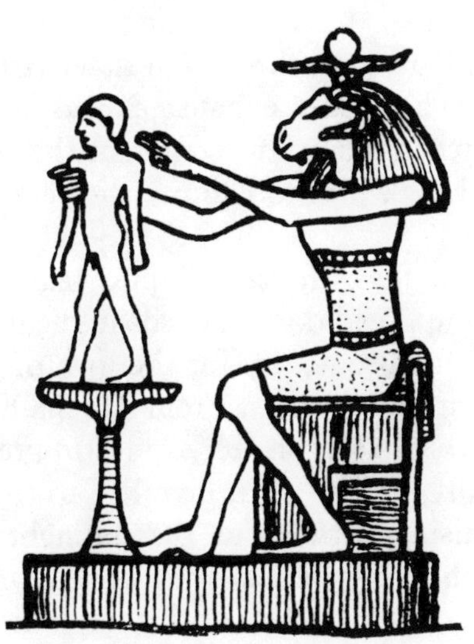

Egyptian god modeling a man.

Everyone knows, of course, the legends of some of these fabled heroes: Jason, who went in search of the Golden Fleece; Hercules, the mighty son of Zeus, who accomplished the twelve great tasks; and Achilles who could be wounded only in the heel. But the story of Æsculapius is less well known, and so here is one of the many versions of his life, the myth found in the works of the Greek poet Hesiod, who lived twenty-seven hundred years ago.

According to the story, Apollo was the father of Æsculapius; his mother was Coronis, a maiden from Thessaly. Coronis was secretly married to the god, and being unable to divulge the secret, was finally forced by her father into a wedding with her cousin Ischus.

Apollo heard of the marriage from his spy the raven. In anger the god first took vengeance upon the bearer of evil tidings. The raven, which had been white, he turned black, and ever since black has been the sign of mourning. Next he turned to the luckless but innocent husband, Ischus, and slew him with one of his far-reaching arrows. The unhappy Coronis was killed by Apollo's twin sister Artemis.

Then Apollo, his anger exhausted, was stricken with remorse and snatched his infant son from the funeral pyre of his mother and took him to Chiron, the centaur, on Mount Pelion.

From Chiron, the child Æsculapius learned the healing art. As he grew up, he did great deeds in medicine. But filled with pride—though some say for the love of gold—he ventured too far with his powers. From Athena he obtained the blood of the fabled Gorgon. He could do great magic with it, could cure all disease, even give life to the dead. It was this last, the raising of the dead, that brought him into trouble. Some legends say he accepted bribes, and others that Pluto, the God of the Underworld, complained to Zeus that Æsculapius by his magic threatened to depopulate Hades by bringing all its residents back to earth. Either in anger at his greed and as warning to all physicians to respect their art, or else to maintain the balance of population, Zeus punished Æsculapius. The poem says that great Zeus:

> *Was filled with wrath, and from Olympus top*
> *With flaming thunderbolt cast down and slew*
> *Latona's well-loved son—such was his ire.*

Apollo, who, it would seem, had a very touchy temper, in grief for his son turned and slew those who had forged for Zeus the thunderbolt that had killed Æsculapius. And then he begged Zeus to place Æsculapius among the stars and so make him a god.

Æsculapius, while living on earth, legend says, was married and had a family. In most of the stories his wife was Epione, daughter of Merops, King of Cos. The best known of his children are two sons, Machaon and Podalirius, and two daughters, Hygieia and Panacea.

The names of the sons have not become a part of our language, but those of the daughters have. Hygieia was the Greek goddess of health, and from her name have come all words such as hygiene, hygienic, and hygienist. Panacea was the goddess of the healing powers found in herbs. Your dictionary will tell you that a panacea is a remedy that cures all diseases, a thing which your physician will tell you is quite as mythical as Panacea herself.

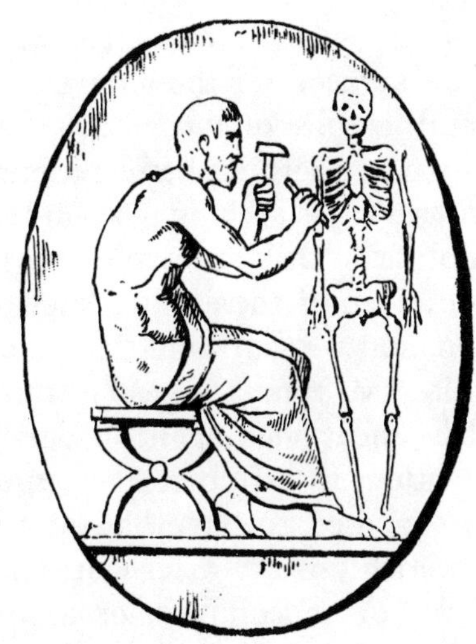

Prometheus carving out man's skeleton.

In the poems of Homer, Æsculapius is called a Thessalian prince; his sons Machaon and Podalirius are mentioned as commanders of sailing vessels and as good physicians practicing their art. In the fourth book of the Iliad, Machaon is summoned to remove an arrow driven through the belt of the King of Sparta:

"When he perceived the wound, where the bitter shaft had fallen, having sucked out the blood, he skillfully sprinkled on it soothing remedies, which benevolent Chiron had formerly given his father."

As would be expected, wounds from weapons were of great interest to the warlike Greeks; the Iliad gives a detailed account of 147 such wounds. It does not speak well for the skill of the surgeons of those days that 114 of these wounds were fatal in spite of the sucking out of the blood and the application of soothing herbs recommended by the great Chiron. Indeed to us sucking a wound sounds like not only a rather unpleasant task but a most unsanitary form of treatment as well. Men of these times knew nothing of the cause of infection, and we shall find this practice of wound-sucking still in use two thousand years after the Iliad was written. It will be mentioned again in our story when we come to the adventures that Robert, the son of William the Conqueror, was supposed to have had at the Hospital at Salerno in the twelfth century after Christ.

The descendants of Æsculapius, or at least those who claimed such descent, controlled the healing art in Greece. Some of them, following the example of Machaon and Podalirius, devoted themselves mainly to surgery as private physicians; others became healing priests in the temples erected to the memory of their godlike ancestor.

Among the early Greeks, wounds were looked upon as being quite different from any other bodily ill. There was nothing mysterious about wounds, everyone could see the cause and effect, and there was no need to attribute them to gods and spirits, so they were treated in a practical if unsanitary manner. But all other illnesses were still held to be a matter of the malign influence of gods, and spirits and demons, and heroes. It was in the interests of the sick, rather than the injured, that the temples of Æsculapius were built.

These temples were sanatoria for the care of sick people. They were often beautiful stone buildings with shady colonnades and olive groves and great courtyards with fountains. The ruins of some of them exist today. The treatment given in them was in principle the same as that used in the Egyptian temple of Imhotep and in the caves of Cro-Magnon men. The priests of Æsculapius were "medicine men." They did not shout and dance like the savage, they did not use the weird magic of the Egyptians, but their results were obtained in the same way—by suggestion.

In each temple was a statue of Æsculapius holding in his hand a staff about which a snake was coiled—the staff and snake are still the emblem of the physician today. With the statue of the god there was often one of Hygieia.

From far and wide the sick came to the temple, but they must not be too ill, for it would be disrespectful to the god to die in his temple. Nor were they treated at once, but instead waited their turn for treatment, living in the meantime in inns outside the temple.

This delay, although they did not know it, was part of the treatment. While waiting, the sick man was made to observe certain rules for purifying himself before he saw the god. He must drink no wine, must rest and diet, and bathe in cold salt water. These practices often of themselves started an improvement in his health, although he probably did not notice it, for his attention was fixed upon something else, something that aroused his keenest interest and made him certain that he would recover.

Each day the waiting crowd assembled to see written on a tablet the list of the cures the god had performed that day. They read of men who had been lame or paralyzed for years and could now walk, of the blind who through the benevolence of the god could see; they heard of men whose pains and aches had left them at the touch of Æsculapius or even his dog.

What these poor people, eagerly anxious to believe, did

not know was that the men who walked and saw and whose pains were soothed were those who suffered from mental disturbances, diseases caused by what some people call "upset nerves" or hysteria. In addition to the fortunate few whose illnesses yielded to suggestion, there were other men and women and even children whose diseases were of the flesh; though they were made to feel better, encouraged, their diseases went on unarrested. But the crowd did not hear of such failures, did not want to know of them.

Perhaps unconsciously the priest of Æsculapius, like the medicine man of primitive peoples, was a good "showman." While people waited for treatment about the temple, he aroused in them the certain conviction that they would be cured. When at last they were led in groups into the sacred grounds each man felt himself nearly well. But the show went on. Led by a priest, the sick man was shown through the temple and told the stories of marvelous cures. The tablets and the mystic symbols that covered the walls were explained to him. An air of sanctity, of deep religious dignity, pervaded the whole temple. The patient was awed and he was certain, without a doubt, that he would recover from his sickness. Already his step felt lighter, his pains were soothed; and the mysterious events of the night to come would complete his cure.

At dusk the patient, dressed in white, lay down on a couch. Prayers were offered to the gods. The lamps were extinguished. Everyone was silent. Sleep came to the sick man as the priests had told him it would, and with sleep, just as they had promised, came dreams of Æsculapius and Hygieia, who stood before him, ministering to him. In the dim light of morning he awoke, and there beside his bed he saw a priest dressed in the costume of the god. With the priest were a snake and a dog. The snake crawled across the bed, the dog licked his hand, and the priest asked him questions about his illness, gave advice, prescribed medicaments, and assured him that he would become well. The priest, the dog, the snake, passed to the next couch. A cure was completed.

Arising, with his pain gone, his lameness cured, the man rejoiced in the goodness of the god. He was convinced of his cure and in his enthusiasm he had the priests write his

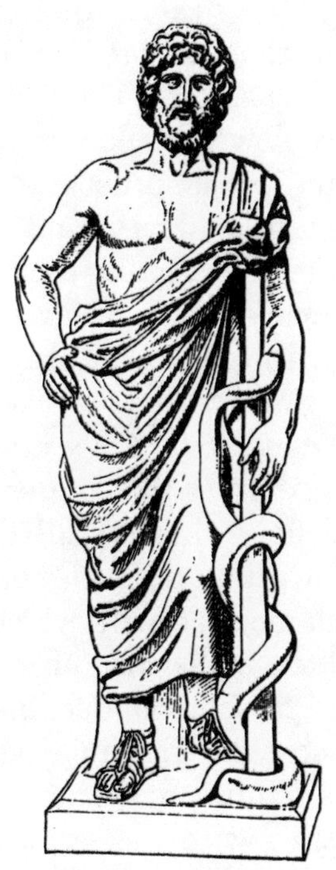

Æsculapius.

story on the tablets while the eager crowd watched. He gave a testimonial. And often he also gave a votive offering to the temple—a little statue of metal or of clay showing where pain had been or in what part his body had been diseased. When he returned home he told his friends of the glory of Æsculapius. And they, too, in time of need, came to the temple.

The cult of Æsculapius spread in Greece. His temples throve. There were not enough descendants of Æsculapius to provide all the priests needed for the temple and all the physicians needed to treat the wounded in private practice. Young men were adopted into the families of the descendants and trained as healing priests and physicians. But the Æsculapian families were jealous of their reputation and fearful that someone thus adopted would bring discredit upon their good name as healers. There had been a warning, you remember—Zeus slew Æsculapius himself because he had become greedy and presumptuous.

When a young man was adopted and took up healing he had to swear to lead a life becoming to the family of Æsculapius. This oath in many different versions has come down through the centuries. In some medical schools of our country today the students on graduation take this same ancient oath. There could be none better for a young man who takes over the grave responsibilities that the practice of medicine brings, for this oath defines what are called "medical ethics." Ethics are concerned with moral duties or moral principles, and the ancient Greek medical oath, which is usually called the oath of Hippocrates, is the code of moral duties for the physician. It tells how he shall conduct his life and perform his duties so as to deserve the trust and confidence of all men and the respect of his fellow physicians.

A physician is trusted with the secrets of the people he treats, and these he must never tell. He is trusted with poisons, and these he must never use except to cure. Any beneficial treatment that he discovers he must make public for the aid of all sick people; he must not keep it secret in order to obtain money for it, like the inventor of a mechanical device who may patent his discovery and sell it. All these things and many more are dealt with in the code of medical ethics—established by the early Greek physicians and followed by the physicians of today. Here is a portion of the ancient oath, and you will see not only that it is a moral code but also that the medical art in those days was a "family affair."

"I swear by Apollo the physician, and Æsculapius, Hygieia, and Panacea, and all the gods and goddesses that, according to my ability and judgment, I will keep this Oath and this stipulation—to reckon him who taught me this Art equally dear to me as my parents, to share my substance with him, and relieve his necessities if required; to look upon his offspring in the same footing as my own brothers, and to teach them this Art, if they shall wish to learn it, without fee or stipulation; and that by precept, lecture, and every other mode of instruction, I will impart a knowledge of the Art to my own sons . . . and to disciples bound by . . . oath according to the law of medicine, but to none others. I will follow that system of treatment which, according to my ability and judgment, I consider best for the benefit of my patients, and abstain from whatever is harmful and mischievous. I will give no deadly poisons to anyone if asked, nor suggest any such counsel. . . . With purity and with holiness I shall pass my life and practice my Art. . . . Whatever . . . I see or hear, in the life of men, which ought not to be spoken of abroad, I will not divulge, as reckoning that all such should be kept secret. While I continue to keep this Oath unviolated, may it be granted to me to enjoy life and the practice of the art, respected by all men, in all times! But should I trespass and violate this Oath, may the reverse be my lot!"

Since the days when the Greeks defined the conduct of the doctor, the ways of treating disease have changed; indeed, as we shall see in the next chapter, the whole principle of medicine was to change at the hands of the Greeks themselves—but the oath, the ethics, remain unaltered. It was the Greeks who gave the physician his most priceless possession: not worship, not veneration as the priest of a healing god; but honor. They saw the physician as an honorable man, as did also the ancient Hebrews. These words strongly expressing the sentiment of the ancient oath were written in the Bible:

> *Honor the physician according to thy need of*
> *him with the honors due unto him . . .*
>
> *The skill of the physician shall lift up his head:*
> *And in the sight of great men he shall be admired.*

CHAPTER VI

Hippocrates, the Name

IN the fifth century before Christ, among the Greeks, there occurred the most important event in the history of medicine—perhaps in all history. It marked a change in the tide of battle against disease; from then on man, and not disease, was to be the victor.

This great discovery was not itself a cure or a means of preventing disease; it was merely a new way of studying disease. It was a belief, a philosophy. It told where the enemy was to be found and fought.

For a hundred centuries and more men had struggled against disease, but always with their attention fixed on spirits, ghosts, and demons; they had fought with shadows. Never once had they seen or touched the enemy in reality. In these years disease had flourished almost uncontrolled.

But now in the fifth century B.C. men at last turned from the supernatural in their search for the cause of disease, and sought it where it really is—in nature, in the workings of the body, in the earthly surroundings of man.

This turn in the battle against disease marks the beginning of modern medicine.

In the days when this great event occurred Athens was the supreme city of the Greek states; yet it was not there that the change had its beginning, but in Asia Minor, in the Greek colony called Ionia. And what a seemingly insignificant event it was! A man named Thales, who had been in Egypt studying with the priests, had returned to his home in the town of Miletus. The Athenians who gathered in crowds about the temple of Æsculapius would have laughed in derision if they had been told that Thales was shaping a force that was to destroy belief in the gods of healing and in the demons and spirits as causes of disease. And Thales himself did not realize it. What he was doing was predicting that in the year 585 there would be a day of darkness, an eclipse.

Men were always foretelling things, predicting events by looking at the livers of slaughtered animals and by listening to the mysterious mutterings of oracles. But Thales said he could foresee a day of darkness by studying the position of the stars and sun and moon. There was no telling what sort of queer ideas might grow in the mind of a philosopher; such men were to be laughed at unless too many foolish fellows, deceived by words, began to believe their theories. It was time then to punish them for disrespect to the gods, who, as every reasonable man knew, were responsible for all the things that happened in the world and in the sky as well.

But the eclipse occurred. Surely some god must have whispered to Thales that the darkness was to come. Yet there he was, the foolish one, trying to tell men he had figured it out by himself.

Equally absurd was his idea that water was the primary element from which everything, even man, was derived. Surely the Ionians—so the good Athenians must have thought—were stupid to listen to such words. Everyone knew that Prometheus, the Titan, had created the first man out of clay, had breathed the spirit of life into him, and for his use had stolen fire from the heavens.

But other men in Ionia caught the fever of speculation; they were forming new philosophies of life in a most sacrilegious manner. They were beginning to doubt that the gods were responsible for what went on in the world; they were talking of things called nature and numbers. Empedocles of Akragas was saying that everything in the world was composed of four things: earth, air, fire, and water.

Pythagoras of Samos was trying to solve the riddle of life with mathematics. Ten was the perfect number; it included everything in the whole universe. Three and four were also important numbers, especially four. There were four elements in the universe; earth, air, fire, and water. There were four conditions, or states, which all things might possess: heat, moisture, dryness, and coldness. There were four fluid substances in the body called humors: blood, phlegm, yellow bile, and black bile.

Here, most sacrilegious of all, the philosopher had pushed the gods and spirits and demons aside and said that disease was due to natural causes. When the four humors were in proper proportions, a man was healthy. But when the humors were out of balance, when there was too much or too little blood or bile, or phlegm, or when their condition was too wet, or cold, or dry, or hot, he was diseased. The way to treat disease was not to ask aid of the gods or to drive away the spirits, but to try to restore the humors to their proper balance.

Of course, you and I today, like most Athenians of the fifth century B.C., but for very different reasons, would say that such theories were silly. Yet these beliefs were destined to be the great guiding theories of medicine for centuries after the time of the Ionian philosophers. We shall meet the theory of humors and the theory of numbers again and again in our story. The important thing is not the theory but the fact that in the new ideas concerning disease the gods and spirits and demons were nowhere mentioned. Men for the first time in all the ages had stopped looking for the cause of disease in the air and the heavens and were searching for it in the flesh of man. They were hunting for a reasonable, a natural, explanation of disease. Their explanations, we know now, were wrong, but the direction in which they sought was the right one.

The new philosophies that were taking shape in Ionia, although perhaps men did not recognize the fact, were destined to place a great responsibility on human beings. When spirits and gods and demons were believed to be the cause of disease, man took no responsibility for his misfortunes.

He was merely the plaything of a host of creatures that might injure or help him. Disease was no fault of his, it was just bad luck.

But if what these philosophers were saying was true, then

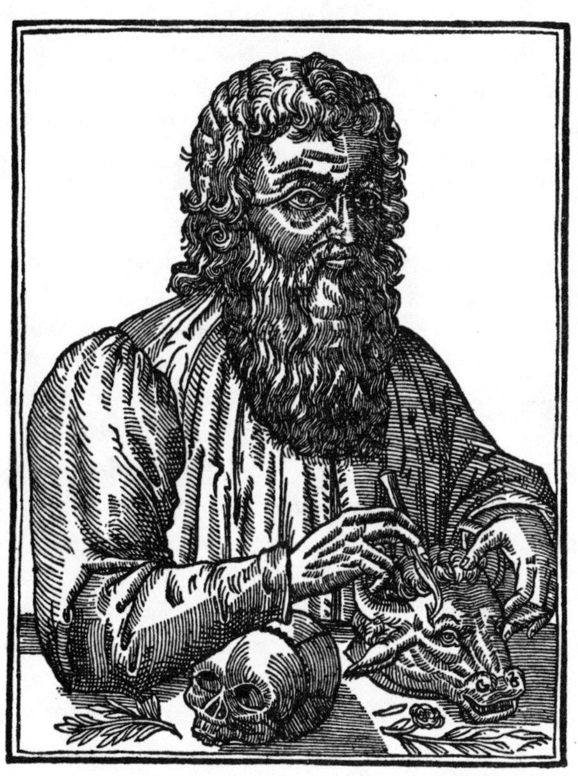

Hippocrates as shown in the surgical works of Ambroise Paré.

man was responsible for disease. If illness was caused by natural forces, then it was man's responsibility to discover these forces, learn the laws of nature, and find out how to control them.

As we have pointed out in Chapter II, where we talked

about egotism, most men are anxious to blame their misfortunes on something other than their own ignorance. That is, they are eager to avoid taking responsibility for their own faults. It was a hard road that the philosophers were pointing out for men to follow. It meant putting aside the childish, dreamlike myths like those of Apollo and his chariot, Æsculapius and his snake, Zeus and his thunderbolts, and all the host of gods and demons and spirits which had saved men from taking responsibility.

In the centuries that follow, as we shall see, men often strayed from this narrow road and shifted the responsibility back to the gods. But in the fifth century before Christ there were courageous men, keen and curious.

The new idea of a rational philosophy spread. It reached Athens at a fortunate time when the Greek cities were more closely united than they had ever been before. They had been driven by necessity to join forces against a common enemy, the Persians, who were led first by Darius and later by Xerxes. In the battle of Salamis in 480 and of Platæa and Mycale the following year, the Greeks had been victorious. Then followed a half century—very different from the past—in which the Greek cities were at peace among themselves.

In this period of prosperity Athens was governed by a wise statesman, Pericles. Men had leisure to think and study.

It was then that a philosopher named Anaxagoras came to Athens from Ionia. He attempted to explain to men the nature of eclipses, and of the rainbow, and of the stars and meteors. He told them that the earth was round. Quite naturally his teachings brought him into conflict with the religious beliefs of the Athenians. He could talk of any god he wished, believe in any one he cared to, but he must be respectful to all gods and not deny their deeds. He was arrested and tried. Pericles himself defended him. Anaxagoras was forced to leave Athens, but his ideas remained behind.

In and about the city of Athens there soon formed the greatest group of thinkers that has ever existed. You know the names of some of them—Socrates, Plato, Aristotle. These men and many others sought behind the myths for truth.

Some of the philosophers were physicians, and they treated disease according to the explanations for its cause which they had developed from their speculations. They tried to correct the balance of the humors, or to work with numbers, or to apply the theory of heat and cold and wetness and dryness. They failed in their efforts. Their patients were not cured.

The philosophers could theorize about the movements of the planets, the origin of man, and the nature of matter, but their speculations, right or wrong, had no effect upon these things. The sun rose and set as regularly and shone as warmly, whether it was thought of as a chariot driven by Apollo or a burning mass around which the earth revolved. But disease was different. Merely to tell a man that he was ill because the humors were unbalanced, or that he had too much black bile, or that his blood was too warm, stopped no pain. Speculation alone cures no diseases. Men wanted their pains relieved, their children cured of illness.

Theories, as we have said before, are useful, indeed necessary, guides in finding or arranging facts, but the facts and not the theories are the important thing. When men only speculate, they often become so interested in their theories that they forget realities.

It is to the speculation of philosophers that we are indebted for the separation of disease from the supernatural, and medicine from religion. But after speculation had pointed the way to look for the cause of disease, it ceased to be useful. What was needed was fact. The facts of nature had to be found out and recorded. When, and only when, the facts had been accumulated, could sound theories and explanations result.

It was a physician and philosopher named Hippocrates of Cos who rescued medicine from speculation and began the collection of facts about disease. Today we call him the father of medicine.

Hippocrates did what no physician had ever done before. He examined sick men carefully and recorded honestly the signs and symptoms of disease, without theorizing. He was not looking for spirits; he was not trying to show that the humors were out of balance; he was attempting to find out exactly how the sick man differed from the well man and how one sick man differed from another.

The chief importance of the work of Hippocrates lies in the fact that he observed and recorded the symptoms of disease. He began the accumulation of the facts concerning disease upon which the knowledge of modern medicine rests.

When the physician of today is called to visit a sick man, he follows the same general method that Hippocrates followed 2300 years ago. You have seen a doctor at the bedside of a patient—probably your own bedside. The first thing that he does is ask questions—how you feel, how old you are, what illnesses you have had before, what diseases you have been exposed to recently.

Next he examines you—looks in your throat, your eyes and ears, feels about your body for sore places, taps your chest, and listens to your heart.

The modern doctor is seeking, with the symptoms as clues, to find out from what disease the patient is suffering. He is making what is called a diagnosis. From his knowledge of the various diseases he is then able to prescribe the proper treatment.

Diagnosis is one of the important steps in dealing with disease, for without diagnosis there can be no sound basis for treatment. But diagnosis also depends on the knowledge that there are separate and distinct diseases which may affect man. Physicians did not know this in the days of Hippocrates; it was not discovered until more than two thousand years after his time. But it was learned then by the method that Hippocrates originated—careful study of sick men, the recording of symptoms, and the accumulation of knowledge from actual observation.

Hippocrates believed, as indeed all men did until the seventeenth century A.D., that no matter what form the symptoms took, disease arose from some common disturbance in the body. Nevertheless he recognized that when a certain combination of symptoms appeared the illness seemed to follow one course and when another combination appeared it seemed to follow a different course. He wrote down the symptoms and the course of the illness in the cases he studied. Such records of how men appear and behave when affected by disease are called clinical histories. When he had collected many of these records, Hippocrates could draw general conclusions. He could say that when certain symptoms appeared the disease would follow a certain course.

He wrote down what he learned in the form of aphorisms or proverbs, such as these:

When sleep puts an end to delirium, it is a good sign.

Consumption comes on mostly from 18 to 35 years of age.

Apoplexy is commonest between the ages of 40 and 60.

Old persons bear fasting most easily, next adults, and young people yet less; least of all children, and of these least again those who are particularly lively.

Weariness without cause indicates disease.

Hippocrates was not able to make a diagnosis as the modern doctor would, but he was able to give a prognosis, a feature of medicine in which the Greeks were especially interested. Prognosis means a foretelling. It is the answer to the questions that the sick man always asks: "What is going to happen to me? How long am I going to be in bed?"

And Hippocrates carried medicine beyond mere prognosis; he laid the basis for sound treatment. His clinical records showed him the benefit or lack of benefit derived from the various treatments given, and he was able to select from among them those treatments that were most beneficial.

But it is not because of the prognoses he made or the treatments he gave that we call Hippocrates the father of medicine. It is because of his method of studying disease, of describing and recording. He was the first to use the principle of science in medicine.

All the knowledge that physicians have gained of disease since the time of Hippocrates has been acquired by following the principle he laid down—careful observation. Hippocrates clearly expressed the difference between speculation and guesses on the one hand and on the other knowledge gained from observation of facts. He said: "To know is one thing; merely to believe one knows is another. To know is science, but merely to believe one knows is ignorance."

Now much has been said here of what Hippocrates did for medicine; more will be told as we go on with our story. But we have said nothing of Hippocrates himself. All that we actually know of him as a man can be told in a few short sentences. He was born on the island of Cos about 460 B.C. He was a member of the Guild of Æsculapidiæ, those men who claimed descent from Æsculapius or who were adopted into such families. He is said to have died about 360 B.C.

If so little is actually known of Hippocrates, how does it happen that we credit so much to him? The records of his own time make little mention of him: Plato and Aristotle name him merely as a prominent physician, no more. But in the centuries following his death Greek physicians, and later those of Rome, said he was the author of the writings in which appeared the principles we have discussed.

The manuscripts were written in his time and they were

written in the region where he lived and taught. But we have no way of knowing whether or not he was the sole author of them; certainly it would seem that he did not write all the books credited to him. And really it makes little difference.

Hippocrates exists as a name rather than as a man. Under that name we group all the great and now forgotten men of Greece who in the fifth century B.C. founded the scientific basis of medicine.

Hippocrates lived and died, but his name alone among perhaps many who lived and worked with him has come down through the years to symbolize the ideal physician. Each stage of medicine in each civilization has had its ideals and its god who personified these qualities. Imhotep with his magic expressed the ideal of Egyptian medicine; he became the god of healing. Æsculapius with his divine powers was the model for the healing priests of ancient Greece; he became the god of medicine. Hippocrates with his honesty, his insistence upon clear reasoning and upon observation of facts rather than speculation, expresses the ideal of our medicine; he is the demigod of modern medicine.

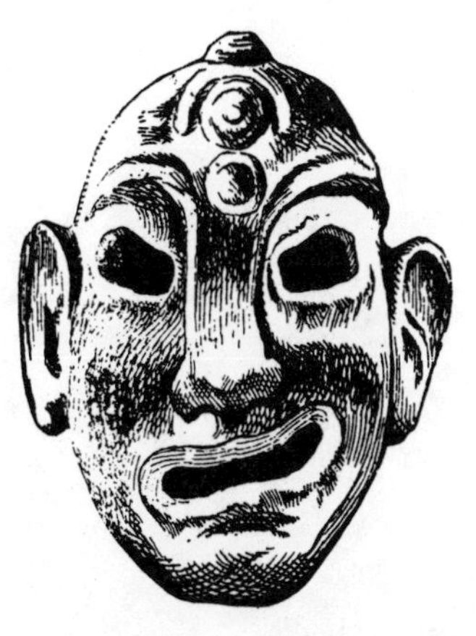

Part Three

THE PATH OF MEDICINE

THE BEARERS OF KNOWLEDGE

THE WAY DIVIDES—EAST AND WEST

CHAPTER VII

The Path of Medicine

IN 430 B.C. an epidemic of some grave infectious disease broke out in Athens and lasted five years. Pericles, his power broken by political intrigue, saw first his sister and then his two sons contract the disease and die. Then in the year 429, he too fell victim to the epidemic.

In spite of changing local politics, in spite of epidemics, in spite of the loss of a powerful ruler, the medical advance started at Athens went on.

Ahead of the country itself lay tragedy. It was doomed to political extinction before a rising civilization to the west —Rome.

Except for chance, the example set in medicine by Hippocrates might have perished and all records of his work been lost in the ruins of war and conquest. No doubt many discoveries that would be of vast importance to us have been made in the past and have disappeared. But the principles laid down by Hippocrates were destined to be spread to the farthest corners of the ancient world and were finally to be carried in the stream of civilization down to our own time. They guide the medicine of today.

In the turmoil of changing politics, of war and conquest, through shifting scenes, we can trace the path that Greek medicine followed.

Almost in the year that Pericles died, two boys, who were called Plato and Xenophon, were born in Athens. Their destinies led them to widely different careers. Plato became a great philosopher and teacher in Athens. Xenophon as a young man joined with other Greeks in a war that Cyrus was waging against his brother, Artaxerxes II, ruler of Persia. The army of Cyrus was defeated in the year 401, and the Greeks returned home under the command of Xenophon. He describes this expedition and the famous retreat of the "10,000" in his book, the *Anabasis*. Back in Greece the disbanded soldiers told their townsmen that Persia was a rich country for plunder and ill-prepared for war against a strong invading force.

Presently in the little country of Macedonia, north of Athens and beyond Thessaly where, according to legend, Æsculapius was born, two other young men embarked on careers as widely different as those of Plato and Xenophon. One was Philip, the son of the King of Macedonia; the other, Aristotle, the son of the king's physician. Aristotle went to Athens and there studied with Plato. Philip became King of Macedonia.

Each of these men made amazing progress in his chosen field. Philip spread the boundaries of his country wider and wider by conquest and finally united all the Greeks in a great war against Persia. Aristotle conceived the idea of studying nature in the way that Hippocrates studied disease—not by speculating about it, but by observing and describing it, and arranging his information in orderly fashion. He became the first natural historian. The tremendous task that he began of taking stock of the whole world goes on today; after all these years the study is still far from completed, although it has given us the vast fund of knowledge that we now have.

Philip was the greatest warrior of his day; Aristotle the greatest scientist. The careers of the two were united by a third young man, Philip's son Alexander. Philip asked Aristotle to return to Macedonia to tutor Alexander, and Aristotle taught his young pupil science and philosophy and developed in him a love of natural history. Philip proposed to the Athenians and the inhabitants of the other Greek towns that they join in a war against Persia. Some of the townsmen, remembering the stories told by the soldiers of Xenophon, were willing to go with him, but the Athenians refused. Demosthenes, the orator, denounced Philip and his plans in his famous speeches, the Philippics. But the matter was not to be settled with words; the armies of the Macedonians and the Athenians met in battle, and Philip won. The conquest of Persia was to start under his leadership.

In the year 336 B.C., as the army of the united Greeks began its march, Philip was assassinated. Alexander, the pupil of Aristotle, became king, and the conquest went on under his command. Alexander did not forget the teachings of his famous schoolmaster. With the army went scientists to collect information from every country for Aristotle's great books of natural history.

Thirteen years later Alexander the Great had completed the conquest of Persia and the whole of the ancient world as far east as India. Then at the age of thirty-two he died of fever in the city of Babylon. After his death the empire he founded fell to pieces, but in each land he had left Greek rulers, Greek settlers, and Greek scholars.

Greek knowledge was thus scattered over the civilized world. But in one place particularly it took root and flourished. That was in Alexandria, in Egypt, near the delta of the Nile. Alexander had founded the city and left one of his companions, a man named Ptolemy, to govern it. The succeeding Ptolemies became the Greek rulers of Egypt; the famous Cleopatra, who was defeated by the Romans, was the last of them.

Under the guidance of the earlier Ptolemies a great museum and a library were erected at Alexandria, and a vast number of manuscripts of Greek scholars were collected. The museum was really the first university in the world. With its founding Athens ceased to be the center of learning. Students went instead to Alexandria. Euclid worked there upon his geometry; and it was there that Eratosthenes measured the size of the earth and came within a few hundred miles of being correct in his figures. It was at Alexandria also that Archimedes studied his problems in engineering, and Heron built the first steam engine.

Not only literature, mathematics, and engineering flourished at Alexandria, but also medicine. In the third and second centuries before the Christian Era the leading doctors of all countries gathered there. They developed something new in medicine, and made the greatest advance since the days of Hippocrates—although it was to be forgotten. It was the study of human anatomy through dissection of the human body.

Such a thing would not seem unusual to us today, for we realize that a doctor cannot carry out his work unless he knows the structure of the body and all its organs. But in ancient times, and in fact until only about a century ago, there was intense opposition to dissection; one of the most lurid chapters in the history of medicine concerns, as we shall see, the "anatomy murderers," the anatomy riots, and grave robbers in the early years of the nineteenth century, before the present anatomy laws were passed.

In ancient times the Egyptians had held the body far too sacred, as you could guess from the care they took in embalming it, to allow dissection. The religious beliefs of the Greeks likewise forbade it. Hippocrates knew very little about the actual structure of the human body and though Aristotle, perhaps, knew more, he had never seen a human dissection. Both these men had studied only animals, and they drew their conclusions concerning human beings from what they found in animals.

But in Alexandria in the third and second centuries B.C., people from every part of the world met, beliefs were mingled, old religions were discarded, and new ones grew up. Traditions were changing, and for a short time dissections of the human body were performed without opposition.

One doctor at Alexandria, Herophilus, wrote a textbook of anatomy, telling what he found in the body and comparing human structures with those of animals. Although we call it a book, it was really a hand-written manuscript, a roll of papyrus. There were, of course, in those days before printing, few copies of any work, because of the great labor involved in writing out each one by hand. The anatomy book of Herophilus was known to the men who lived in his time, but only fragments of it have come down to us.

It was Herophilus who discovered the nerves in the body; Aristotle had erroneously thought that nerves and tendons were the same, just as he had thought that arteries held air instead of blood. The word "artery" means a passage for air.

Knowledge of anatomy is the first step toward the discovery of the cause of disease. That step was made, but forgotten; and progress stopped for nearly 1800 years. Ancient medicine had reached its peak and was about to start on a period of decline.

The medicine of the Greeks, as we have seen, was spread widely by the conquests of Alexander. In the various countries changes were made in it. At Alexandria it was improved; in other cities queer local beliefs concerning the influence of stars, of colors, and of numbers on disease were added to it. Some of these notions were eventually to find their way into the medicine of Europe in astrology and other superstitions, but for a time our story does not concern them; rather we shall follow the stream of civilization that carried Greek medicine on to our time. And so for a moment we turn again from medicine to politics.

To the west of Greece lay a strip of land extending like a great boot out into the Mediterranean—the Italian peninsula. When Alexander was making his conquests, the foot of the peninsula and the island of Sicily next to the toe were inhabited by Greeks; their main cities were Tarentum and Syracuse. On the mainland of Africa, divided from Sicily by a narrow strip of water, was the city of Carthage, founded long before by the Phœnicians.

The greater part of Italy belonged to a people called the

Latins, or Romans, from their principal city, Rome. They were mainly farmers. For a long time they had struggled with a neighboring people, the Etruscans, and with the barbaric Gauls who lived in the north. In 290 B.C., thirty-three

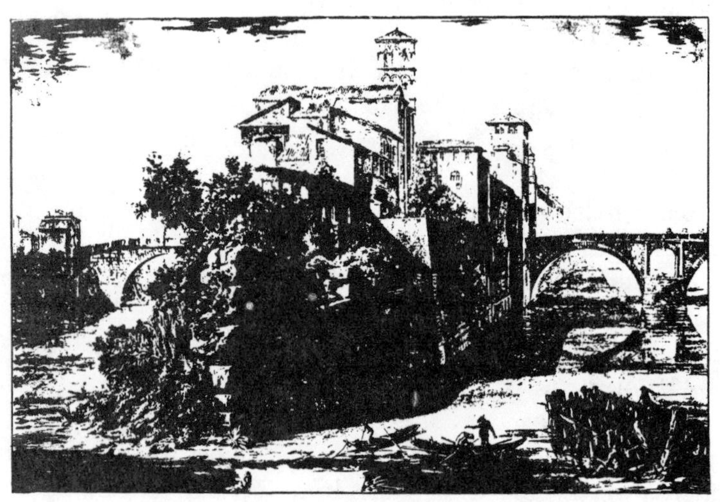

Site of the Roman Temple of Æsculapius.

years after Alexander had completed his conquest, Rome became mistress of the whole central region of the peninsula.

The Romans at this time were far less civilized than their Greek neighbors; they were more like backwoodsmen. They worshiped gods that were almost the same, except in names, as those of the Greeks. Their medicine was still religious in character; indeed they had a god or goddess for nearly every symptom of disease. They had no physicians as did the Greeks.

In 293 B.C. a severe epidemic like the one that had occurred at Athens more than a century before, broke out in Rome. The Roman gods seemed powerless to control it, and so a messenger was sent to the Greeks to borrow one of their gods for the occasion. A temple of Æsculapius was erected on an island in the river Tiber opposite the city of Rome. This temple is of importance in our story, for it was to become the first true hospital.

The Romans up to this time seem to have attracted little attention from their Greek neighbors. But during the next hundred years the farmers of Italy, successful in their battles against Carthage—the famous Punic wars—became a conquering people thirsty for land, for power, and for booty. Eventually they extended their conquests as far west as Britain and east over the countries that Alexander had ruled.

The Romans as conquerors were a far different people from the Greeks. They did not put men of science in the countries they defeated; indeed they had no scientists, for the Romans were "practical" people and regarded law and war and politics as the only honorable careers. Instead Greek physicians came to Rome, some as slaves and others as free men to make their fortunes there. It was after the fall of Corinth that Greek medicine finally reached Rome.

With the coming of Greek physicians, Greek medicine together with Greek customs and luxuries became popular at Rome. There were many of these physicians whose names have come down to us for the cures they wrought, the wealth they accumulated, and the public monuments they erected, but none, until the first and second centuries A.D., is important to our story. Let us see what the Romans themselves gave to medicine, for although they had no physicians of their own, they did contribute to the progress of medicine. Their contribution was in the field of what we should call public health, or sanitation.

The Greek cities were not equipped with sewers, nor did they always have good supplies of fresh water. For lack of sanitation they could not grow to any great size. The practical Romans, however, put in sewers and built aqueducts to bring fresh water to their city. When Rome was in her prime, nearly two hundred million gallons of fresh water flowed into the city each day. No modern city of equal size has a greater water supply than Rome had nearly 2000 years ago.

Sewers and water supply are not the only contributions to medicine made by the Romans—the greatest gift was the hospital. It was during the reign of the Emperor Claudius, from 41 to 54 A.D., that the first public hospital was founded.

When in an earlier chapter we told of the temples of Æsculapius, we did not call them hospitals. Sick people spent in them only a single night and that for religious reasons. The temples were not places where men, women, and children when seriously ill could be cared for over a long period of time. In Rome, before the days of the Emperors, there were no hospitals in the cities; some of the Greek physicians had offices where they performed operations, but the sick were cared for at home. If they had no relatives to look out for them, they received little or no attention. There were no nurses, in our sense of the word, who could be summoned into the home. And merely to give sick people clean, comfortable surroundings, to care for their wants, to provide them with proper food are some of the most important measures in treating disease.

The first institution of which we know that can be correctly called a hospital grew up on the island in the Tiber on which the Romans in 293 B.C. had erected the temple to Æsculapius.

In the intervening years it had been a cruel custom to put on this island slaves who were old or ill. The Roman author Suetonius says: "On this island of Æsculapius certain men exposed their ill and wornout slaves because of the trouble of treating them." The word "exposed" has, as he uses it, an unpleasant meaning. When a baby was deformed or simply not wanted in the home it was exposed on the steps of some temple. "Exposed" meant that it was left until it had died of starvation.

Suetonius has more to say of this island and the practice of exposing sick slaves there: "The Emperor Claudius, however, decreed that such slaves were free, and, if they recovered, they should not return to the control of their masters."

In time the island became a place of refuge for all poor people who were ill. Care was given to them there. The old temple became a crude sort of hospital.

Soon other hospitals were built, and even free Roman citizens began to use them. The greatest development of the hospital, however, took place in the Roman army. Before the idea had originated, sick and wounded soldiers were sent home for treatment. But as the Roman Empire and the Roman army extended over wider territory, the journeys became too long, and so hospitals were erected at convenient places. The ruins of many of them still exist. They were planned and arranged in a manner far in advance of any subsequent hospitals until modern times.

These Roman hospitals were not charity hospitals. There are few indications indeed that the pagan Romans felt it their duty to provide medical care free of cost for poor people. But it was at Rome, after the rise of the Christian religion, that a lady named Fabiola founded the first charity hospital. We shall tell more of her later.

In this chapter we have followed the progress of medicine over a period of more than four hundred years. We have seen the origin of the study of natural history, the spread of Greek learning, the development of the school of Alexandria, the rise of the Roman Empire, and the founding of sanitation and the hospital. But we have said little of any medical heroes. So before we leave the Roman Empire to its gloomy fate at the hands of the barbarians, we shall turn in the next chapter to three men, two Greeks and a Roman—Dioscorides, Galen, and Pliny. There have been greater heroes of medicine than these three men, greater by far, but their importance lies in the fact that they seemed to the people of the next ten centuries and more, the greatest. Each of these men wrote books on medical subjects. These books, rather than the original works of Hippocrates or Aristotle or Herophilus, became the guiding influence of medicine in the following centuries. Medicine was Greek medicine as interpreted by Pliny and Galen.

CHAPTER VIII

The Bearers of Knowledge, Dioscorides, Pliny, and Galen

IN the days when Alexander made his conquests, and even later when the Roman Empire rose, some men believed in science, but more believed in magic.

Greek medicine and science, although they followed the army of Alexander and later came to Rome, did not rid people of superstition or of belief in spirits and demons and ghosts as a cause of disease. The medicine that we have described was practiced by only a few men. The great masses of people still clung to their age-old beliefs in healing gods and in the magic wrought by spells and charms.

In illness they did not turn to the Greek physicians, but to the remedies their forefathers had used, or else they went to the shops of the rhizotomists or "root cutters" for magic herbs. A "root cutter" was a man who gathered roots and herbs and sold them to people to use in treating disease. With the drugs he gave magic rituals to be carried out when the medicaments were taken. Likewise, when he gathered his herbs, he performed certain rites which were supposed to add to their healing powers.

The mandrake was a popular remedy with the rhizotomists. The plant had a root like a carrot, though it frequently was split into two parts so that by using one's imagination very vigorously it could be seen to resemble the body and legs of a man. This human shape was supposed to give it a special healing power, and according to the rhizotomists it was a dangerous plant to gather. When the mandrake was pulled from the ground, it gave a terrible shriek; anyone who heard the sound fell dead. Of course the question one asks is: How did anyone know this to be so, if everyone who heard it died before he could tell anyone else? That we ask means simply that we are better educated and hence more critical than were the customers of the rhizotomists. They did not ask; they simply believed what they were told and marveled at the powers that such a wonderful drug must have over disease. The rhizotomists told people that the only way this root could be gathered was by tying one end of a string to the plant and the other to a dog. The owner of the dog tightly stopped his ears so that he might not hear the shriek of the mandrake and then called the dog. The dog pulled; the mandrake came from the ground and presumably shrieked, whereupon the dog died. No wonder such a drug brought a very high price.

In Shakespeare's *Romeo and Juliet*, in the fourth act, Juliet says, "And shrieks like mandrakes' torn out of the earth, that living mortals, hearing them, run mad." So we know that the legend of the mandrake was still current 1600 years and more after the time of the most famous of all the Greek rhizotomists, Crateuas.

Crateuas was private herb doctor to Mithridates VI, King of Pontus, in the last century before the Christian Era. He was famous, not for the medicines he prepared, but because, as far as we know, he was the first man to use drawings to illustrate descriptions of plants. His book, or rather the remnant of it that has survived, was filled with the usual magic spells that all rhizotomists used—but it differed in having pictures in it.

There had been men before Crateuas who had described plants, notably Theophrastus, a pupil of Aristotle, but none had used pictures to aid in recognizing them.

About a hundred years after the time of Crateuas, a surgeon in the army of the Emperor Nero named Dioscorides classified plants in a new way; he listed them under the diseases for which they were supposed to be beneficial and gave a short account of each plant, where it grew, what it looked like, and how it was to be used as a remedy.

We know little of the life of Dioscorides himself. Probably he was not an exceptional physician and certainly he would have been forgotten entirely if he had not hit upon this useful way of classifying medicinal plants. He founded what we call today *materia medica*, the materials of medicine, or the list of remedies to be used in treating disease.

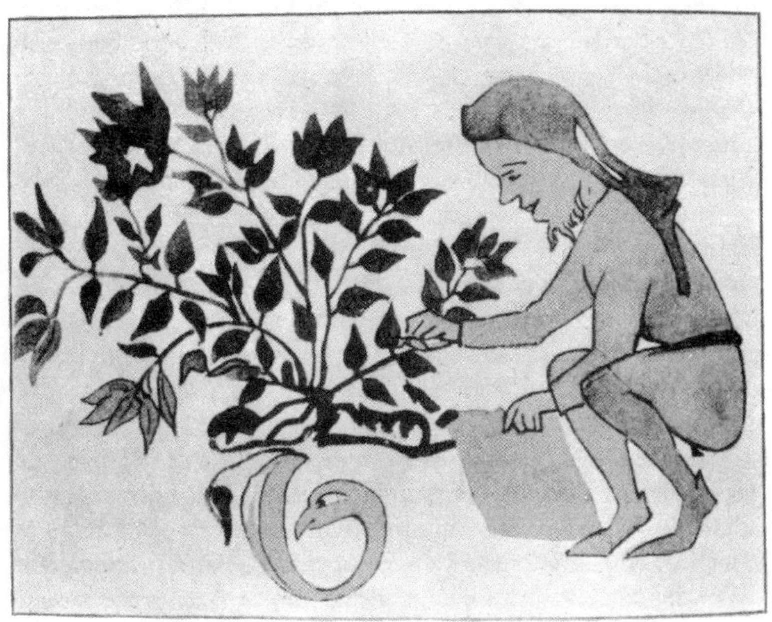

A rhizotomist.

In his travels with the army, Dioscorides had the opportunity to study plants native to many countries, and his book contains descriptions of some six hundred plants and plant products. About one hundred and fifty of these were known to the Greek physicians in the time of Hippocrates; perhaps ninety of them are still used in medicine. It was not the plants he chose that made the work of Dioscorides important, but the manner in which he classified them.

His book, because of its practical nature, quickly became popular. Copies of it were prepared and illustrated as Crateuas' book had been.

The *materia medica* of Dioscorides came to be called an herbal, which means a book of botany. It was used by the physician, and also kept on the shelf in homes to be referred to in case of illness as a guide to the sort of remedy to be taken.

The pictures in some of the early copies of the book are really excellent works of art. But with each copying little errors crept in and tiny omissions were made, until finally after several centuries the pictures no longer had much resemblance to the plants they were supposed to represent.

Translated into nearly every language, the herbal continued in use for more than 1500 years. During all these centuries no one took the trouble to make the drawings fit the plants. This slavish copying of the old, regardless of error, is characteristic of the unprogressive state into which medicine passed during the years following the fall of the Roman Empire.

The herbal of Dioscorides and the *Natural History* of Pliny were the great sources of scientific information in the first 1400 years of the Christian Era.

Pliny was one of the few Romans who wrote on science. He was born at Como about 23 A.D. He was a learned man, and very well educated in the humanities and subjects considered essential in his time; that is, he had studied rhetoric and was familiar with the popular philosophy of his day, he was well versed in military and legal matters and had even studied botany in the gardens of Antonius Castor at Rome. But from our point of view Pliny was learned rather than well educated. He accepted without criticism everything that he heard or read, and wrote things down as facts without attempting to prove by trial or observation whether they were true or false. He had a great curiosity, and his curiosity took him into every field of knowledge. But somehow as we read his writings the words of Hippocrates come to mind: "merely to think one knows is ignorance." Unfortunately the men who came after Pliny were as credulous and as uncritical as he was, and they too believed all that he had written.

If you wish to know how an energetic, studious Roman

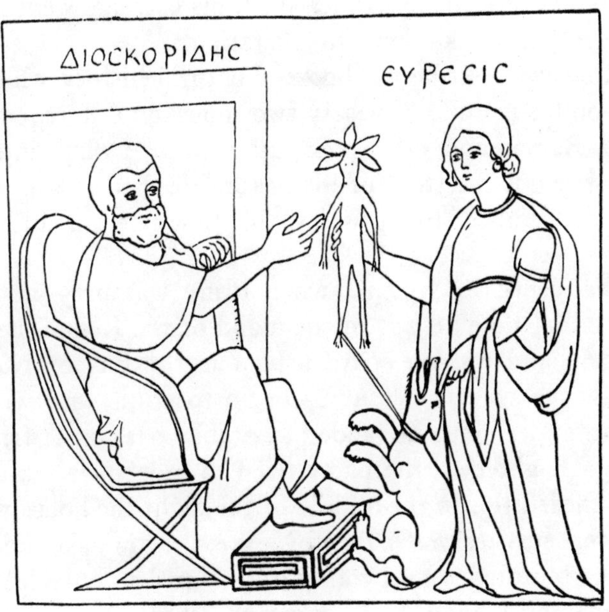

The legend of the mandrake.

like Pliny spent his days, you can turn to the account which his nephew, Pliny the Younger, has left of his uncle's habits. He called upon the Emperor before daybreak (the Romans had no adequate artificial lighting and so, except in the case of a banquet or celebration, they went to bed early and rose before dawn). Pliny's call of ceremony over, he performed the necessary duties of the various government offices he held. These completed, he went home and had a slave read to him or else take down in a kind of shorthand what he dictated. Next came luncheon, after which, unless official duties called him, he lay down and again listened while his slave read. Later in the afternoon he bathed, ate a light lunch, and took a nap. Then he often continued his studies until dinner time, which was just before dark. He rarely walked, so the nephew says, but was usually driven in a conveyance to save time. With his carriage went a secretary ready to take down his dictation.

Before we describe the book of natural history which he based on his reading of nearly two thousand different works by 146 Roman and 326 Greek authors, it is perhaps interesting to recount the story of his death. He died in a peculiar way, as a result of his curiosity, this time not to read but to see.

It happened in 79 A.D., when Pliny was fifty-six years old. At that time he was in command of the Roman fleet at Misenum and was on board a boat in the Bay of Naples. He saw the volcano Vesuvius begin to erupt, and wishing to get a closer view, he landed at Stabiæ with some friends. Though frightened, the party tried to hide their fears and dined cheerfully. In the middle of the night the house where they were staying was shaken by a great earthquake. Fearing that the building would collapse, they rushed outside; they were met by a shower of rocks and ashes. Hastily seizing cushions, they bound them over their heads and stumbled about in darkness lit now and again by flashes of flame from Vesuvius. They waited for morning, but no sunlight could penetrate the cloud of dust and smoke. With lighted torches they made their way to the shore. The sea was too rough to embark in small boats. Fumes of sulphur began to fill the air. Pliny, weak and choking, lay down and asked for water. Threatening flames shot through the pall of clouds. In fear the men roused Pliny; two slaves lifted him, but he collapsed. The slaves fled. The eruption grew more violent.

Molten lava flowed down the mountain sides and covered the famous city of Pompeii.

This great upheaval of nature which Pliny had seen with his own eyes he could never describe in his *Natural History*. When, two days later, his companions came back in search

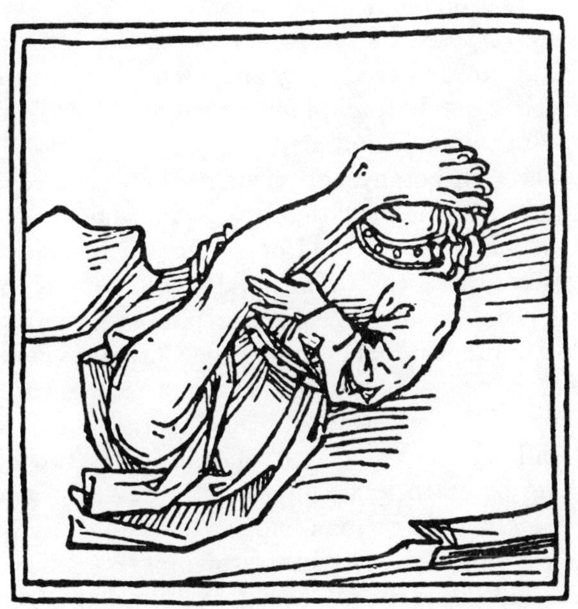

A man from the country of one-footed people.

of him, they found him in the very spot where the slaves had left him. There were no injuries on his body, but he was dead.

His great *Natural History* was copied and recopied and became the storehouse of knowledge for the men of fifty generations after his time.

The book, or rather books, for it is divided into thirty-seven parts, was intended as an encyclopedia of all physical knowledge. It contains much sound information, but mingled with fact is fancy and legend and what is for us superstition.

The book begins with a description of the universe. Pliny, like all learned men of his time, knew that the earth was round; but in spite of the general belief in his writings the men who came after him often doubted whether he was correct in that opinion.

Having disposed of the formation of the earth and the stars, Pliny covered geography and the rise of man; next he dealt with animals and plants, then with medicine, and finally with minerals and art.

The parts on botany and medicine are what concern us here. Pliny held the view that every plant had some special medicinal value if we could only discover it, and that for every disease there was a plant that would cure it. Indeed it was this peculiar sort of belief, or philosophy, of his that made his writings popular among the Christians, who in his day were gaining strength and who in a few centuries were to dominate Western Europe. The Christians held what we should call teleological beliefs. That is, they thought that everything on earth had a useful purpose and was created for the sole benefit of mankind, an idea that, as we shall see later, greatly influenced medical progress. Pliny wrote: "Nature and the earth fill us with admiration . . . as we contemplate that they are created for the wants or enjoyments of mankind." Pliny, although a pagan, seemed thus to hold Christian views and so his works were in great favor among the Christians.

The *Natural History* contains marvelous tales of men (living of course in a far distant country) whose feet turned the wrong way, of men who had no mouths but fed entirely on the fragrance of flowers, and of men whose feet were so large that they could hold them over their heads like parasols to shade themselves from the sun. Side by side with sound facts and science are stories of winged horses, unicorns, mermaids, and the almost human dolphins. Such fanciful tales would be merely amusing if it were not for the fact that they were implicitly believed by later men. We find them scattered through the stories of the *Arabian Nights*, and in the folk tales of Europe and the beliefs of ignorant people of today, and we shall encounter them again

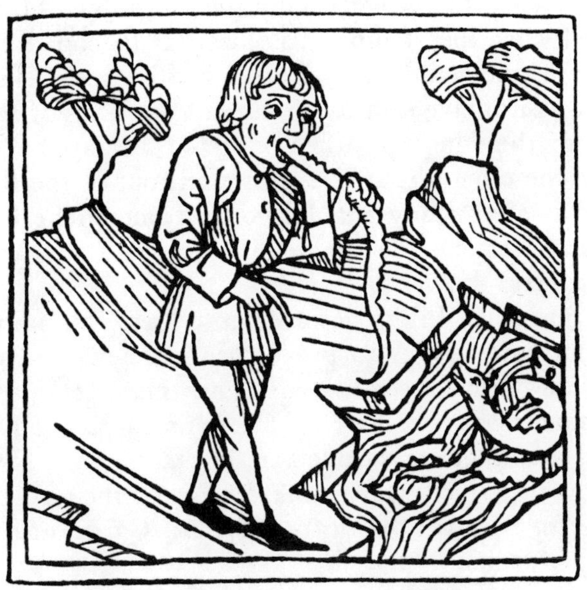

A man from the country of snake eaters.

and again in the medical beliefs of Europe as late as the sixteenth century. A famous king of France once paid an enormous sum of money for the horn of a unicorn to be used as a medicine. What the unscrupulous dealer sold him was probably the horn of a narwhal.

Pliny had a great influence on medicine after his time, though unfortunately he really knew little about the subject. He did not trust in theories; he was rather a "practical man," and believed in what he called "experience." But like so many "practical men" what he meant by experience was what he had heard and what he himself believed. Untrained as he was in science, he often took for proofs of facts things that were neither proofs nor facts. He did not test his experience with experiments.

Here is one of his typical "proofs." "The herb dittany," he writes, "has the power to extract arrows. This was proved by stags who had been struck by these missiles which were loosened when they fed on this plant." If he had really desired proof, he could easily have tested his idea. With arrows he could have shot say a dozen stags but not fatally. To six of these he could then have fed dittany, but given none to the other six. If the arrows fell out of the flesh of those that ate dittany but did not fall out of the flesh of those that ate none, then he would have had a real proof of his statement.

It is unfair to Pliny, however, to criticize his failure to carry out experiments to prove theories. Few men before and equally few for centuries after his time, attempted any such thing. Today we look upon experiment as the natural way of finding out and demonstrating facts.

Of the three men whose work dominated the medicine of Europe for nearly 1500 years only one, Galen, attempted any experiments.

The story of Galen takes us first to the year 133 B.C., when there occurred one of the extraordinary events in history. In the rich Greek colony of Pergamum in Asia Minor the king, Attalus III, when he died, bequeathed his kingdom, for no known reason, to the Roman people. All its riches and its lands were to become the property of the citizens of Rome.

Imagine if you can the same thing being done today: the King of England, let us say, presenting Great Britain to the people of Italy! Of course today no king has such absolute power over his dominions as to be able to do anything like that. But Pergamum at the bequest of Attalus became Roman property.

In this Roman land of Pergamum a boy was born 264 years later who was destined to perhaps the greatest reputation that any physician, save Hippocrates, has ever achieved. His name was Galen, which means the calm, peaceful one. He was the son of Nicon, an engineer.

The boy Galen was carefully trained to be a philosopher. But when he was eighteen his father had a dream which led

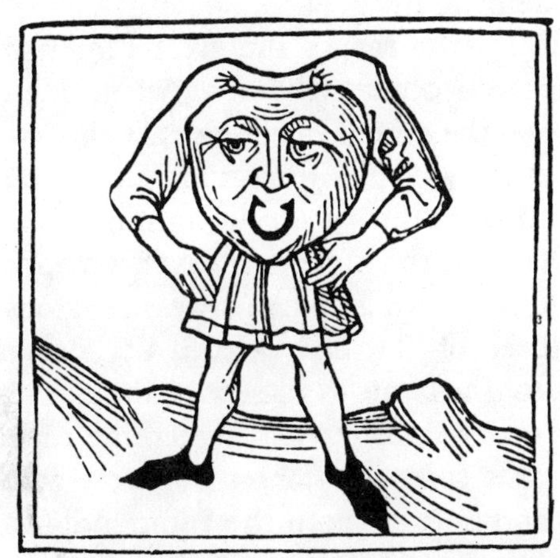

A man from the country of headless people.

him to have his son study medicine. Dreams, as you know, were taken as omens in those days. Today telling the future from dreams is a practice limited to not very bright or well-instructed people, who read what are called "Dream Books," supposed to tell the significance of every sort of dream. Dreams may tell a great deal about the past and the dreamer's thoughts, but they tell nothing of the future. Yet in 149 A.D., when Galen was eighteen, even the most intelligent and educated men shaped their lives according to their dreams. Because of his father's dream, Galen turned from philosophy to medicine, and a great and influential physician was given to the world.

When Galen was twenty, his father died; but already the young man had acquired all the medical knowledge which his teachers were able to give him. There was nothing to keep him in Pergamum. And since it was the practice then for physicians who wished to gain wide experience to go from country to country studying with the leading doctors, Galen set out on his travels. For nearly ten years he wandered, staying here awhile and there awhile, but steadily nearing Alexandria, his goal.

Alexandria was no longer the great center of learning it had been nearly 500 years before when Herophilus and Archimedes and the other Greek scientists had worked there. But the skeletons used for dissections in the old days were still there, and from them a physician might learn the shape and arrangement of the human bones. This opportunity was lacking in the Greek and Roman cities; religious beliefs forbade such abuse of the body. Even at Alexandria Galen could not obtain a body to dissect, although he must have seen skeletons there and learned something of human structure. But he was forced to content himself with the dissection of hogs and apes to learn the form and arrangement of the internal organs. He assumed that man's organs were similar. This assumption, as we shall see later, had an unfortunate influence upon medicine for many centuries after Galen's time, for men believed that the human anatomy was like that of apes and hogs.

In 157 A.D. Galen returned to his native city of Pergamum, ready to start on his career as a physician. It was an amazing career, one that almost forces us to believe in luck.

Of course, many wise people tell us that there is no such thing as luck, that success and happiness in life come to those who work hard for them and seize their opportunities. It is certainly true that many people try to cover their own deficiencies and faults by calling them "bad luck." But that is not the sort of thing we mean. We mean that some men have the ability to seize fortunate opportunities. Galen was a well-trained physician, he was highly intelligent, and he had, perhaps most important of all, a remarkable personality; people liked him and were impressed by him. He was very, very sure of himself—too sure, in fact. And he was willing to assume responsibilities. No doubt there were many other men of Greece and Rome as gifted as he. But fortune was with Galen.

When he returned to Pergamum, the summer gladiatorial shows were about to begin, but no one had been appointed to fill the important position of surgeon to the gladiators. Welcomed as the returning son of an honored man, Nicon, Galen was given this position. That was good fortune for a young man. Many gladiators were wounded, and wounded seriously, in the contests, but under Galen's care not one died. Galen was credited with their recovery. No doubt he was a good surgeon for his time, but often gladiators were so badly wounded that no medical care could save them. And for three years in succession Galen was appointed surgeon to the gladiators.

A man less ready to seize the opportunities of fortune might have stayed on in this important post, training, directing, treating the athletes and acquiring a great reputation in Pergamum. But Galen in the midst of his first success continued to study philosophy and medicine, trying to perfect himself; and he wrote, practicing the art of expressing himself in order that he might influence people.

In 161 A.D. he gave up his position in Pergamum and went to Rome, the great city which drew every ambitious man of the Empire. Rome for young Galen was a far different place from his home country, Pergamum. In Rome no one knew of him or of his father, Nicon. It must have seemed to him that there were countless physicians in the great city. Some were good, some bad, some modest and honest, some shrewd and self-exploiting, and every one of them fighting for his own success. Galen was an almost friendless country boy in a big city.

A lesser man than he might have failed and returned to Pergamum, but Galen watched for his chance. He called on fellow countrymen from Pergamum who had come to Rome and were established there. One of them, Eudemus by name, fell ill; he called in a famous physician to treat

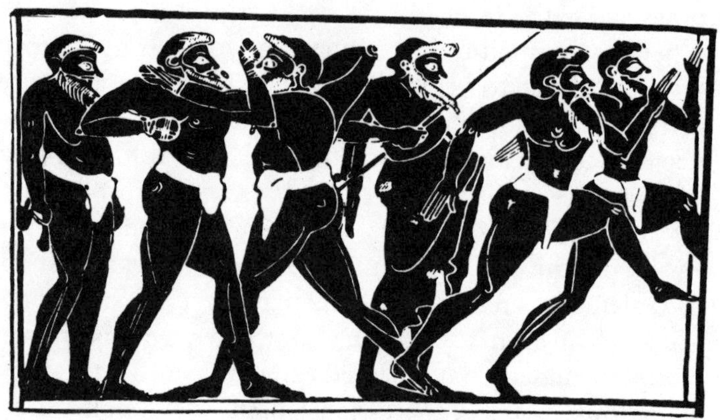

Gladiators training.

him. But each day he grew worse, until at last his life was despaired of. Thinking he was soon to die, he sent for Galen. That young man with amazing courage disagreed with the great doctor who was in charge of the case. He said that the treatment was wrong, but that if Eudemus followed his advice, he would live. That was a grave responsibility to take, for if Eudemus died, Galen would be a ruined man.

It may have been Galen's skill, or his good fortune, or both—but at any rate the patient lived. And that Eudemus happened to be a prominent man at Rome, with many admirers, was certainly Galen's good fortune, for Eudemus told all his friends how the young doctor from Pergamum saved his life when the leading physician of Rome had given him up as hopeless.

Patients flocked to Galen. Jealous, the physicians of

Rome turned against him. He defended himself in speeches and with pamphlets. His patients believed in him and trusted him.

The wife of the Consul, Flavius Boethius, fell ill. Galen treated her, and she too recovered. Her husband became a firm friend and admirer of Galen. He set aside a room for the young physician where he might dissect animals and prepare a book on anatomy.

In four years the country boy who had come to Rome had reached the height of success in medicine. Only one step remained, and that was about to be taken. The Consul Boethius and another friend, Marcus Barbarus, son-in-law of the Emperor Marcus Aurelius, wished to have Galen appointed physician at court. Everything was in readiness for this last success when Galen did a peculiar thing. Probably no one will ever know why, but suddenly he left Rome, returned to Pergamum, and took up the practice of medicine there.

Many people have speculated as to why he left. Perhaps they wondered then, for a second curious thing occurred, and some men have said that his departure was closely connected with it. Within a few months a great epidemic of some infectious disease broke out in Rome, killing thousands of people. Did Galen leave to escape the approaching epidemic —did he run away? We can hardly blame him if he did, for his medicine, his skill could be of no avail against this great outbreak of disease which for sixteen years was to fill the streets of Rome with funerals and the homes with sorrow. But to run away is a thing that few physicians have ever done, as we shall see when we come to the story of the epidemics of the Black Death in Europe years later. Physicians stay and treat and comfort people even when they know they are giving their lives to their calling. It has been suggested that Galen went home to Pergamum because he felt that he would be needed there if the epidemic spread to that city.

He had been in Pergamum two years when a messenger from the Roman Emperor arrived there searching for him. Galen was ordered to join the army of the Emperor Marcus Aurelius and to become the court physician. He reached the army at Aquileia, then a large city situated near the upper end of the Adriatic Sea. The epidemic of disease, still spreading, swept down upon the Roman army. The Emperor Marcus Aurelius fled toward Rome, and with him went his adopted brother, the Emperor Verus. Marcus Aurelius reached Rome; Verus died on the way; Galen stayed at Aquileia.

Again Marcus Aurelius sent for Galen. He was to accompany the Emperor as his personal physician on a campaign against the barbarians to the north. But Galen convinced the Emperor that it would be better if he, the great physician, stayed in Rome to take care of the Emperor's son, Commodus.

Marcus Aurelius died some ten years later, still fighting the barbarians. Galen remained at Rome, writing, studying, and lecturing. Commodus came to the throne, and Galen was his court physician. Twelve years later Commodus was murdered, but Galen remained on at court, still working. Pertinax and Didius Julianus became emperors, and then Septimius Severus, and Galen continued as court physician —still writing, still studying. Finally in 200 A.D., in the reign of Septimius Severus, he died.

The volumes he wrote have lived as have the writings of few other physicians. As we read on in our story we shall find the name of Galen occurring again and again. It will be Galen this, and Galen that, and Galen said, and Galen can't be wrong.

Even in the sixteenth century when the Belgian, Vesalius, wrote the first true anatomy of the human body, men said he was wrong because Galen had not found things in the body as he found them. In the seventeenth century when William Harvey, physician to King Charles II of England, discovered how blood circulated in the body, men said that he was wrong because Galen had found it otherwise.

Why were Galen's writings so popular? What was it

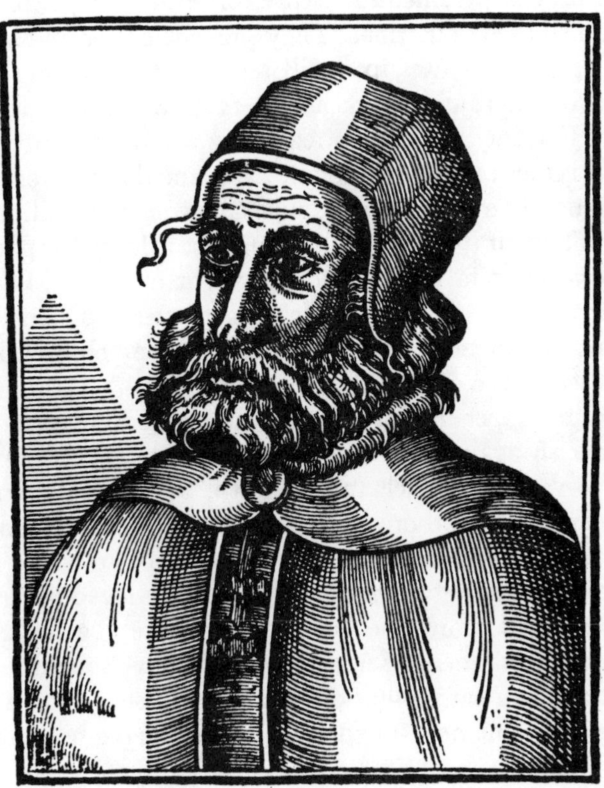

Galen as shown in the surgical works of Ambroise Paré.

about them that made men believe in them? Certainly there had been greater physicians than he; Hippocrates was far greater.

There were two reasons. The first was his positiveness, and the second his love for systematizing everything. Galen was very sure of himself, very certain that he was always right. There was never any doubt in his writings. He had an explanation for everything that might occur, and he was clever enough to make his explanations plausible. People, unless they are trained in science, often have a great liking for plausible explanations. They prevent doubt and so save thinking. Hippocrates, you will remember, was never really certain of anything except actual facts which he could observe. He knew that human reasoning was often faulty. One of his sayings on this very point has come down through the ages in nearly every language. Perhaps you are familiar with the first half of it: "Life is short and art is long." It goes on: "Experience is fallacious and judgment difficult." Hippocrates avoided explanations. He said in effect, "Observe and find out for yourself, and prove it so by many observations." Galen seemed to say, "I'll explain it for you."

Now it happened that after the time of Galen, science did not flourish again for many centuries; men turned passionately to religion, which taught faith, belief in the written word, belief in authority. And Galen was accepted as the supreme authority in medicine. His very positiveness made him so. He said he was right—and men believed him. Here are his actual words: "Never as yet have I gone astray, whether in treatment or in prognosis, as have so many other physicians of great reputation. If anyone wishes to gain fame . . . all that he needs is to accept what I have been able to establish."

Galen's purpose in writing was to bring system into all medical knowledge and to prove that everything was created for a useful purpose for man. He started with the works of Hippocrates, which he admired greatly, but which he felt were badly out of date. He intended to add to them all the knowledge gained in the six hundred years since Hippocrates' time. Then he would bind the whole together into a system, a theory, an explanation of everything that might happen to a man.

Not only did he bring together all the medical knowledge he knew of, but he included all the theories and speculations that had been evolved. To sound facts and observations he added the number lore of the Pythagoreans which we spoke of in the chapter on Hippocrates, the theory of the four humors, and the theory of the qualities. You will remember that the body of every man was supposed to have four qualities, heat and cold and wetness and dryness, and that it was believed that in health these qualities were balanced in the body. In disease they were unbalanced. If a man had fever, one need only say he had too much heat and not enough coldness—that was what ailed him. Everything in the world had one or more of these same qualities. Thus some vegetables were hot, some cold, some wet, and some dry. Cucumber seeds were cooling to the fourth degree—"cool as a cucumber"—and so Galen might give a man with fever cucumber seeds to balance with their coolness the excess of heat which made him sick. It was a simple system—and, as we see it, a foolish one.

We could perhaps laugh at it, if it were not for the sad fact that for fourteen or fifteen centuries after Galen's time sick men and women and children were dosed with the useless "herbs" that Galen had recommended. They were the sort of medicaments that old women in the country sometimes use even now for home remedies—horehound water and onion syrup, sassafras tea and tansy stew. Many of the prescriptions that the followers of Galen used contained hundreds of different herbs. They were what the modern physician calls "shotgun prescriptions"—many drugs shot at the disease in the hope that one of them may hit it. Even now herb drugs—and some few of them are of course very valuable in medicine—are called Galenicals.

If ever any man committed what Hippocrates called the sin of ignorance—"to know is science; merely to believe one knows is ignorance"—it was Galen. And great harm resulted from his "ignorance" spoken with the voice of authority! He said that pus, matter that forms in infected sores, is a necessary part of the healing of wounds. Of course he knew nothing of bacteria or of infection—no one did in those days—but he made a positive statement. There were physicians, nine centuries and again thirteen centuries after his time who said that wounds should be treated so that pus did not form. But men paid no attention to them, for the great Galen had said otherwise. It was only late in the nineteenth century, almost in our time, that a great physician, Lister, showed that Galen was entirely wrong and that antiseptics could be used to prevent infection and the formation of pus.

When one thinks of all the thousands upon thousands of men and women and children who have suffered and perhaps died needlessly of infection because the great Galen had said that pus was necessary to healing, it is difficult to be sympathetic toward his work. But there was one side of it that deserves not only our sympathy but also our admiration.

Galen was the first experimenter in medicine. Men before him had observed facts, but Galen went further; he demonstrated facts. Thus men had observed that injury to the back sometimes led to paralysis of the legs. Galen by cutting the spinal cord showed that this paralysis was due to the injury of the nerves that went to the legs. By experiment he showed that the heart pumps blood and that the lungs draw in air when we breathe. These were great and important discoveries, and he used a great and important method for making discoveries—experiment.

The sad fact is that the men who came after him forgot his experiments, ignored the very thing that would have unlocked for them the secrets of nature, and remembered instead his useless theories and his foolish systems. Whom shall we blame? Galen held out the shiny dross of speculation and the dull gold of true science; men chose the dross.

CHAPTER IX

The Way Divides—East and West

THERE were evil portents in the city of Rome.

When Galen in his old age laid down his pen, he had written *finis* to a chapter in medical progress. Men were no longer concerned with the search for facts, or with science—even the kind of science that Pliny had followed. It was not the diseases of men, but the diseases of society that held their attention. An empire was dying.

The greatest physicians of the ancient world had once come to Rome. But now there were few left in the city whose names are worth recording.

On the streets where Galen had walked proudly there were peddlers of drugs, magicians who pretended to cure disease with charms, fortune tellers, stargazers—fakers all. There are always men willing to profit from the ignorance and the necessities of the most pitiful of all people, the sick and the infirm. When civilization declines, when poverty reigns, when life seems darkest and hardest, people turn more and more to the false prophets of medicine who promise most and do least. And so it was in Rome. The peddlers, magicians, and astrologers were practicing the kind of medicine that savage people had used. Civilization was moving backwards.

We could turn from these scenes of a declining civilization and close the book upon Roman medicine if it were not for one fact. The roots of our own civilization are buried in Roman soil.

The events of those closing years of the Empire left their impression on medicine for centuries to come. The kind of lives people in Europe were to lead, the diseases they were to have, the beliefs they were to hold, and the doctors they were to employ were influenced by things that were occurring in the days when Rome was going to her ruin.

In Galen's time the Roman Empire had expanded to the greatest size it was ever to attain. The Roman eagle held sway over all the lands that touched on the Mediterranean Sea. On the map you will see a ring with Rome at its center, a ring made up of North Africa, Egypt, Palestine, Greece, Italy, France, and Spain. To the north and west the legions had pushed into the British Isles, and there the Romans had erected a wall to hold back the barbarians. Ruins of this farthest outpost of the ancient Empire still stand today in England.

From the conquered lands tribute poured into Rome—taxes and levies, slaves and plunder.

Outside the land held by the Roman Empire, in the great expanse to the north, were the tribesmen of the forests and plains whom the Greeks and Romans called barbarians—the Goths, the Vandals, the Angles, and the Saxons, and to the east the Huns. Although primitive in their way of living as compared to the luxurious Roman nobles, the barbarians loved liberty and freedom and admired strength and courage. The Romans had defeated some of these tribesmen, as Cæsar tells us in his story of the conquest of Gaul, and had made soldiers of them. In the Roman army the barbarians learned Roman ways of fighting. And now like a circle of hungry dogs eying another dog with a juicy bone, they eyed Rome. It was the age-old situation—the city dweller growing fat and soft, the virile nomad watching for a chance to seize and plunder.

But Rome was not only fat and soft; Rome was diseased, sick with the worst of social disorders, injustice and oppression.

The Roman Empire contained perhaps as many inhabitants as does our country today—a hundred million and more. The vast majority of these people were neither free nor independent; they were completely subject to Roman rule; they worked and slaved and paid so that a comparatively few men, Roman citizens, might live in luxury. Wealthy Romans often bought their way into high office; they controlled the Empire; with part of the money they collected they built great stone roads extending from county to county; they erected magnificent public buildings; they

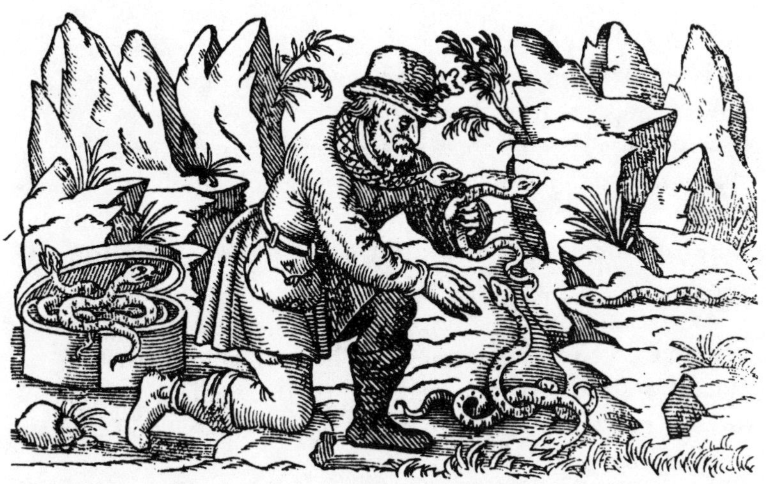

An illustration from one of the translations of Dioscorides.

hired an army to hold back the barbarians; they gave elaborate gladiatorial shows and circuses for the people; to the multitude of restless adventurers and ne'er-do-wells who migrated to Rome they handed out doles of oil and grain.

None of these things brought contentment or prosperity to the people of the conquered lands, who were little better than slaves. The poor and oppressed far outnumbered the Roman citizens. If they had risen under some great popular leader, they might have overthrown the government in a civil war. Such things have happened often in history. But He who had risen to unite the common people in a single cause was not a warrior counseling bloodshed. His message was, "Love your enemies." His fame grew widely in the centuries after he had been condemned to death by the Roman judge of Palestine, Pontius Pilate. The words he had spoken to his disciples in the brief years when he walked the dusty roads of the Holy Land became full of meaning for the oppressed. He had said that all men were brothers; the Roman patrician and the slave were equal before God. He had preached peace and submission, with promise of reward in a future life.

The Christian religion was a solace to the oppressed. It offered hope to the downtrodden; it made a man of the slave. It grew and spread. Every effort of the emperors to stamp out the growing menace to Roman rule brought converts to the Christian fold. Men by thousands and millions were turning from the Empire of Rome to the Empire of God.

Among a people whose minds were fixed upon heaven, who looked for miracles and the help of God, there was no place for science or for medicine of the kind that Hippocrates or even Galen had known. Faith and hope and prayers were taking the place of science.

Among such a people, united in their misery by religion, there could be no patriotic fervor for the Empire of Rome. When the barbarians turned upon the legions, defeated them, and advanced on Rome, the common man did not rise to defend the state. To him the barbarians were merely other masters; none could be worse than the Romans. What did it matter to him if the rich were plundered, the pagan temples burned, and the gladiatorial amphitheaters ruined?

The capture of Rome by the Visigoths in 410 and its destruction by the Vandals in 455 were not events of enormous importance; they were merely announcements that the Empire in the west, long ill, was at last dead. Already the Vandals had settled in Spain, the Angles and Saxons had moved into Britain, the Huns from the east had migrated into France.

A century before the fall of Rome, the capital of the Roman Empire was transferred from Rome to a city to the east called Byzantium.

It was not the approach of the barbarians that drove the emperors to Byzantium, but the unsuitable position of Rome. The Romans were not seafaring people; they traveled by land and not by water. Italy projects far out from the mainland and a journey half the length of the peninsula was necessary when troops or messengers or the emperor himself wished to go from Rome to other provinces. Because of this fact the emperors in time of war had often set up temporary headquarters at some place more conveniently located. Constantine the Great, who ruled from 306 to 337, finally transferred the imperial power permanently to Byzantium, and the name of the city was changed to Constantinople.

Constantine was the first emperor to be baptized a Christian. In three centuries Christianity had spread from the hovels of slaves to the imperial court.

With the removal of the capital, the Empire split in two great divisions: a Greek-speaking eastern half and a Latin-speaking western half. The Western Empire fell to the barbarians, and that portion included southwestern Europe.

Our story of medicine divides now and runs for many centuries in two channels—one to the West, one to the East. In the East it will be the record of medicine in the Byzantine Empire and among the Arabs, who are soon to come in a conquering horde. In the West it will be the record of medicine in a barbaric civilization, but a civilization from which our own has sprung. Far along in our story the medicine of the East and of the West will finally meet and go on together.

First let us see what the conditions were in the Western Empire. The barbarians had entered the Roman towns; the tribesmen and the men who had lived under Roman rule occupied the same lands. There was a great mixing of the population; barbarians and highly civilized men intermingled. The tribesmen from different regions spoke different languages, which gradually blended with the Latin of the Roman inhabitants. New languages were evolved, modifications of Latin which we now call French, Italian, Spanish, and Portuguese. And when Europe was in the making there was little communication and little travel between the small settlements of people, and so many different variations of the languages—dialects—grew up.

With the fall of the Roman Empire, Europe was left with no general controlling power. The scattered tribes of barbarians had for a time been united under leaders in their conquests, but as they settled they again broke into small groups, each one independent of the others. It was in effect a condition which still persists in some uncivilized countries, such as parts of Africa, where each town is the home of a tribe and each tribe is an independent unit. Conditions in Europe were in many ways similar to those in our own country during the gold rush of 1849, when rough and lawless men as well as worthy citizens migrated to the West and set up new towns. Because of the lack of a governing power, the strong preyed on the weak, and brigands made the lands between the towns unsafe for travelers. You will remember how in our own newly settled West, under the influence of the men who saw the need of law and order, vigilance committees were organized to stop crime, and officers were elected, laws drawn up, and order finally established.

Similarly in Europe in the early days there were, mingling with the barbarian invaders, men who had been under Roman rule and had ideas of civilization. Under their influence a form of government grew up that came to be known as the feudal system. Someone, because of his strength or cunning, became the feudal lord. The people on the neighboring farmlands swore allegiance to him; he became ruler, protector, and military leader. As a result of the growth of this system, Europe became a network of feudal domains. Each had its lord with his castle and men at arms; in the surrounding lands over an area large or small, depending on the strength of the lord, the lesser people acknowledged his rule. In theory the feudal lord was the owner of all the land under his domain.

In time another ruling power appeared—the king, who, so it came to be believed, held all the land by divine right. The kings at first were usually feudal lords who had become powerful and expanded their domains by conquering other feudal lords and forcing them to acknowledge their overlordship.

The matters we discuss here may seem to be far more political than medical, but we cannot follow the course of medicine in the early days in Europe unless we know the conditions under which people lived.

The part that Christianity played in medicine was important, too, and to study it we must return for a moment to Rome in the closing years of the Empire. Christianity, as we have said, had spread among the people and even reached the palace when in the fourth century after Christ the Emperor Constantine was baptized. Now there was one feature of Christianity that linked it to medicine. Christ had taught self-sacrifice. Some of his followers interpreted this as mortification of the flesh. That is, they tried in every way to abolish all their earthly desires by tortures which they imposed upon themselves. Many of them left their families and their friends and went into desert regions to live alone in caves. They rarely ate, they whipped and tortured themselves, and they prayed long hours at a time. They thought that this mortification of the flesh, this suppression of all earthly pleasure, would make them pleasing in the sight of God and so assure them a place in heaven.

Men and women who gave a broader interpretation to the meaning of self-sacrifice, instead of becoming hermits, devoted their lives to caring for the poor, and the ill. The Roman Empire at this time needed such men and women badly; century after century great epidemics of disease had been spreading among the inhabitants. In the next chapter, we shall describe one such epidemic, but here we are concerned only with the way the Christians behaved in the presence of disease. The pagan Romans, when epidemics broke out, had often fled in fear and left the sick to die

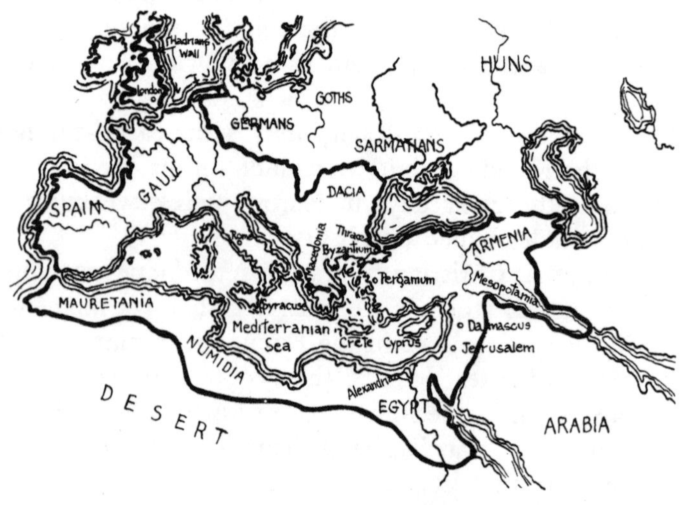

Map of the Roman Empire.

without care. Many of the Christians felt it a religious duty to stay and nurse the sick, to sacrifice their own lives if necessary in the service of the helpless.

Fabiola, whose conception of self-sacrifice inspired the founding of the first charity hospital at Rome was a Christian.

In another chapter we told how the Romans founded the first public hospital, built on the island where sick slaves were left to die. But so far as we know, food and shelter and medical care were not given there free of cost. Only those who could afford to pay were welcomed. Fabiola created a hospital where free care was given out of charity, as a Christian duty.

About a century after she had founded her hospital, when the feudal system was in its infancy, a young man whom we know as St. Benedict decided to become a Christian hermit. He went to a place fifty miles from Rome where Nero had once had a summer home, crawled into a cave, and scourged his flesh with whip and hair shirt. For three years he lived there; and during this time his reputation as a holy man spread over the countryside. People flocked to see him. Finally he emerged from the cave, gave up his self-torture and established monasteries in which young men were educated to be priests of the Christian religion. The monks in these monasteries extended charity and help to the poor and needy, and cared for the sick. The monasteries grew in number and spread throughout Europe. They were the sole centers in which education was kept alive; they served as hospitals; the monks, who were the only educated men—indeed the only men who could read and write—acted as physicians.

The Western Empire—Europe—as we leave it now to turn to the eastern channel of our story, was a country of feudal rule and monastic medicine. Its civilization was primitive, and so was its medicine. There were no medical schools, and no trained physicians. The well-meaning priests did what they could to help ailing people, but too often all they could do was pray and comfort.

In contrast to the primitive conditions in the West, the luxury of Roman life continued in the East. The emperors in their palace at Constantinople carried on the customs of Roman rule. But these people of the East were different from the Latins of Rome.

The traditions of the Eastern, or Byzantine Empire, were older than the Roman. They came from Egypt and Syria and Greece.

In the Eastern Empire there was a mingling of Greek

culture, Roman law, Christian religion, and Egyptian and Syrian magic.

In one respect, and it is a very important one for medicine, this Greek civilization differed from that of the time of Alexander. The Greek love for learning lasted, but the spirit of the search for truth was lost. The learned men of the Eastern Empire were mere copyists—repeating what other physicians had said, especially Galen and Dioscorides and Pliny. And into their writings crept beliefs that were held by the Christians of those days, belief in miracles and the effectiveness of prayer in curing disease, and belief in magic. This influence you can see in the writings of the doctors of the times. Aetius, physician to the Emperor Justinian I, prescribed as the best method for removing a bone from the throat saying in a loud voice to the bone, "As Jesus Christ drew Lazarus from the grave, and Jonah out of the whale, thus Blasius, the martyr and servant of God, commands, 'Bone come up or bone go down.' " The author of these foolish words occupied the same position in the Roman court of the East that Galen had held four hundred years before in Imperial Rome.

Beyond the description of the symptoms of a few diseases, there was no advance made in medicine in the Eastern Empire, no lives of medical heroes to record. But the scholars of Byzantium performed one service to medicine. In the palaces and in the monasteries the men who admired Greek learning but could not use it collected and copied the ancient medical books. The books were preserved—a store of knowledge which would be available when men knew how to use it.

Medicine, as we leave it here at the close of the sixth century, had declined far below the level to which Hippocrates raised it. It survived, but feebly, in the monasteries of the West; it was preserved in the documents in the libraries of the Eastern Empire, in the works of Galen, of Pliny, of Dioscorides, and in a few scattered manuscripts of Hippocrates and Aristotle. Before medicine could progress again, it had to regain the ground it had lost. A thousand years and more had elapsed since the days of Aristotle and Hippocrates; a thousand more must pass before medicine would revive fully. And it is to the first of the quickening influences in this revival that we now turn. Our story leads us next to a people who have not yet crossed our pages—the Arabs. But before the Arabs descend to ravage the cities of the East there is another event to record—a tragic event—a great outbreak of a deadly disease.

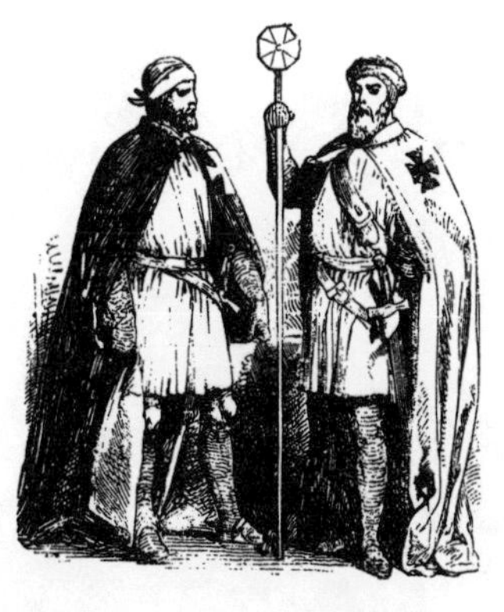

Part Four

DISEASE AND CONQUEST

SCIENCE UNDER THE CALIPHS

MEDICINE FOLLOWS THE CRUSADES

CHAPTER X

Disease and Conquest

PLAGUE and pestilence dealing death in the home and in the street, or a barbaric enemy killing on the battlefield and plundering in the town—which is the more terrible? Both were to fall upon the Eastern Roman Empire.

The pestilence came first—a product of trade and commerce.

When people live in small communities isolated one from another, there can be little diffusion of acute infectious diseases. By an acute infection is meant one in which the illness develops quickly and is severe; it lasts a few days or weeks and then the man affected is either dead or on his way toward recovery. In either case he can no longer spread the disease. You are familiar with the milder forms of acute infectious diseases—tonsilitis, the head cold, measles, and chicken pox, and perhaps scarlet fever. There are others which are serious and deadly: smallpox, bubonic plague, and typhus fever.

There are also infectious diseases that are not acute, but that are called chronic. They may persist for years, during all of which time the sick man may spread the disease. Leprosy and tuberculosis are diseases of this kind. They can be spread even by slow commerce, but the acute infections cannot.

In a sparsely settled district where weeks or even months of travel lie between the towns, epidemics of acute infections rarely occur, for they are spread only by the contact of the sick man with the well. If, then, travelers with smallpox, let us say, started out for a distant city, they would be ill on the way. Some might die, but those who finally reached their destination would have recovered so completely that they would no longer spread the infection.

When large groups of people hold active commerce with

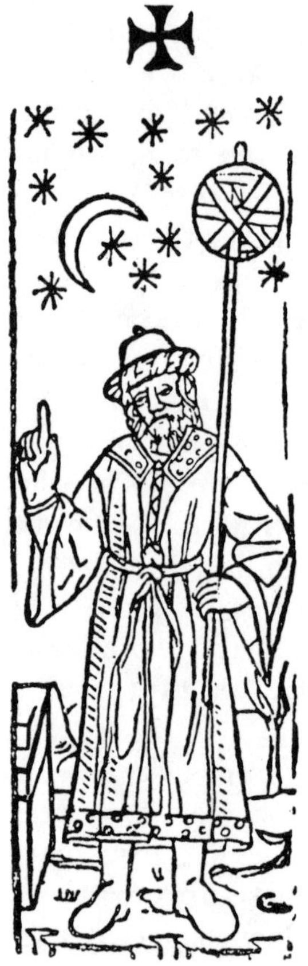

The planets that caused the plague.

each other, when cities are close together and means of transportation rapid, then acute infectious diseases travel along the same routes that men travel.

The Romans built paved roads throughout the Empire.

Their trade extended even to China, where Roman gold changed hands for silk. Trade and travel grew up before medicine had developed the means for controlling the more serious epidemics of disease. In the Empire extending along the shores of the Mediterranean, plague and typhus rode in the caravan of the traveler and in the ranks of the legions. Reaching the cities, disease would advance like a great conflagration, sweeping everyone before it. The population would flee in panic, leaving the sick to die unattended. Finally, when, like a fire that had burned out, the disease died down, the refugees would return. Many of their friends would be gone; some would have survived, crippled and broken in health. Again travel and commerce would begin and flourish. Then after a pause, perhaps a decade, perhaps a century or more, the plague and pestilence would again ride in the caravan of the traveler and in the ranks of legions and would wreak their frightful mortality upon the cities.

We have mentioned some of these epidemics of disease in earlier chapters. Pericles and his sons died in a pestilence that occurred at Athens. The Romans before their conquest of Greece suffered from epidemics; it was then, you will remember, that they erected on the island in the Tiber the temple to Æsculapius that was to become the first hospital. Again at Rome when Marcus Aurelius was Emperor there was another outbreak, the one that men said frightened Galen away and that killed the Emperor Verus. There were other epidemics in the closing years of the Western Empire, and unquestionably they contributed to the decline and eventual fall of the Empire. But when the barbarians conquered the Western Empire, trade and travel everywhere except in Italy itself slowed and stopped. The epidemics ceased.

In the Eastern Empire, commerce, war, and travel went on uninterrupted. The epidemics continued.

In the year 542, travelers coming to Constantinople, where the Emperor Justinian reigned, brought word that an epidemic was raging in lower Egypt. Slowly the disease spread, following the coast line where traffic was most active. In 543 it reached Constantinople. There at its height it killed ten thousand of the inhabitants in a single day.

Justinian was at war with the barbarians who had migrated into Italy. He expelled the barbarians and in doing that he spread the plague. For fifteen years it tarried in the border regions of the Eastern Empire and then it moved slowly back toward Egypt. Again on its return it struck at Constantinople. This time the havoc was even greater than during the first outbreak. There were so many dead that the bodies could not be buried. Finally the roofs were taken off the towers of the walls that surrounded the city; into the space below were crammed thousands upon thousands of bodies. Then the roofs were replaced and sealed. Gibbon, who wrote *The History of the Decline and Fall of the Roman Empire*, says of this epidemic:

"No facts have been preserved to sustain an account, or even a conjecture, of the numbers that perished in this extraordinary mortality. I only find that, during three months, five and at length ten thousand persons died each day in Constantinople; that many cities in the East were left vacant, and that in several districts of Italy the harvest and the vintage withered on the ground."

For fifty-two years this outbreak of plague attacked the tortured people in recurring epidemics.

If the modern physician could control plague no better than the physician in Greek or Roman days, we too should suffer from the great epidemics. The diseases still exist, smoldering today in the Eastern lands from which they arose and spread in ancient times. Although we have commerce, active commerce, with those countries, the diseases do not reach us, for in the intervening centuries physicians have learned how to control them. But before that triumph was achieved, Europe only five, four, and three centuries ago was to suffer outbreaks of plague and pestilence greater even than those which occurred at Constantinople in the years beginning with 543.

Now for a time we leave the Byzantine Empire, weakened by disease, and, following the retreating wave of the plague, we go eastward, although it is not disease or even medicine we are to consider, but politics again.

Our interest now is Arabia, a great tract of land lying between the Red Sea and the Persian Gulf and separated from the Mediterranean by Syria and the Holy Land. This country of Arabia is mostly rough pasture lands dotted here and there with fertile tracts; in the center is a great sandy desert. There are in the whole country only a few small walled towns, and of these only two are of any importance; one is Medina and the other Mecca. In the sixth century most of the inhabitants lived a nomadic life in tribes, knowing only the rule of their own chosen leader and worshiping among their gods an idol—a meteorite, built into a temple at Mecca.

In Mecca in the years when the great plague was still sweeping over the Eastern Empire, a man was born who was destined to unite the wandering tribes in a common cause. His name was Mohammed. His force for union was religion. He was the prophet of a living god, Allah.

Arabia was stirred by his words. Arguments were waged and battles fought over the gods of Mecca and the god of Mohammed. Slowly Mohammed's god won the allegiance of the people.

The outside world paid little attention to the turmoil in Arabia, a domestic row among flea-bitten riders of the desert. The rulers of the surrounding countries smiled when in 628 the envoys of Mohammed ordered them to surrender to his cause. But they did not smile when, less than ten years later, the forces of a united Arabia stormed their gates. The Arabian conquest was under way. Syria and the Holy Land fell before troops of horsemen shouting their war cry of "Allah, Allahuakbar."

The Persians under Rustam went down to defeat amid a stampede of their own trained war elephants. Egypt, Armenia, Turkestan, North Africa, and Spain were brought under Arabic rule.

Allah triumphed.

Constantinople survived the attack of the Arabs as it had survived the attacks of plague. But shorn of its great Empire by one and weakened by the other, it was dead so far as progress was concerned.

The great library at Alexandria was burned by the Arabs because the leader of the expedition said that there was no need of any books except the Koran, the bible of Arabia.

The glory of Athens had passed years before and little was left of the glory of Rome. But the stream of medical progress flowed on, no longer through Athens and Alexandria and Rome, but through Bagdad, Damascus, Cairo, and Cordova.

The center of progress and the center of medical advance in the eighth, ninth, tenth, and eleventh centuries lay among the Arabs.

CHAPTER XI

Science Under the Caliphs

THE story of Arabian conquest is again the story of the nomad and the settler. In the span of a single century the virile Arabs had engulfed the wide lands of an ancient civilization and had themselves been swallowed by that civilization.

They had come out of Arabia, a crude and ruthless people, simple and primitive in their ways of living, a people of tents and horses, subsisting on goat's milk, mare's milk, and dates.

Unlike the Romans they did not make slaves of the people they conquered. All that they demanded was acceptance of the words of Mohammed as written in the Koran. The men under their rule were of many nations and languages, but translation of the Koran was forbidden. The people must learn the Koran; hence they must learn Arabic, and so this language became the universal one of the lands ruled by the Arabs—the Moslem Empire.

Their conquests accomplished, the Arabs had time to take stock of the new and strange things they found about them. They were full of curiosity. They saw castles and bridges, aqueducts and engines of war; they tasted the sweets of a luxury unknown in their simple way of living; they found men of medicine whose potions stopped pain more surely than did the magic words of the wise men of the desert; they learned that the wisdom of great men was set down in books —but the writing was in a language unknown to them.

The Arab conquerors had gained great wealth from their plunders; wealth unlocked the secrets that had aroused their curiosity. Learned men—Jews, Persians, and Syrians—were offered gifts to translate into Arabic the books of the Greeks and Romans. Persians, Jews, Syrians, and even

Greek Christians, rather than the Arabs themselves, were the scientists of the Eastern Empire. It was indeed from the Christian followers of Nestorius, a priest of the Byzantine Empire, that the Arabs first obtained knowledge of Greek and Roman medicine. Nestorius had been a bishop in Constantinople, but he had been driven from that city with his followers because he differed with the accepted doctrines of the Eastern Church. He and his band finally found refuge in Persia. Strangers in a strange land, they turned to the care of the sick and so to the study of medicine—medicine of the kind that had survived in the Byzantine Empire. Under the patronage of the Arabs such men of science and medicine were not content to stop with the mere copying of the ancient books of the Greeks and Romans; they went further. Science flourished in Arabia as it had at Alexandria under Greek rule. The sciences of chemistry, geology, and algebra were founded. The numerals we use today in our arithmetic are the Arabic form. A great many herbs native to the Orient were put into medical use in addition to the remedies of Dioscorides. These substances were mainly spices, such as camphor, nutmeg, cloves, and musk; but at that time they were used to treat diseases, and so they have a place in our story.

Later, as we shall see, the medical knowledge of the Arabs passed into Europe. It was through the civilization of the Eastern Empire that the stream of knowledge flowed on to our own day and our own country. That is the reason why we have stopped here to talk of the Arabs and their medicine. We have said nothing of the medicine of China or of India, for it lay outside the channel in which ancient knowledge came on down through the centuries to us.

Because the medicine of Europe followed that of Arabia, the spices used as medicaments by the Arabic doctors were also used in Europe. Centuries later in our story we shall see King Charles II of England on his deathbed dosed with spices, with nutmeg, camphor, mace, and cloves.

A spice trade was established between the East and West, but it was really a drug trade. When Columbus tried to find a shorter route to India to obtain spices, and discovered America by a blunder, the spices he sought were not to be used by the cook but by doctors to treat sick people. It has often been said, but erroneously, that the spices of the East were used to preserve food in those days before ice boxes and the invention of canning. In reality they were too expensive to be used as preservatives; salt was cheaper and quite as effective.

Clear evidence of the fact that a great deal of our knowledge came from Arabia is seen in the words of our own language. Later in our story we shall find that men in Europe turned for information to the books written in Arabic—translations made from Greek and Syrian books by the learned men employed by the Arabic rulers. Because the Europeans could not read Arabic, they too employed translators to change the Arabic into Latin. But there were no Latin words for many of the things mentioned in the Arabic books and so the Arabic terms were kept. In our language the words alcohol, alfalfa, admiral, arsenal, azure, cipher, algebra, zero, zenith, syrup, julep, and many, many more are Arabic.

Nor are words the only things in everyday life we owe to the Arabs; like the Chinese they invented fireworks; they were the first to use windowpanes, to cultivate fruit, and to use street lights. As we have said, they were the founders of chemistry, and chemistry has since continued to be closely associated with medicine. The Arabian chemists discovered such important substances as alcohol, sulphuric and nitric acids, silver nitrate, and bichloride of mercury; but it was the philosophy behind their chemistry that influenced men of later times more than the chemicals they discovered.

Their chemistry was combined with astrology, and belief in the elixir of life which bestowed perpetual youth and cured all disease. According to their ideas, the seven heavenly bodies—the sun, moon, Mercury, Mars, Venus, Jupiter, and Saturn—corresponded to the seven days of the week and the seven metals that were known at that time: gold, silver, iron, mercury, tin, lead, and copper. All these metals were born in the earth from a common substance under the influence of the planets. The chemists, or rather alchemists, sought to find the secret of the birth of metals so that they could change lead and iron into gold. And further they sought to dissolve gold so that it could be eaten or drunk, for potable gold was an elixir of life.

Absurd as these ideas seem now, they nevertheless were considered serious matters up to a time within three centuries of our own. Men spent their lives and their fortunes trying to change lead into gold and to find the secret of perpetual youth. In their search and their experiments they discovered, by accident, many useful chemicals—but no one found the universal remedy or the secret of eternal life.

From Arabic chemistry grew in time some of the weirdest of all medical beliefs, particularly the idea that the seven planets ruled seven vital parts of the body. In antiquity, a planet was any heavenly body which appeared to move. Thus the sun was a planet; it ruled the heart, the moon the brain, Jupiter the liver, Saturn the spleen, Mercury the lungs, Mars the bile, and Venus the kidneys. The influence of the stars on diseases fills a great chapter in medical history and one that we shall deal with when we come to the beliefs current in Europe centuries later. Even today some almanacs, as you may have noticed, show pictures of the planets that rule the organs of the body; and some people still believe in astrology.

Early in this chapter we said that the Arabs came out of Arabia a rough and simple people, eager for knowledge. We have mentioned some of the things they learned and some of the things that were accomplished under their rule. The Arabs themselves were changing. Within a short time they had given up their desert ways. After a century they were living in great cities, Cairo, Damascus, Bagdad, and Cordova in far-off Spain. The streets of these cities teemed with the traffic of caravans and were lined with the shops of merchants displaying beautifully woven cloth and rugs,

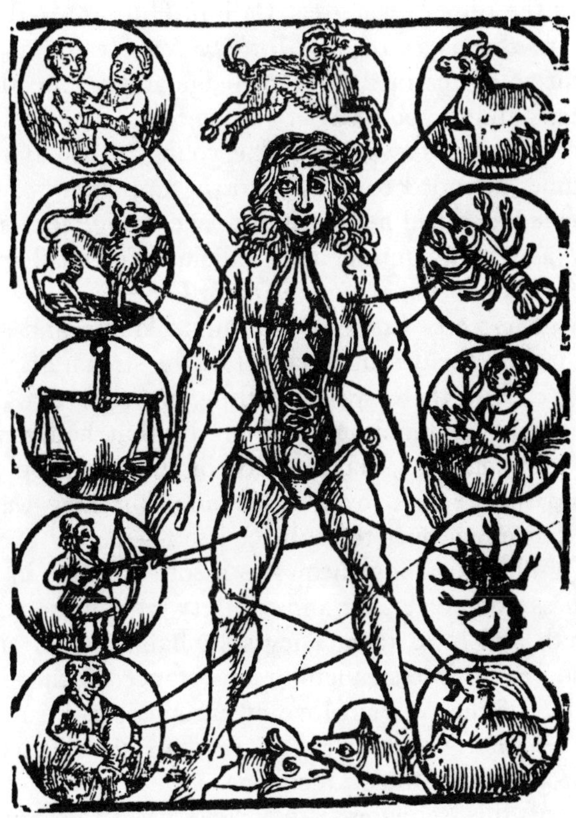

Astrological influence.

delicate metal work and jewelry, glassware, pottery, and sweetmeats. Under the shade of canopies the merchants and their friends sipped what was to become our lemonade and "soda water," for the Arabs were the first to use drinks flavored with essence of rose and lemon and spices. In the shaded courtyards of private homes were wealth and luxury and comfort. There were beautiful public buildings, hospitals, schools, and colleges. These were the times told of in the *Arabian Nights*, the times of merchants, and princes, and emirs, and viziers, and caliphs, and wizards, and genii. This was the time of the great Caliph, Haroun Al-Raschid.

Turn to the pages of the *Arabian Nights* and you will find mention of the medical knowledge and science that we have been talking about. There is the tale of Abu Al-Husn and his slave girl Tawaddud. The young man, having lost his fortune, intended to sell her to the Caliph, who, to test her knowledge, asked her questions concerning religion, philosophy, astronomy, music, and medicine. The medicine that she glibly told of was the medicine of Galen.

Through Greece, Rome, Byzantium, Arabia and so into Europe wound the devious channel of the stream of medical knowledge. But there was one thing peculiar to Arabian medicine that distinguished it from all that had come before; it grew out of a characteristic of Eastern people. The Arab and the Persian loved to dispute, but they were not greatly concerned over the subject itself—merely the argument. Quibbling among them was a sort of game in which shrewdness and cleverness and subtlety were more admired than truth and solid fact. They split hairs, but often they made no real impression on the substance of the matter. Something of the Arabian love of argument as a substitute for the search for facts was, as we shall see, carried over into Europe with Arabian medicine.

Some of this showiness, this cleverness, this trickiness even, was admired in their doctors. And so we find that many Arabian physicians were tricksters who puffed up their own reputations by pretending to perform marvelous cures on men whom they hired to pose as patients. Sometimes a physician sent around confederates to find out what they could about sick people so that when he came, he would appear to have profound knowledge.

But along with the ostentatious Arabian physicians there were also many who were sober, earnest, sincere men. The names of two of them in particular have come down through the centuries. One was Rhazes and the other Avicenna.

Both these men were Persians and their real names were Abu Bekr Mohammed ibn Zakhariya Ar-Razi and Abu Ali al-Husain ibn Abdullah ibn Sina. But we shall continue to call them by Latin names—Rhazes from Ar-Razi, and Avicenna from ibn Sina.

Rhazes lived between the years 860 and 932. He devoted his youth to studying philosophy and music, and turned to medicine many years later. But his fame as a physician grew rapidly, and soon we find him called from his native city of Raj (the Razi of his name) to take charge of a new hospital that was to be built at Bagdad. His first task was to select the place where the hospital was to be erected. In making his choice, so the story goes, he hung up at many points about the city large pieces of meat and then watched them to see which would be the last to spoil. That place he chose for the site of the hospital, in the belief that the air there was better than at any of the other sites. Of course he knew nothing of bacteria or infection, but he must have realized that putrefaction and disease had something in common. The realization that this common element was bacteria came nearly a thousand years after the time of Rhazes, and with it came modern sanitation, the use of antiseptics, and all the sterile procedures that make modern surgery possible.

Rhazes is remembered only in legend for his association of disease and putrefaction; his contributions to medicine were his descriptions of the symptoms of disease. He was the first to thoroughly describe those of smallpox. He also wrote a book on the treatment of disease, following Galen's methods closely. It was in wide use in Europe as late as the seventeenth century.

Avicenna, called later "The Prince of Physicians," lived between the years 980 and 1037. He was, according to story, one of those phenomenal young men whose brilliance seems almost superhuman. At ten he knew the Koran by heart; next he perfected himself in philosophy, law, and mathematics. At sixteen he turned to medicine; at eighteen he was famous as a physician. Thereafter his way led through the courts of the emirs; sometimes he had good fortune, sometimes bad; sometimes he was vizier and chief minister of state; sometimes he had to flee for his life in political turmoils.

Avicenna wrote extensively on medical matters. Galen was his authority, and like Galen he wished to make medicine into as sure and exact a system for treating disease as mathematics is for solving a problem in its field. His system had all the defects of Galen's and more besides, but since people like systems, even wrong ones, his writings were widely popular in Europe for centuries after his time. Indeed the medicine of Europe was to become very largely Galenic medicine interpreted by Avicenna.

None of the Arabian physicians dissected the body; their religious beliefs forbade this practice. Nor did they undertake surgery when they could avoid it. Indeed Avicenna taught that surgery was inferior to medical practice and was to be carried on by men of lower social rank.

This belief of his was also widely accepted in Europe years later, and so surgery was left to barbers, executioners, bathhouse keepers, and strolling fakers. The distinction between the superior physician and the inferior surgeon persisted until well into the seventeenth and eighteenth centuries.

Another thing that Avicenna taught and that was widely accepted was that the cautery—a red-hot iron—should be used in surgery instead of the knife. It seems a rather brutal thing to burn wounded and injured people, and that is exactly what a famous surgeon of the sixteenth century thought when he discarded the practice. We shall tell the story of this man, Ambroise Paré of France, and his adventures in war in a later chapter. But perhaps Avicenna was right and Paré wrong. The fire hurt frightfully and made terrible wounds, but it also killed the bacteria that caused infection, in a time when no one knew of the use of antiseptics. It is probable that more men died of infection when cautery was given up in surgery than when it was in use.

It is curious that Rhazes should, without knowing the reason, connect putrefaction and disease, and that Avicenna, also without knowing the reason, should strongly advocate a kind of antiseptic against infection, heat. If only they or the men who followed soon after them could have seen deeper and recognized the truth that lay just behind these two things, medical progress might have been hastened by centuries.

But the men of Europe to whom we now turn saw only what was written in words—the words of Galen, Rhazes, and Avicenna.

CHAPTER XII

Medicine Follows the Crusades

WE have told how the followers of Mohammed, sword in hand, fought for the glory of Allah. They conquered an ancient civilization; they united it; they stimulated it to progress.

And now in the West much the same sort of change was taking place, but more slowly. Religion there also was turning to the sword to drive men into union.

The Christian religion in the days of the Western Roman Empire had taught submission—"Love thine enemies." But centuries had passed since then; in the intervening years the Cross had passed from the hands of the martyr to be borne as the banner of the warrior.

Let us trace briefly this changing attitude and see its consequences.

When Constantine moved the capital of the Roman Empire to Byzantium, the center of the Christian church remained behind at Rome. The Bishop of Rome was recognized as the head or patriarch of the Church, the Pope.

Although the Western Empire fell, the center of the Church still remained in Rome. Indeed the patriarch of the Church took over added powers and dignities as the representative of all the spiritual forces of Christendom. From the Pope in Rome emanated the influence which controlled the monks of the monasteries scattered over feudal Europe. Missionaries preached the Christian religion to the barbarians. Christianity spread, slowly, steadily. The barbarian rulers became converted to the faith; with them the Pope held overlordship as the leader of all Christians.

Thus Christianity gradually became the unifying force, the one thing in common, the controlling power over the scattered domains of Europe.

With religious unity there grew political unity. Kings were rising. The lands from Belgium to the Pyrenees were united in the Frankish kingdom, which was steadily becoming a Christian domain. But in one respect the Franks failed to develop the unity of the followers of Mohammed in the East. The universal language of the Mohammedans was Arabic; in the Frankish kingdom the people of the western half, present-day France, spoke dialects of Latin; those of the eastern half, now Germany, retained the language of the Germanic barbarians. Language was in time to be the insurmountable barrier to complete unity of the countries. But in those years from the fifth to the middle of the ninth century the different lands were held, though not very firmly, under the rule of the Frankish kings.

In the year 800 there came to the throne a man named Charles. On the day of his coronation he was crowned by the Christian church not as king but as emperor of the whole of Christendom. His only superior was the Pope. Charles the Great—or Charlemagne—was the warrior of the Church. His wars of conquest were wars for Christianity; with the sword he converted the barbarians. Christianity had become a warlike religion. What the followers of Mohammed had done in the East, the followers of Charlemagne were now doing in the West. The Arabs had said to the peoples of ancient civilizations, "Yield to Allah or die"; the Christians of the West were saying to the pagans of the Rhinelands, "Become Christians or die."

While Charlemagne conquered in the West, the Caliph Haroun Al-Raschid ruled in the East. These two, so stories tell us, were friendly; it is even said that Haroun Al-Raschid sent Charlemagne the keys to the Holy Sepulcher.

But friendship was not the force that was to bring the East and West together, to cut the channel for the westward flow of medical knowledge. It was to be war, and war in the cause of religion.

Haroun Al-Raschid allowed Christians, if they wished,

to visit the Holy Land, the early home of their religion. The stern rule of the followers of Mohammed had become relaxed; luxury, riches, political strife, had weakened a once rigorous, stern people. The Arabs had been nearly swal-

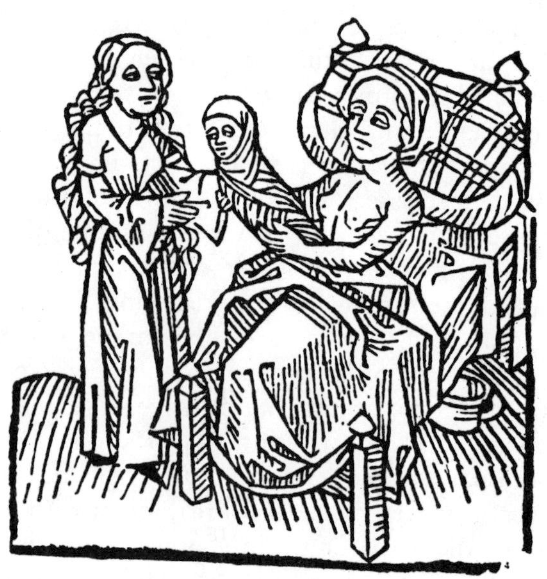

The medieval way of wrapping a baby.

lowed by the civilization they had seized. But off to the northeast, in Turkestan, Mohammedanism throve in the vigorous warlike form that Mohammed had preached. The Turks were far less civilized than their fellow Moslems of Syria, Palestine, Egypt, and Spain.

The closing centuries of the first thousand years after Christ were times of shifting populations and constant migration. So also were the opening years of the next millennium. In 1066 William led the Norman conquest of England; five years later the Turks descended upon Asia Minor and stormed the very gates of Constantinople.

The Holy Land was now in the hands of an intolerant

people, unfriendly to the Christians. No longer could Christian pilgrims visit Jerusalem; the Sepulcher was desecrated by the infidel. So the forces of militant Christianity turned for the first time to the East. A religious war was to be organized; all strife among Christians was to cease, and they were to unite under no political rule but under the banner of all Christendom to seize the Holy Sepulcher from the infidels.

Princes and knights were to put on their armor and followed by their men at arms go to war with the Moslems. Chivalry in its flower was to strike at the Saracens.

But that is not quite the way the matter turned out, for a peculiar character appeared among the people, preaching not a war but a true crusade. Into town after town of Germany and France there rode on a donkey a barefoot man clad in rough garments and bearing on his shoulder a huge cross. This was Peter the Hermit. He described the tortures of Christians who attempted to make pilgrimages to the Holy Land, and the profanation of holy ground.

During 1094 and 1095, the years that Peter the Hermit preached, there had been a famine and an outbreak of an infectious disease in Germany. People were excited; his words wrought them to a fever pitch. In great bands, without leaders, without food, without arms, with no plan except to reach the Holy Land, multitudes of people started eastward. The first two bands reached Hungary and were massacred there by the inhabitants. A third broke up in the same country. The fourth and fifth led by Peter reached Constantinople; they crossed the Bosporus and were slaughtered by the Turks in 1096.

The following year the first organized crusade moved in military fashion eastward and took Antioch after a long siege and then Jerusalem.

The Turks, aroused, fought to recapture the conquered lands; new crusades went forth. For two hundred years the

Knights of Christendom struggled back and forth across the Holy Land.

We need mention here only one crusade, and that formed no part of the channel through which the medical knowledge of the East came to the West. But it gives an idea of

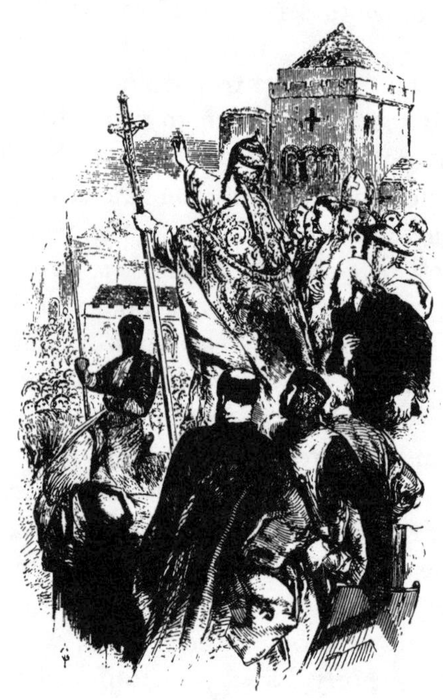

Pope Urban preaching the Crusades.

the excitement of the times and the barbarity of the people. It was the Children's Crusade—a dreadful affair. A crowd of many thousands of boys from France and Germany left their homes to conquer the Turks and rescue the Holy Sepulcher. Those from France were lured on board ships by slave traders at Marseilles and sold in Egypt; some of those from Germany reached Italy, but most of them died on the way. It may have been from the story of the Children's Crusade that there has come down to us the legend of the Pied Piper of Hamelin Town who, to the tune of his pipe, led the children away in a great crowd.

The Crusades were directly and indirectly responsible for the first feeble revival of medicine in the West. But not all the changes that resulted were favorable to medical progress, and we pause first to tell of two things growing out of them that retarded rather than advanced medicine.

You will remember that in the West after the fall of the Roman Empire medicine became monastic; that is, the monks acted as best they could as doctors, and the monasteries were often places of refuge for the sick. Among the barbarians of Germany healing was largely in the hands of the women of the tribes. In the towns of the Frankish kingdom there were strolling peddlers, mountebanks, who pretended to be surgeons and dentists; but there were really no good doctors, except occasional ones among the Jews who came as immigrants from Arabia. Unfortunately Christians were forbidden to employ Jewish doctors.

In the monasteries some of the monks studied medicine, but their only textbooks were the few manuscripts that had been preserved. Most of these they could not use, for without special schooling they were unable to understand the complicated works of Hippocrates and Galen.

In their stead the monks used merely books of recipes, herbals, and the simpler sort of medical books intended for home remedying, such as those of the rhizotomists.

As late as the tenth century there was no chance at all in the whole of Western Europe for a man to obtain an education in medicine except at a place in Italy called Salerno, of which we shall tell more shortly. Even if men outside the Church could have become trained doctors, they would have had difficulty in practicing. These were rough times and poor ones; the common people had little money with which to employ physicians; the knights, the feudal lords, and the members of royalty were uneducated and often intolerant of failure. If a physician did not succeed in effecting a cure he often had to leave town quickly. Many a peddler who pretended to be a doctor lost his life, or, what was more common, had his eyes put out for rashly promising to cure some irritable nobleman, and failing.

In 580 Gutram, King of Burgundy, killed two surgeons because they could not save the life of the queen when she had plague; in 1337 John of Bohemia threw a surgeon into the river Oder because he failed to cure him of blindness.

The priests alone were free from risk in their charitable medical work, but in the year 1163 a law was passed by the Church which limited their efforts and, quite unintentionally, brought surgery into disrepute. The monks sometimes performed crude operations; there was, so the officials of the Church thought, a possibility that by accident a monk might, in his efforts at surgery, cause the death of some man—a very unpleasant responsibility for a Christian monk. Therefore, with the good intention of preventing such an occurrence, an edict was issued beginning with the words, *Ecclesia abhorret a sanguine*—the Church abhors the shedding of blood.

The edict went wide of its mark and was interpreted as meaning that surgery was not approved of, was not respectable—an idea, you will recall, that the Arabs also held.

In 1300 there was another edict, equally misread, that brought opposition to anatomical dissection. Pope Boniface VIII decreed that whoever dared to cut up a human body or boil it should fall under the ban of the Church. The ruling was intended to prohibit a practice which the crusaders occasionally used. When one of their number died in a far off country, his companions sometimes cut up his body and boiled it in order to obtain his bones, which could be easily carried back to friends at home for burial. The rule of the Church against this custom was understood to mean that there should be no dissection for medical study.

These two edicts, detrimental as they were, were more

than compensated for by benefits to medicine that arose from the Crusades. The greatest of these was the founding of many hospitals.

Men were wounded in the battles in the Holy Land; many more became ill during the journeys. You will remem-

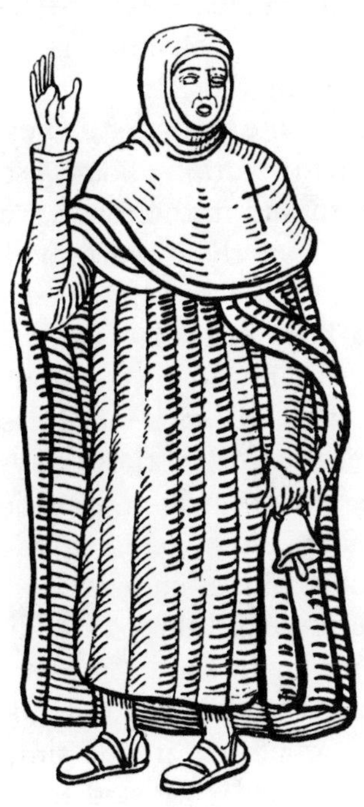

A Hospitaler.

ber that Christians had peculiar ideas in regard to the sick and injured. In primitive times, in Greece and in Rome the diseased were looked upon with some contempt; they were disregarded, they were unlucky people, often outcasts. The strong and healthy man did not help the feeble and ill; it would have been a sign of weakness if he had. But the Christians believed that illness and pain brought man nearer to

God. The sufferer was a privileged person; he who helped him shared in his privilege and made himself more Christ-like. Christianity established the principle that to help the sick and needy is a sign of strength, not weakness.

To care for the men diseased and wounded during the Crusades, religious orders were founded, such as the Knights Hospitalers, and the Teutonic Knights. The men of these orders wore distinguishing costumes, and, like the Benedictines of recent times in the Alps, sometimes used dogs to help in their rescue of the wounded. They did valiant work in the Holy Land, and returning home, established hospitals on the lines of march and in the towns where they stopped.

We must not think of these places as being like modern hospitals—far from it. They were usually rough buildings with straw on the floor instead of beds. Food and shelter were given to the people who entered, but very little medical care. Patients with all sorts of illnesses or with none were mingled together, for in those days there was little knowledge of the way in which infectious diseases were spread. Eight diseases only were regarded as contagious: bubonic plague, tuberculosis, epilepsy (which is not contagious), the itch, erysipelas, the cattle disease—anthrax—the eye disease—trachoma—and leprosy.

Leprosy was connected with the Crusades. In speaking of the great epidemic of plague in the time of the Emperor Justinian of Constantinople, we said that a chronic disease such as leprosy could be spread even by slow travel. It can of course be spread still faster by rapid travel. Leprosy had come into Europe from the East at an early date, but now, with the passage of men back and forth from the Holy Land, it became widely prevalent. It spread just as it did among the Hawaiian Islanders after they began to trade with China.

Hospitals were erected by the monks to care for the lepers and to keep them from coming in contact with well people. These hospitals were called lazarettos, after Lazarus, the leper of the Bible. How widely prevalent leprosy became you can judge from the fact that in France alone there were 2000 of these lazarettos and in England more than 200. The isolation of lepers which began 800 years ago eventually wiped out the disease in Europe, save for a few small centers of infection which still persist, mainly in the countries of Scandinavia.

Hospitals thus grew up as a result of the Crusades, and so did medical schools.

Earlier in this chapter we said that when the Crusades began there was only one place in all Europe where any medical education could be obtained and that was Salerno, a town near Naples.

Just how or why or when that tiny school was founded there no one knows. The only certain records we have of it are of a time when it came into prominence during the Crusades. It happened to be on the line of march to the Holy Land.

The School of Salerno was not part of a monastery; it was probably the first nonecclesiastical center of education in all Christian Europe. There in that little seashore town, known to the Romans as a health resort, a spark of Greek and Roman medicine had persisted in spite of the fall of the Western Empire. It was a feeble spark, but just at the time the Crusaders were marching it was fanned into a meager flame by a man named Constantine of Africa.

Constantine was born in Carthage about the year 1010. He traveled through Arabia and even India and learned the medicine of these lands. When he returned to Carthage, he was looked upon with suspicion because of his knowledge. He was thought to be a wizard, a doer of black magic, and was driven from the city. He fled to Salerno, disguised as a beggar. The King of Babylon, so the story says, passing through Salerno, recognized him and raised him from his lowly position. At any event Constantine finally found his way to the monastery of Monte Cassino and became a monk.

Since he knew both Latin and Arabic, he set himself to the task of translating the Arabic works of medicine into Latin.

Thus it was that some of the books of Galen and of Dioscorides made the short journey from Rome to Salerno by the roundabout way of Arabia. But in this journey the Greek and Roman writings had taken on the flavor of the East. The medicaments were spices; the methods of surgery, the knowledge of anatomy, were those which the Syrians and Persians of Arabia had used.

Under the influence of Constantine of Africa medicine began to flourish at Salerno. The doctors there wrote and rewrote the medical knowledge of the past and added to it some of the things they observed.

Even in the days of Constantine of Africa the bands of Crusaders began to pass through Salerno. The town's fame spread. Wounded knights and nobles came there for treatment. They carried away tales of the new medicine, and soon schools were started in other cities, recruiting their teachers from Salerno.

There are many legends, more indeed than facts, surrounding the history of the School of Salerno. One of these legends, although it is not at all true, is perhaps worth retelling, for it illustrates the kind of medicine that was practiced in Europe in the eleventh, twelfth, and thirteenth centuries and even later.

According to the story—and remember it is only a story—which we have copied from an old medical book: "Among the visitors of distinction who honored Salerno with their presence was Robert, Duke of Normandy [a son of William the Conqueror] who, having gone among the first Crusaders to Palestine and having been wounded there in the arm with an arrow, came to Salerno for medical advice in the year 1100 accompanied by his wife Sybillia, daughter of the Count of Conversana, a lady of distinguished beauty and accomplishments, for whose sake Robert had sacrificed his chance of succeeding to the throne of England on the death of his brother, William Rufus, by wearing away his time with her in Italy when he should have been on his way to England."

After that long sentence let us say parenthetically that

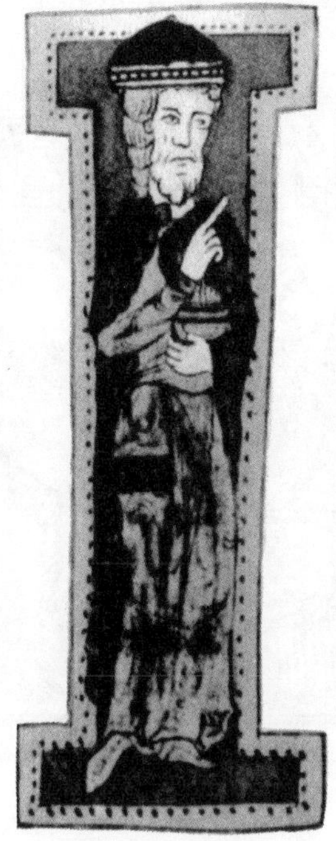

Constantine of Africa.

there were no doctors or surgeons with the Crusaders. Robert was shot through the arm with an arrow and the wound became infected from lack of care. A little iodine put into the sore might have saved him a trip to Salerno, but iodine or any other antiseptic did not come into use until late in the nineteenth century.

To continue:

"Robert's wound had, from neglect, degenerated into a running sore. Upon a consultation among the medical men of Salerno, it was decided that the only means of extracting the poison which prevented the wound from healing was by sucking it out [wound sucking was sometimes a part of the surgeon's trade in those days!] could any person be found bold enough to undertake the office. The high-spirited and

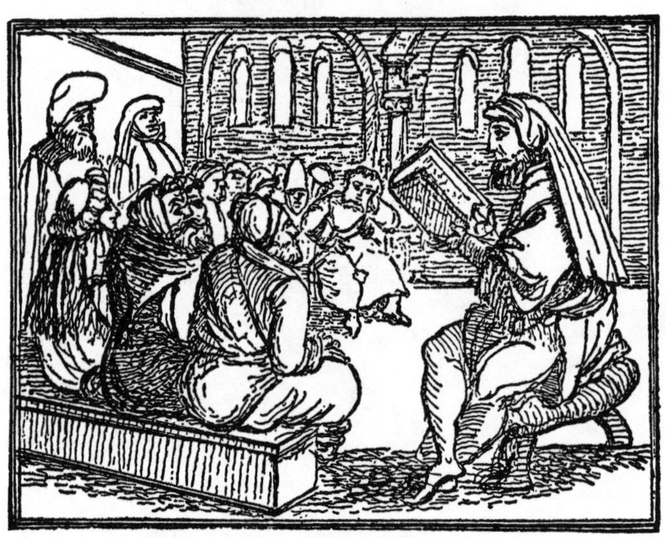

Scene at the medical school of Salerno.

generous prince refused to listen to the proposal of a remedy which threatened the operator with danger; but the advice of the physicians coming to the ears of his wife whose affections were wedded with her hand to her husband, she resolved not to yield to him in generosity; and, taking advantage of an opportunity when his senses were locked in slumber, she extracted the poison from his wound with her own mouth, and thus rescued from the grave, at the price of her own existence, a husband without whom she felt the gift of life would have been valueless."

Very romantic! But even if Sybillia had carried out this unpleasant task, she would not have died in consequence; the old belief that infected wounds were poisoned has, of course, been given up. The point we want to make with this story is that this was what surgery was like in Europe 800 years ago.

The tale goes on to say that when Robert left Salerno, cured of course, the doctors wrote for him a medical book which he could give to any physician treating him in order that the doctor might have the last word in medicine of the year 1100.

The book actually exists, but it was not written for Robert; in fact it was probably written a century and a half after he died. It is called the *Regimen Sanitatis Salernitanum*, which translated very loosely means: A textbook of hygiene from Salerno.

It was probably the most popular medical book ever written. It was copied and recopied; and when printing came into use, it went into more than two hundred editions. It was still popular as a home health book in the time of Queen Elizabeth, and was in fact translated into English by her godson, Sir John Harington, and probably used in the education of the English royal children.

The book itself was written in Latin, as in the West, for reasons of which we shall speak in the next chapter, Latin was used by all doctors. It was composed in the form of short verses. In the days before printing, books were very scarce and very costly, and so the students were forced to memorize them. And verse is easier to learn by heart than prose.

Even today there are a few lines well worth remembering from this old book. One couplet goes thus:

Joy, temperance and repose,
Slam the door on the doctor's nose.

And another:

Use three doctors still, first Doctor Quiet
Next Doctor Merry-man, *and Doctor* Diet.

Here is a verse that reminds us of Galen and his herbs:

Six things, that here in order shall ensure,
Against all poisons have a secret power,
Pear, Garlick, Reddish-root, Nuts, Rape, and Rue,
But Garlick chiefest; for they that it devour
May drink, and care not who their drink do brew;
May walk in airs infected every hour.
Sith Garlick then hath power to save from death,
Bear with it though it make unsavory breath;
And scorn not Garlick, like to some that think
It only makes men wink, and drink, and stink.

And still another verse:

If in your teeth you hap to be tormented
By means some little worms therein do breed:
Which pain (if heed be taken) may be prevented,
By keeping clean your teeth when as you feed,
Burn Frankincense (a gum not evil scented)
Put Henebane unto this, and onion seed,
And in a Tunnel to the Tooth that's hollow,
Convey the smoke thereof, and ease shall follow.
By nuts, Oyles, Eels, and cold in head,
By Apples and raw fruits is hoarseness bred.

The belief that toothache and cavities are due to worms that eat away and rot the tooth just as worms do apples is a very ancient idea. It probably dates back to Egypt and Babylon; it appeared in the Roman medical books in the first century after Christ; and it was in the hygiene of Salerno a thousand years later. And here finally to complete its course is a line or two from an advertisement for a tooth powder published in the year 1724 in a magazine called *The British Journal.*

"The Incomparable Powder for cleaning the teeth, which has given great satisfaction to most of the nobility and gentry for above these twenty years. Sold only at Mr. Palmer's Fan Shop in St. Michael's Church-Porch, Cornhill, Mr. Markham's Toy Shop, at the Seven Stars under St. Dunstan's Church in Fleet Street and nowhere else in England. It at one using makes the teeth as white as ivory, never black or yellow. It wonderfully cures the scurvey in the gums and kills worms at the root of the Teeth, and thereby hinders the toothache."

Medical knowledge and medical errors flowed through the same roundabout channels—primitive, Egyptian, Greek, Roman, Arabic, and finally European. And now in our story we are approaching the days when in Europe new knowledge is added to the old knowledge which has been regained. But before we leave the Middle Ages to come to the Revival of Learning, and the Renaissance, we must pause to describe life in the medieval cities and in the medieval universities and record another great epidemic of disease—perhaps the greatest—the Black Death and its fantastic companion, the Dancing Mania.

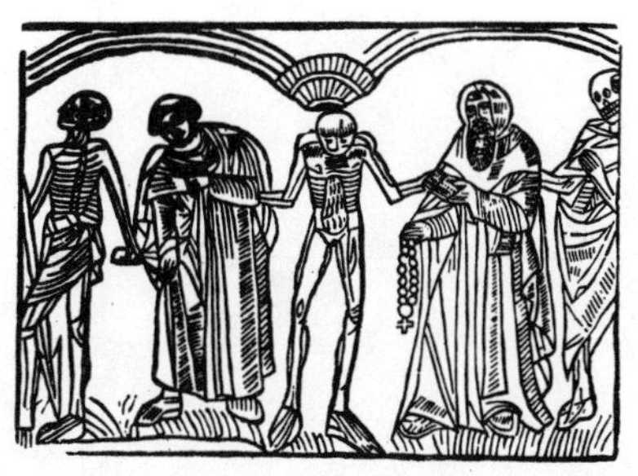

Part Five

TOWN AND GOWN

THE BLACK DEATH

THE MENTAL CONTAGIONS

CHAPTER XIII

Town and Gown

THE Revival of Learning and the Renaissance mark the beginning of a true scientific advance in the West. The Renaissance, which was at its height in the sixteenth century, did not spring up suddenly, fully under way. It grew slowly. There were important events in the twelfth and thirteenth centuries, the centuries of the Crusades, leading up to it. In these years the feudal system gave way to central rule, cities grew in size and number, and the great universities of Europe arose. Each of these events was a step toward the Renaissance from which our own progress has sprung; each had its influence directly or indirectly on medical matters.

You will remember that we mentioned the feudal system when we told of the fall of the Roman Empire. Feudalism arose then because there existed no central government strong enough to protect the common man, the small land owner, the farmer, the laborer, the merchant. Unable to defend himself against robbers, against invaders, against anyone in fact who wished to seize his lands, his goods, or even his family, he was forced to seek aid of some strong, rich neighbor, a great land owner, or a nobleman. In return for protection the feudal lord made lesser people his vassals, if they were gentry; his serfs, if they were laborers. The price of protection was paid by vassals in military service, by serfs in labor and shares of crops. Europe was dotted with these feudal domains, often hostile one to another. Under such conditions there could be little travel, little communication, little trade, and no general education at all.

In time, as we have said, kings gradually gained in power; they conquered the feudal lords, one by one over a period of centuries, and made them their vassals. The kings became the supreme feudal lords.

Slowly central rule was again established; the nobles lost in power, but remained privileged characters of social importance. Their rights passed on from father to son in an hereditary nobility. Likewise the lot of the common man changed; if he had land, it became his own to be passed on to his sons. He ceased to be a serf and became a peasant or a merchant or a free craftsman. He still paid taxes to his lord, but now he paid in money, no longer in personal service. Money could be used to hire soldiers. In early feudal days when the lords went to war, each one, followed by his vassals, had formed a separate army unit. Under central rule the peasants stayed at home and worked their farms, and the fighting was done by professional soldiers.

With the breakdown of the feudal system and the rise of central authorities, trade and travel and communication increased. Cities grew in size and number. They could flourish only with the growth of a merchant class, the free farmer, and free craftsman.

When the Romans had inhabited Western Europe and fought there with the barbarians, they had built cities surrounded for protection by high stone walls. These walled cities and many new ones now became the market places to which the farmers of the outlying districts brought their produce for sale and where they bought in turn the merchandise of the traders and craftsmen. There were, of course, no factories in those days; each craftsman carried on his work in his own home. There were indeed few factories until late in the eighteenth century, when steam power came into use. But great churches were erected in the medieval towns, and the universities so important to our story of the progress of medicine grew up.

The conditions of life in the cities of the twelfth and thirteenth centuries were much the same in the fourteenth, fifteenth, and sixteenth. These conditions have significance for our story of medicine and show us how disease goes with filth and vermin.

Cleanliness was not regarded highly in medieval Europe. The pagan Romans in the time of the Empire, at least those of the wealthy class, had been a cleanly people. Indeed they

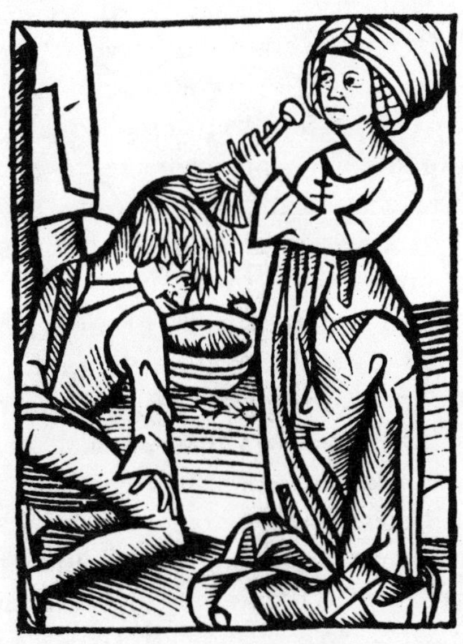

A domestic scene in the Middle Ages—removing head lice.

had made a luxury of bathing. Cleanliness, the care of the body, was to them a matter of comfort and pleasure. The early Christians in opposing the demoralizing luxuries of the pagans had also opposed the idea of cleanliness. Dirt and filth were to some of them indications that they ignored worldly matters and the flesh in order to develop the spirit. There were Christian saints who, to show their holiness, actually boasted that they had never bathed. And cleanliness in the Middle Ages was still looked upon as a sign of weakness and worldliness and luxury. It was not until the modern discovery that bacteria are the cause of infection that there was any scientific reason given for cleanliness. In the last seventy-five years the civilized world has returned to the cleanliness and sanitation of the Romans, not only for the sake of comfort, but for the sake of health.

With our modern ideas of what a city should look like and smell like, the medieval cities—if we could see them now as they were five or six hundred years ago—would appall us. Those walled cities were unbelievably dirty. They were crowded. The streets were crooked and narrow; the second stories of the buildings projected over the sidewalks so far that the shop signs on opposite sides sometimes touched. The windows had no glass in them; some were merely barred, others were covered with oiled paper. There were no fly screens, and multitudes of flies crawled over the walls and ceilings, over the food on the table, and rose in a buzzing cloud when anyone walking on the rushes on the floor disturbed them in their feast of filth. There were no ice boxes in the kitchens, no running water piped to the houses, no bathrooms in the homes, and no sewers in the streets. The streets were the dumping grounds for all refuse. Each year, with the accumulation of filth, their level rose higher and higher. Hogs wandered about, rooting in the bubbling mire for refuse thrown from the shops and houses. Citizens often shared their homes with their horse or cow. In some places there were city herdsmen who each morning rounded up the squealing swine and drove them outside the walls of the town to feed on the pasture land. Pigs and pigpens were a normal part of the domestic scene of the city. The first regulation against allowing swine to wander on the streets was passed in 1281 in London; and the first to prohibit keeping swine in town was passed in 1481 in Frankfort on the Main. Leipzig followed in 1645. It is said that an occasional hog might be seen wandering on Broadway in New York City as late as the middle of the nineteenth century.

If you had gone into a prosperous home in a medieval walled town, you would have found the handsome, courteous, devout, but not well bathed, gentlemen and ladies living, and happily, in the midst of filth. You would have seen rushes strewn on the dining room floor, a few plates on the table. For the most part the food was served on slices of bread and eaten with the fingers and a knife—there were no forks. Refuse from the table was thrown on the floor to be eaten by the dog and cat or to rot among the rushes and draw swarms of flies from the stable. The smell of the open cesspool in the rear of the house would have spoiled your appetite, even if the sight of the dining room had not.

But manners have changed under the influence of modern medical discovery! Because of the danger of spreading disease, to spit on the sidewalk or in any public building is now against the law; spitting is, in consequence of changing custom, regarded as ill mannered. But it was not so in the days we are telling of here. There was no connection known then between the secretions of the body and the spread of disease. Saliva was thought to be a healing fluid. Pliny tells of its use in treating many diseases. And Christ, you will remember, used saliva mixed with dust to cure a man of blindness. In medieval times to spit anywhere and in any place was no more ill mannered than to cough or sneeze, and people then did not cover their mouths with their handkerchiefs when they coughed.

In fact handkerchiefs were not much in use. Neither for that matter were underwear and nightgowns and sheets. Men wore chiefly leather garments; women, dresses of heavy cloth. Only the wealthy had beds; ordinarily people slept on piles of straw. But there was one thing shared by all, rich and poor alike, and that was vermin. The houses and the inhabitants as well were overrun with fleas and lice. By our standards these medieval cities were horrible places in which to live. And the farmhouses of those days were no better.

It is little wonder that in such surroundings disease flourished. In the thirteenth century the great epidemic of the Black Death, which in one great wave was to wipe out nearly half the population and leave the people broken and

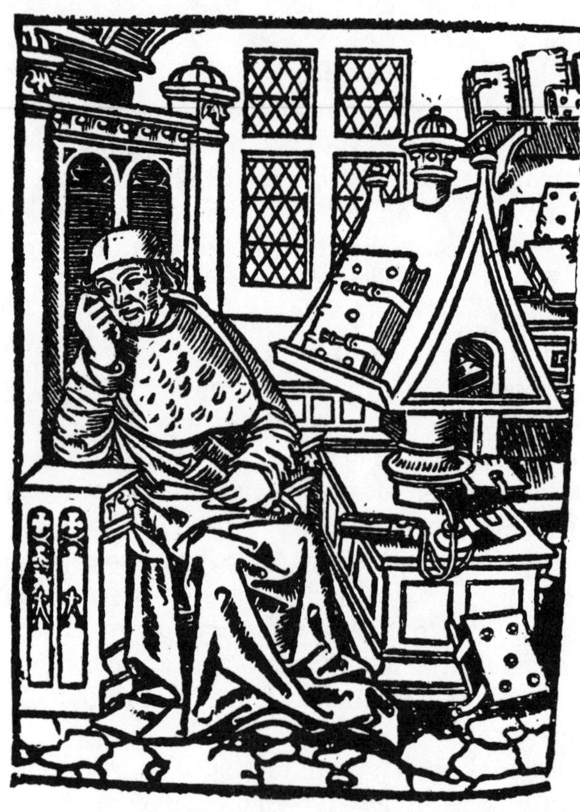

A medieval professor of medicine.

demoralized, was slowly but relentlessly approaching the walled cities. But before the epidemic came, the greatest gift to us from medieval days had been made; the universities had been founded. Education had started to revive.

After the collapse of the Roman Empire, Western Europe sank to the lowest point in the history of its intellectual life.

The period from the sixth to the ninth century has been called the Dark Ages. Europe during this time was isolated from the civilization of Byzantium and the East. Knowledge survived only in the monasteries, and even there education amounted to little more than literacy in most cases.

The monks of the monasteries of early medieval days could read and write. But few other men in Western Europe had mastered even the rudiments of an education. It was Latin that the monks used, for the services of the Church and the text of the Bible itself were in this language. The dialects of Latin and the Germanic tongues had not yet become written languages.

So rare was the ability to read and write in those days that a man with these simple accomplishments was given under the laws special privileges, called benefit of clergy. That is, he had the right to be tried before a Church court for any crime except treason. There were two kinds of courts of justice, one conducted by the Church and the other maintained by the town or state or nobleman. The Church, or ecclesiastical, court did not decree capital punishment, for the Church abhorred the shedding of blood. Except in case of heresy, for which men were burned, its penalties were usually very mild. The civil courts ordered the death penalty freely and for crimes that would seem to us rather minor offenses. As late as the eighteenth century, robbers, pickpockets, and counterfeiters when caught, were hanged; men of noble rank were spared this ignoble mode of death and beheaded instead, but usually only for political crimes.

Benefit of clergy was almost permission to commit murder with impunity. And this privilege, if you wish to call it such, was granted to men who could read and write. In those days the educated man was a cherished citizen.

It was the Emperor Charlemagne, he who united the countries of Europe in the eighth and ninth centuries, who first made an effort to extend education. He could probably read; it is doubtful that he ever learned to write. But he decreed that there should be schools established in the monasteries of his realm. These monastic schools were the forerunners of the universities which sprang up in the twelfth and thirteenth centuries. Up to the time of Charlemagne it had been believed by Western Christians that much education was inconsistent with godliness. Charlemagne broke down this belief and made it possible for young men to study the seven liberal arts. The first three of these, the *trivium* as they were called, were grammar, rhetoric, and logic. Of these, logic was held in highest esteem. The remaining and less important four, the quadrivium, were arithmetic, music, geometry, and astronomy. The astronomy was really astrology; the arithmetic was very simple and elementary.

A teacher of any of these subjects might be called a *doctor scholasticus*, but usually the term doctor was reserved only for the men who taught logic. Finally, when the universities expanded, the degree of doctor was given to students who graduated in law and theology. But it was not until the fourteenth century that the term doctor came into use in medicine. In America as late as the eighteenth century physicians used only the title Mister.

The term university has likewise gone through changes in coming to its modern usage. The Latin word *universitas* was first applied to a corporation or guild of students. Sometimes the group moved from one place to another—and where the group was, there was the university. The actual site of the university, its buildings and its grounds, was called a *studium generale*, meaning a place where students came together from all directions.

As the country was opened up for travel, especially after the Crusades, the students came from many countries, often over long distances, to these medieval *studia*. They spoke different languages and dialects. Partly for that reason, but more because of the association of teaching with the Church, Latin was used as the common spoken and written language in the universities. A boy wishing to enter a university first went to a school of Latin; often his entrance examination to the university consisted in presenting his case to the rector in acceptable Latin and answering in the same language any questions put to him. Once enrolled in the university, he was usually required to speak only Latin, even when at play. Often there were spies, called *lupi*, or wolves, whose duty it was to detect for punishment those students who thoughtlessly spoke in their native tongue.

Students were not very different in behavior from those of today, if one may judge from the regulations of the old universities; there were solemn edicts against bringing bean shooters into schoolrooms, pouring water on the heads of people in the street below, whispering in class, and, as the old rules say, against "heckling the public hangman in the execution of his duty." But there was one thing that the modern student would have missed sorely—and that was games. They were considered irreligious; no student was allowed to play ball, race, or even play chess. Exercises with the sword, the bow and arrow, and the lance were the only manly sports.

The buildings, too, would have given the modern student much to think about—great bare stone halls, unheated, lighted only with torches, and with no glass in the windows. In the dormitories the students slept on straw piled on the floor.

Then as now there were self-supporting students. They earned their way by begging and they also stole. Begging had been made respectable by sects of monks who supported their monasteries in this manner; stealing came naturally to the unruly youths. Anything along the road from university to university that was not nailed down or tied down found its way into the hands of needy students. Fortunately for them they were protected by benefit of clergy.

As a result of the rise of universities, it became possible for men to be trained in medicine. Soon then there were educated doctors, but they rarely practiced among the common people; they were in too great demand with the nobility and the officers of the Church.

As a rule these doctors did not perform surgical operations. Surgery was still of the crudest kind and performed

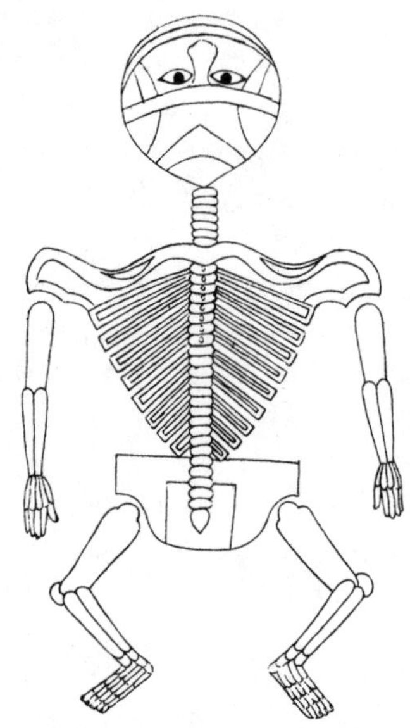

Medieval picture of the skeleton.

only in case of dire necessity. The surgeons used no anæsthetics and no antiseptics, and had little knowledge of the structure of the body, for human anatomy had not been studied since the days of Herophilus at Alexandria.

The physicians looked with contempt upon surgeons; few educated men cared to take up this branch of medical study. During four centuries, from 1100 to 1500, there were perhaps not more than a few dozen educated surgeons in the whole of Europe. These few in turn scorned the uneducated men—the barbers—who did most of the surgery.

The barber surgeons owed their origin indirectly to two

edicts of the Church. Most men of the day wore beards, but in 1092 the Church passed a ruling that monks and priests should be clean shaven. Consequently barbers were trained and kept at the monasteries to serve the clergy. Then in 1163 there came the famous edict forbidding churchmen to perform any surgical operations—*Ecclesia abhorret a sanguine.* So these tasks fell to barbers. They carried out the bleeding so much in use in treating disease, and performed any necessary surgical operations—lanced abscesses, reduced dislocations, splintered broken limbs, and amputated legs and arms. They were even the dentists, for they pulled teeth —there was no other dentistry.

The barber-surgeons, because they did not know Latin and had not studied at the universities, were called surgeons of the short robe to distinguish them from the educated surgeons of the long robe. In a later chapter we shall have much to say of the conflict that eventually occurred between the men of the long robe and the men of the short robe.

The important thing in medicine that resulted from the rise of universities was not the improvement in the practice of medicine, but the fact that medical education had been revived. That step was of itself a great advance over conditions that had existed earlier.

But there were peculiar limitations imposed upon medical study. Men could study Pliny and Dioscorides and Galen and Avicenna, but they were not allowed to question them. Everything in medicine had been settled by those authors; no new facts were to be sought, no new truths found. Under such conditions there could of course be no advance in medical science. And this stationary state of affairs in medicine was only one aspect of the whole approach to learning in the period.

In earlier chapters we have described how philosophy may act as a guiding influence and direct men toward or away from the path that leads to truth. The philosophy of primitive men led them to believe that disease was due to spirits, to supernatural causes—false beliefs. The philosophy of Hippocrates and other great Greeks led to the belief that disease was due, not to supernatural, but to natural causes that could be found out by observation, reduced to almost mathematical rule, and so brought under control. This philosophy guides the beliefs of the doctor and the scientist of today.

The attitude of the Middle Ages, so far as medicine was concerned, lay almost midway between these two extremes. It was an attempt to combine the natural and the supernatural, to work out a system which would explain both. It was not science; it was speculation.

The supernatural was stressed in all medieval scholarship that had its origin in the monastic schools that Charlemagne had founded. The monks depended for knowledge almost wholly on the writings of the Christian saints whose works had become part of the New Testament. These men were concerned with spiritual matters, not with science or natural history. The monks followed them in believing that everything in the world was under the direct influence of divine control. Disease was due to the wrath of God and the sins of men. It was to be controlled by prayer and penance. In spite of the beautiful sincerity of these religious beliefs, the guiding medical philosophy was not at all different from that of primitive peoples. God, the saints, and their opposing force, the devil and his legions, had merely taken the place of the forces which brought good and ill fortune to the savage.

Knowledge of the natural world came almost entirely from fragments of the writings of the ancient Greeks and Romans. In medical matters, the words of Galen, of Pliny, of Avicenna and of Dioscorides became nearly as authoritative as the words of the Bible. It was sinful to doubt Galen even if his statements disagreed with common sense and common observation.

Aristotle had said quite mistakenly that women had fewer

teeth than men; in the Biblical story of creation, Adam lost a rib and therefore men had one less than women. These statements were accepted in spite of the fact that all one had to do to disprove them was to look in the mouth and to run a finger down the ribs. Men did not seek for truth even in this simple way. They viewed the world not with their own eyes but with the eyes of authority.

The task of the medieval scholar was not to add new knowledge to what was given him by his authorities but to codify and systematize their statements. With the help of an elaborate training in logic, all sorts of tricks were devised to make the authorities agree and to explain away their contradictions. Galen said one thing; Aristotle seemed to say the opposite, while Pliny held a third view on the subject, Avicenna perhaps a fourth, and the writings of a Christian father presented a fifth. In reconciling the differences the medieval logician started with a general proposition, let us say: "Plague is an act of God." Then he collected the statements of the authorities on the subject. One had seen plague follow earthquakes; another attributed it to air poisoned by the fumes of volcanoes; a third considered it a Job-like penalty sent for the torment of mortal flesh; a fourth had seen it spread from man to man in an army but spare the inhabitants of an island only a short distance away, and so on and so on. Finally, after he had cited all the authorities the scholar came to the most important part of his dissertation, the argument. He carefully scrutinized and weighed each word, each statement of the authorities. Where did it fit into the scheme of the whole; what figurative interpretation would it yield? In the end, by one way or another, each authority was made to justify the general proposition.

Earthquakes and volcanoes were acts of God, and anything that resulted from an act of God was likewise an act of God. In smiting the men of the army with plague, God, in His infinite wisdom, had taken this means to direct political destiny into the beneficial channels which subsequent events showed that it did take. And so on and on, until the conclusion finally emerged that, as shown by the authorities, the ways of God were manifold; His acts took diverse and infinite forms; the plague was an act of God.

The imperfect observations of ancient doctors had to be reconciled not only with each other but with the prevailing

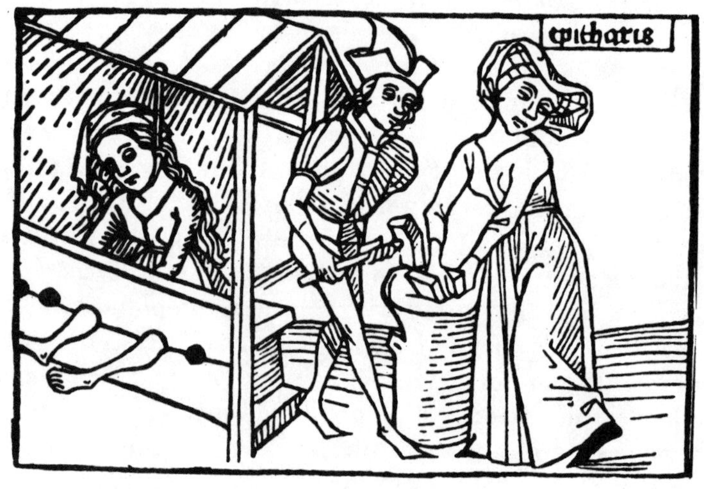

Legal torture.

supernaturalism. Whether or not we now consider such a task worth doing, it was a tremendous undertaking, one which men found so fascinating that for centuries it entirely occupied their attention. They were too preoccupied with speculation of this sort—their system of scholasticism—to check the truth of ancient observations or to make new ones for themselves. Medical study in the Middle Ages was largely a matter of recapturing the knowledge of the past; only the spirit of observation which had made this knowledge possible was still lacking.

As time went on the medieval scholar obtained more manuscripts, more authorities, sometimes from an occasional traveler and translator such as Constantine of Africa who went to Salerno. And on the Crusades, the men of the West met at first hand Eastern scholars versed in the science of the time. They marveled at the science of the Moslems. They obtained badly garbled translations of the *Natural History* of Aristotle; they secured more of the works of Galen and Pliny. But the writings of these men had passed through many hands before they reached the Christians; in the copying, recopying, and translating they had been altered and mixed up. To the West also came the medieval writings of Avicenna and with them his astrological beliefs. All these things had in turn to be worked over and made to harmonize with the general propositions.

The greatest mills were the universities. There the authoritative beliefs which were proper for Christians to hold were ground out by the clever argument and refined by the hair-splitting logic of medieval scholasticism.

To us, with our freedom of thought and our skepticism, such an attitude is almost incomprehensible. But remember that these men were not trained as we can be today; their beliefs were very different. All education from childhood onward, in the home, the school, and the Church, was dominated by the belief that life on earth was only a brief preparation for a future that might be vastly better or vastly worse. A heaven of infinite peace and security and a hell of everlasting torment were vividly real and ever-present in their minds. It did not follow that they were well behaved and free from vice—far from it. They were often turbulent, immoral, and cruel. But sins of the flesh could be forgiven if penance were done; such sins were mere individual weaknesses of frail mortals for whom God had compassion. Sins of thought were a different matter. To doubt, to disagree, was heresy. Heresy threatened the security of the Church, and undermined the very foundation of Christian faith. It must be met with the severest penalties. For heresy men were excommunicated, even burned—and assured of hell everlasting.

Ignorant of methods of observing and recording facts such as Hippocrates used, men felt that magic and sorcery were the only ways of winning power over nature and securing knowledge of its secrets. But sorcery and magic were heresy, they were sinful.

The fact that medical matters, and indeed everything scientific, became involved in the theological beliefs of the times made medical progress impossible. When as late as the sixteenth century Andreas Vesalius, a Belgian of whom we shall have more to say later, showed the true anatomy of the human body, a great cry was raised against him for daring to disagree with Galen—the great "authority." When in the same century the astronomer Copernicus dared to say that the earth revolved about the sun, he was made to recant by Church dignitaries who knew from their authorities that the world was the center of the universe. When a whole century later William Harvey of England showed that the blood circulated through the arteries and veins, his work was denounced: Galen and Aristotle—the authorities—had said otherwise!

If progress in the science of medicine could not be made in the days when the minds of men were fixed exclusively on spiritual matters, it was equally impossible in those later years when they looked to the past and believed firmly in established authority.

From the fall of the Roman Empire until beyond the thirteenth century—nearly a thousand years—there is no advance in medical science to record in Western Europe. There were humanitarian advances like the hospital. There were scholastic advances like the university. But medical advance, no. It was a period in which the men of the West, with their eyes in turn on the heavens and on the past, sought to adjust themselves to the world they were living in. And now even the slow process of accumulating the knowledge of the past was to be interrupted, for in the fourteenth century there reached the walled cities, the monasteries, and the universities that great sweeping wave of death—the bubonic plague.

CHAPTER XIV

The Black Death

ONE of the great marvels of the universe—so it seems to us—is that man appeared upon earth. It is an even greater marvel that he has managed to survive. Stronger, tougher animals than he have been exterminated in the hard struggle for existence, yet he has lived on and multiplied. He has survived not because of his physical strength but because of his superior intelligence.

The world that early men met, as we have said in an earlier chapter, was rough and terrifying. Life was severe, because man was ill suited physically to cope with its hardships. There were great beasts to prey upon him in his comparative defenselessness; there was uncertainty of food supply; there were diseases.

Man conquered the beasts; his physical strength was less, but his intelligence was greater than theirs. To defend himself he used what no other animal has ever used—weapons: the club, the knife, the spear, the bow and arrow, and, finally, the gun. And he was successful. His only unconquered "enemy" still existing is his fellow man, on whom he has so many times turned his weapons in the useless slaughter of war.

The same superior intelligence that prompted mankind to the invention of weapons led to the discovery of means for insuring his food supply. Man domesticated animals; raised crops, mastered the principles of husbandry.

Of the three great hazards to human existence only one then remained beyond control. That was disease. Man's intelligence failed to lead him to success against it as rapidly as against the other hazards. Disease was an invisible enemy, far harder to cope with than the great beasts that roared in the forests. The spear and the club and the bow and arrow were of no avail against it. The only weapon with which it could be fought was knowledge, the knowledge of how disease is caused and how it can be controlled. It was far simpler to learn the ways of the land, the rudiments of agriculture, the planting of grain, the tilling of crops, than to learn the nature of the thing called disease.

The winning of that knowledge has been slow. What we have been telling and have yet to tell are the steps by which it has been acquired and is still being acquired. It is a story of false paths followed and of obstructions that man has put in the road to his own salvation. The philosophy of supernatural causes of disease was a false path; medieval scholasticism was an obstruction to progress. Fortunately for us, we live in a time when slowly gained, hard-earned knowledge is finally conquering disease. From our position today we can look back over the past and marvel that man has survived on earth. And we can look ahead to the future knowing that if he continues to seek and find knowledge he will win greater and greater victories over disease. His only weapon is knowledge.

As we tell of some of the diseases that afflicted men in the thirteenth and fourteenth centuries, let us at the same time look forward and see when the method of controlling them was discovered and precisely what it was. Often it was a simple thing, seemingly obvious now that we know it, and yet in its absence men suffered and died.

The diseases we shall speak of here are those that came in great terrifying epidemics—almost world-wide outbreaks—called pandemics. We are not yet ready to deal with the diseases that were always present, such as head colds, appendicitis, pneumonia, cancer, and the like. In medieval days there were epidemics of which most people nowadays have never even heard. One of them was called St. Anthony's fire. Sometimes this name was given to the disease erysipelas but more often to a cruel and crippling malady that appeared oftenest among poor people. There would be a season when the rains were heavy and the summer damp and foggy. The harvest of grain, the rye from which the

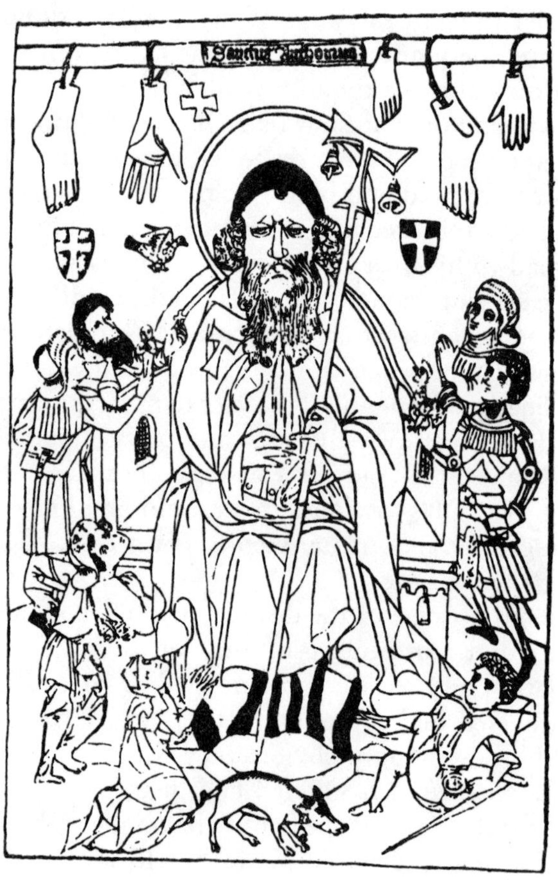

St. Anthony and the victims of the "fire."

black bread was made, would be scanty and the seeds spotted with a mildew blight. Then late in the fall, perhaps at the gate of the town, some poor fellow would be found with his legs and arms black and shriveled, trying pitifully to crawl to the monastery. People would run from him in terror; only the monks of St. Anthony would come to him and carry him to their monastery; they had devoted their lives to aiding such sufferers.

That day the town was quiet; men and women stayed indoors; no children played in the streets. In hushed voices they whispered that the fire of hell, St. Anthony's fire, moved through the land.

Soon in one house and then in another and another a child, a man, a woman would be stricken with the disease. Scarcely a home would escape.

The legs and the arms of the sufferers would grow cold and become frightfully painful. Then they would turn black. Some of the people would die; some would recover; but many of the latter would have lost an arm or a leg which had withered and dropped off. From a few the vicious disease would take both legs and arms, leaving nothing but the maimed trunk and head. It is small wonder that people feared the disease.

But what knowledge did they have with which to fight it? Some men believed that wet weather poisoned the air. The idea that disease was due to evil smells and bad air was very prevalent then; it was one that was to persist until well into the nineteenth century. The disease malaria, common then in Italy and spreading into Western Europe, got its name from the words meaning bad air, *mala aria*. Other men thought that epidemic disease was due to eclipses and falling stars and earthquakes. Some believed that it arose from the anger of God at the sins of men, and some were certain that the Jews had poisoned the wells. In the year 1161 the Jewish physicians in the town of Prague were accused of this crime and burned.

What did men do to control the disease? They prayed; they wore blessed charms; they took the medicines that Dioscorides had recommended in his herbal. But the disease swept on; it maimed and killed in spite of prayers and charms and medicines. It would last for a year at a time; then the next fall with the new harvest it would cease, unless that year too had been wet and foggy.

We have said that St. Anthony's fire is held in check now by knowledge; it no longer occurs. The cause of it lay before the eyes of the people of those bygone days—lay in a fact already mentioned. It was not until 1597 that men guessed the cause, or until 1630 that they were sure of it. It took two more centuries for that knowledge to be put fully into effect. Then the disease ceased to occur entirely. And the knowledge was simply this: rye with mildew blight from the wet season is poisonous. The blight is a fungus growth of a kind called ergot. Ergot like some toadstools is a poison. Taken in large enough quantities it shrinks the blood vessels for a time until so little blood can flow to the arms and legs that they become starved and die. All men needed to know was: to avoid St. Anthony's fire do not eat blighted rye. Without that simple knowledge they prayed—and were crippled or died. With it today we face a world safe in a victory over one disease—and a rapacious one.

In the Middle Ages the epidemics of disease uncontrolled by knowledge made the average length of life far shorter than it is today. Some men, of course, escaped disease and lived as long as any people live today; but many more died young, while they were still babies or small children. The average length of life then was only about eight years; today it is nearly sixty. In the six hundred years that have passed since then, medical knowledge has added half a century to the average length of life.

In this connection one peculiar fact concerning human behavior has been true in all ages. When life is short and hard and uncertain, it seems to be valued least. In the last six hundred years, really in the last one hundred, men have grown far more humane than they were. We value life more highly today; we attempt more, far more, to prevent suffering, perhaps because we know now that it can be prevented.

In the days when St. Anthony's fire was common, many men and women lost legs and arms. There are old pictures and old wood carvings showing these crippled people. With the victims of the fire are those deformed by leprosy. But in

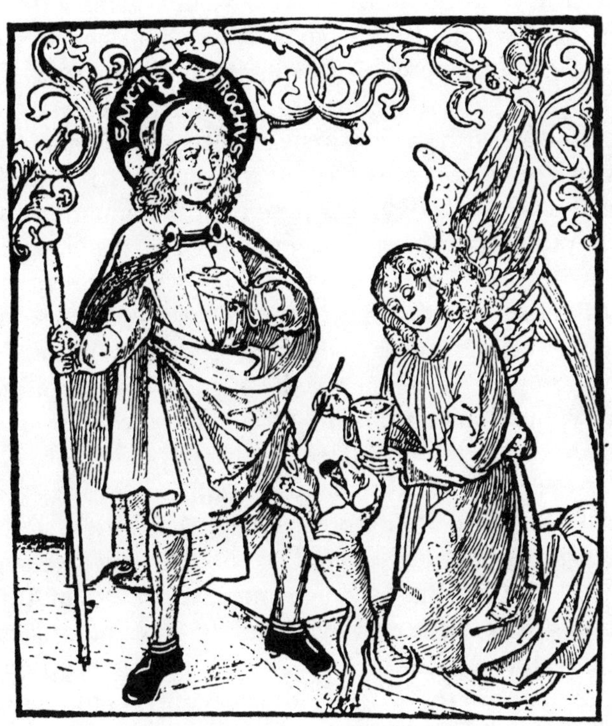

St. Roch treating plague sores.

that procession of the maimed were many who had been crippled deliberately at the will of men. Wars went on century after century. And those too were the days when the penalties of the law prescribed cutting off a hand or an arm for even slight crimes, and on mere suspicion of crime men were tortured with rack and boot. Next to disease, man has always had himself as his worst enemy.

St. Anthony's fire and leprosy were both great scourges of the Middle Ages, and there were others. What disease would you add to the list? The smallpox that killed its millions? That came later. Its great onslaught was after the fifteenth century; the knowledge for its control came in the eighteenth century. Perhaps you would name diphtheria, which once wrought such havoc throughout the world and killed Napoleon's wife Josephine, and perhaps George Washington. But that disease made its greatest ravages from the sixteenth to the twentieth century. The knowledge by which it is controlled came within the lifetime of the older of us living today. Again you might name tuberculosis, consumption, the disease once called the "captain of the men of death." Yes, it was present, always present, taking toll of the population year in and year out, but it never came in sweeping waves as did the "great mortalities."

Typhus fever was one of these pandemic diseases. The word typhus comes from the Greek and means smoke or a cloud, hence a dimness of consciousness, a stupor. Typhus fever was once confused with another disease—typhoid fever—which is quite different except that in it also there is fever with stupor. The word typhoid means "resembling typhus." But typhus is much more serious than typhoid. Typhus was a disease of war and famine, of prisons and jails and ships and of medieval cities. In war it killed more men than were ever killed with shot and sword. Its cause? People of the Middle Ages thought it an affliction from God; we know now that it is due to a germ carried from the sick man to the well man by body lice. The little typhus, typhoid, is spread by food or water contaminated with sewage. Medical science takes the glamor, the dignity away from the enemy disease and shows it in its crude reality. That bit of knowledge—that typhus is carried by the louse—was gained only in the twentieth century. It came barely in time to prevent the spread of the disease in the World War, the first great war in which typhus failed to take its thousands and perhaps hundreds of thousands. In the East, in Serbia, there was typhus fever during the War. But the measures of medical science kept it from spreading in an epidemic to the men in the trenches on the Western front. And the means that medical science used was simply the establishing of delousing stations through which all travelers from the East to the West must pass and leave their lice behind. Disease often loses its terrifying aspects when medical knowledge points out its humble lurking places.

But there are still some infections which defy even modern knowledge. One of these came in repeated epidemics in the Middle Ages, and in all the centuries since the pandemics have continued, twenty or thirty years apart. It is a disease that we all know—influenza, the mildest of the great pandemics.

The term influenza is a clue to beliefs concerning its cause in bygone days: *influenza coelestia* was its full name, heavenly influence. Storms and earthquakes, shipwreck and war, comets and rains of blood were given as the causes of influenza. Those occasional rains of blood especially excited the imaginations of the people. They occurred in very rainy seasons; food and linen and even the walls of the houses were marked with tiny red spots like drops of blood. We today, less prone to look to the supernatural for the cause of everything unusual, should say that those drops of blood were a red moldy mildew—nothing more.

But this mildew, unlike that of St. Anthony's fire, had nothing to do with the disease. Influenza is caused by a germ passed from the sick to the well by coughing and sneezing. That we know, but we do not yet know how to prevent the spread of the germ. We still have epidemics of influenza.

It is the mildest of the great pandemics, but if you think of the last great epidemic, the one in 1918, you may be doubtful of its mildness. That year in the United States alone nearly forty million people had the disease; almost three hundred thousand died. Yet that was mild for a pandemic. Compare the figures with those that would have resulted if instead of influenza we had had an epidemic of the oriental bubonic plague like the one in the fourteenth century. Instead of three hundred thousand, fifty million people would have died. Every town, every city, every state would in the course of a few weeks have shrunk to half its population. Whole families would have been wiped out. We would not have been able to bury the dead. Bodies would have lain in the streets and in the fields and in the homes.

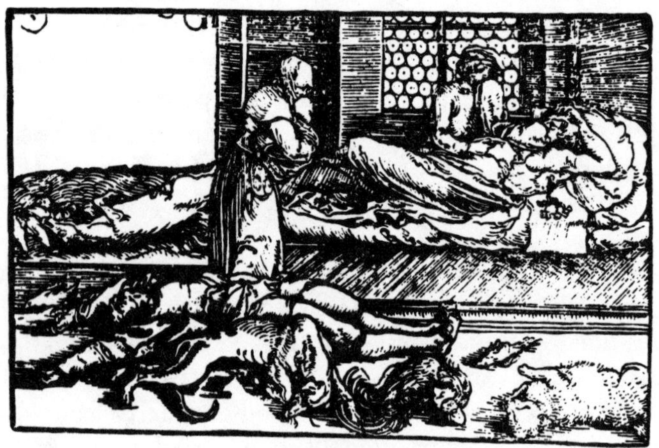

The Black Death.

If such a pandemic should strike our country, our social and business life would be paralyzed. For want of men the factories and the railroads would stop; the fire companies could not respond to calls, fire would spread in the cities. Schools and stores would be closed, the streets deserted; the sick and dying would call for doctors. But half the doctors would be dead. It would take us a century, perhaps longer, to build our country up again after such an outbreak of disease.

This disease was the "great mortality" of the Middle

Ages. Uncontrolled by knowledge, it threatened to exterminate the human race.

We have told of the epidemic of bubonic plague that came to Constantinople in the year 543. But that epidemic did not spread far into Western Europe. At that time, soon after the fall of the Roman Empire, travel and commerce were almost at a standstill in the West. The disease was held in check by the isolation of the people. But by the fourteenth century travel and commerce were active. The countries were overrun with vagabonds; the students of the universities wandered from city to city; bands of soldiers moved across the countryside. It was a warlike century. Gunpowder was first used in battle in 1330; the Hundred Years' War began in 1336. Conditions were ideal for the spread of plague.

In the spring of 1347 the disease, coming out of Asia, reached Constantinople as had the epidemic of 543. By the autumn it had spread to Sicily, and by December to Naples, Genoa, and Marseilles. Early in 1348 it had extended over southern France, Italy and Spain. In June it reached Paris; in August, Britain and Ireland. It took the plague fifteen months to travel from Constantinople to London. But it did not stop there; it spread in all directions into the Netherlands, Germany, Scandinavia, and Russia.

Terror moved ahead of the ruthless march of the plague; its passage left the countries broken, demoralized, nearly depopulated. In the face of overwhelming calamity the customs that held men together grew lax; law and order almost disappeared; human nature followed its own dictates. Some men in panic fled from their families, gave their possessions to the Church, hid in the cathedrals, and prayed until the disease reached and killed them there. Others dashed to boats, sailed out to sea and died on shipboard, and the boats drifted derelict with crews of corpses. A heroic few gave their last days to comforting the sick and dying. Still others gave themselves up to revelry, drinking, feasting, and dancing. Such was the behavior of the people of Jerusalem when threatened with an attack by Sennacherib and his army. It is described in the Bible. "The Lord God of Hosts called to weeping and to mourning and to baldness and to girding with sackcloth: and behold joy and gladness, slaying oxen, and killing sheep, eating flesh and drinking wine: let us eat and drink for tomorrow we shall die."

The Italian author Giovanni Boccaccio, who was one of the first men to write in Italian prose, was living in Florence at the time of the epidemic of the Black Death in 1348. He survived, and in one of his books, the *Decameron*, gives this description of the outbreak in Florence: "Such was the cruelty of Heaven and perhaps of Men [He believes, you see, in the divine origin of disease and yet his story is about a merry group of young people who hid in seclusion in the hope of escaping the disease. Ideas were mixed; God caused disease, but that the disease spread by infection seemed obvious.] that between March and July following it is supposed and made pretty certain that upwards of a hundred thousand souls perished in the city only, whereas before the calamity it was not supposed to contain so many inhabitants. What magnificent dwellings, what noble palaces were then depopulated to the last person, what families extinct, what rich and vast possessions left, and no known heir to inherit, what numbers of both sexes in the prime and vigor of youth —who in the morning Galen, Hippocrates, or Æsculapius himself would have declared in perfect health—after dining with their friends here have supped with their departed friends in the other world."

Disposal of the dead was one of the great problems for the survivors during outbreaks of the plague. At Avignon the Pope consecrated the river Rhône so that corpses could be sunk in it instead of being buried. In other cities they were thrown into the sea—often to be washed back on to the shores with the returning tide.

In these years, because of strife within the Church, the

Pope lived in the city of Avignon instead of Rome. This particular Pope, Clement VI, had in his service the most famous surgeon of the Middle Ages, Guy de Chauliac. At the outbreak of the plague Guy had the Pope lock himself

The Diseases and Casualties this Week.

Abortive	4	Impostheme	8
Aged	45	Infants	22
Bleeding	1	Kingsevil	4
Broken legge	1	Lethargy	1
Broke her scull by a fall in the street at St. Mary Woolchurch	1	Livergrown	1
Childbed	28	Meagrome	1
Chrisomes	9	Palsie	1
Consumption	126	Plague	4237
Convulsion	89	Purples	2
Cough	1	Quinsie	5
Dropsie	53	Rickets	23
Feaver	348	Rising of the Lights	18
Flox and Small-pox	11	Rupture	1
Flux	1	Scurvy	3
Frighted	2	Shingles	1
Gowt	1	Spotted Feaver	166
Grief	3	Stilborn	4
Griping in the Guts	79	Stone	2
Head-mould-shot	1	Stopping of the stomach	17
Jaundies	7	Strangury	3
		Suddenly	2
		Surfeit	74
		Teeth	111
		Thrush	6
		Tissick	9
		Ulcer	1
		Vomiting	10
		Winde	4
		Wormes	20

Christned: Males — 90, Females — 81, In all — 171
Buried: Males — 2777, Females — 2791, In all — 5568
Plague — 4237

Increased in the Burials this Week — 249.
Parishes clear of the Plague — 27 Parishes Infected — 103

The Assize of Bread set forth by Order of the Lord Maior and Court of Aldermen,
A penny Wheaten Loaf to contain Nine Ounces and a half, and three half-penny White Loaves the like weight.

A bill of mortality during the epidemic of bubonic plague in England, 1665.

for the duration of the epidemic in a room in which there burned continuously an open fire to purify the air.

Here is Guy de Chauliac's description of the disease from which millions died. He says, "The great mortality appeared at Avignon, January, 1348, when I was in the service of Pope Clement VI. It was of two kinds. The first lasted two months, with continued fever and spitting of blood, and people died of it in three days. The second kind was all the rest of the time, also with continuous fever, and with swellings in the armpits and groin; and people died in five days. It was so contagious, especially that accompanied by spitting of blood, that not only by staying together, but even by looking at one another, people caught it, with the result that men died without attention and were buried without priests. The father did not visit his son, nor the son his father. Charity was dead and hope crushed.

"I call it great, because it covered the whole world, or lacked little of doing so. . . . And it was so great that it left scarcely a fourth part of the people. . . .

"Many were in doubt about the cause of this great mortality. In some places they thought that the Jews had poisoned the world: and so they killed them. In others, that it was the poor deformed people who were responsible: and they drove them out. In others that it was the nobles; and they feared to go abroad. Finally they reached the point where they kept guards in the cities and villages, permitting the entry of no one who was not well known. And if powders or salves were found on anyone, the owners, for fear that they were poisons, were forced to swallow them. . . ."

The swellings that Guy de Chauliac mentions as appearing in the armpits and groin were enlarged and infected lymph glands. A gland so infected is called a bubo—hence the term bubonic plague; plague itself means a blow. In many infections, often in mild ones, lymph glands became enlarged, as do those in the neck from sore throat. When a person had the bubonic plague the glands were not only swollen, but if the patient lived long enough, they also became filled with pus, broke, and made running sores—plague sores.

The name Black Death was given to the plague because in its victims there appear little hemorrhages under the skin looking like tiny black and blue places—tokens of the plague, they were called.

Guy de Chauliac in his brief description makes one very important statement concerning control of the disease. Perhaps the line caught your attention—"Finally they reached the point where they kept guards in the cities and villages, permitting the entry of no one who was not well known." This was the first time that measures of the kind were put into effect—the first use of quarantine.

The idea of a quarantine which grew out of the epidemic persisted after the plague began to subside. Isolation was for various lengths of time; but beginning in 1383 travelers in ships suspected of infection were held for forty days in the harbor of Marseilles before they were allowed to land in that city. Quarantine means forty. We still use the measure and the name although the term has lost its original significance of forty days; the time of isolation now varies with the disease.

Bubonic plague still exists in the world today; thousands have died of it in this century in Asia. It has even reached our shores, and a few cases have occurred here. But the disease can be held in check, for we now know how it is caused and how it can be controlled. We have knowledge!

The tragic thing about the bit of knowledge that alone keeps us free from plague is that Avicenna, the great physician of Arabia in the tenth and eleventh centuries, came close to guessing it. He observed that before the plague spread, rats and mice came out of their burrows and staggered about as if drunk, and many died. Only late in the nineteenth century did the meaning of his observation become clear. The knowledge by which the bubonic plague can be held in check is this: it is a disease of rats and mice and ground squirrels—of rodents. It is caused by a germ which rat fleas spread. The fleas bite the sick rat and acquire the germ. They leave the dying rat and with their bite infect other rats—or men.

The great difference between medieval times and our own is not so much in ways of living and acting as in ways of thinking and acquiring knowledge, the knowledge that makes us victorious over disease. We often pride ourselves on our material things: our great inventions, such as the radio and the aëroplane, our great cities with streets filled with automobiles, our great buildings lighted by electricity and heated with steam. But such things would be of no advantage if epidemics like the Black Death could sweep over us. The aëroplanes, the automobiles, the buildings, even the cities would be deserted in the face of the Black Death. We would behave just as did the people of the fourteenth century. Knowledge, medical knowledge, is man's most priceless possession; it is his greatest triumph in his struggle for existence, the struggle for safety, food, and health.

CHAPTER XV

The Mental Contagions

THE fourteenth century was the period of that great pestilence, the Black Death. The fifteenth century was the time of the Dancing Mania, the queerest emotional disorder that has ever affected large groups of human beings. It was a curious prelude to a period of contradiction. The century gave birth to Joan of Arc, and to her strange companion, the monstrous Gilles de Rais, to Leonardo da Vinci, the genius of art and science, and Christopher Columbus, the discoverer of America. The century opened with an epidemic of a horrible emotional disturbance; its close marks the beginning of modern times, for during that century printing was first used in Europe and the Revival of Learning and the Renaissance occurred.

We have said little in our story of how the diseases of individual men may affect the course of history. Everyone's behavior is influenced by physical infirmities and by mental peculiarities, and each of us recognizes that fact in his own actions. But we see it perhaps more clearly and certainly more critically in the actions of others. Usually the behavior of the individual affects only a small number of people, his family and those he meets in daily life. But some men are raised to positions of great influence as generals during a war or rulers or popular leaders, as was Peter the Hermit, who incited the people to the Crusades. Then their peculiarities may affect whole nations, even whole civilizations. The indigestion of a king may influence his policies more than the advice of his counselors; his toothache, occurring at a critical moment, may precipitate a civil war; his mental peculiarities may lead his country to ruin or triumph.

We could speculate on the infirmities of the great and wonder what the course of history would have been had they been healthier—if Alexander the Great had not died when he was thirty-two; if William of Orange had not had tuberculosis; if Queen Anne's eyes had been stronger; if Louis XIII had not been feeble-minded; if Joan of Arc had

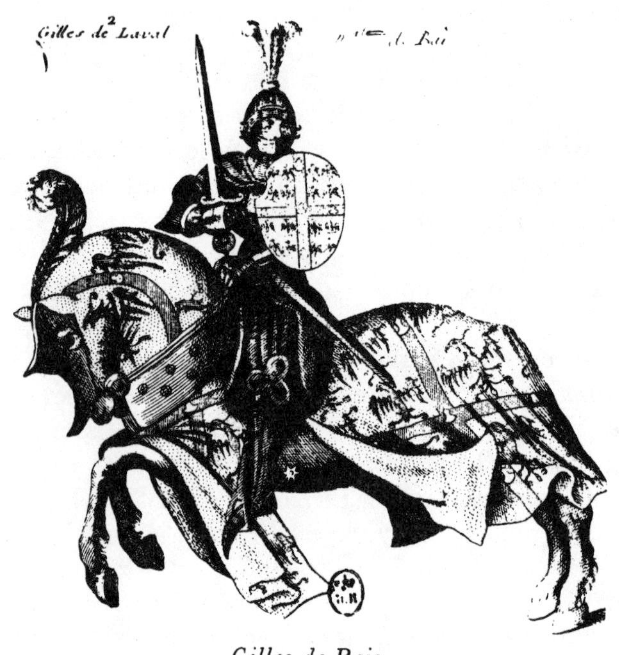

Gilles de Rais.

been a normal-minded peasant girl instead of one who had visions.

Joan of Arc, you remember, was finally burned as a witch, an act characteristic of the times. And Gilles de Rais? It sounds like an anti-climax, but if he had not had his mental peculiarities we, probably, should not have had the story of Bluebeard.

There have been monsters like the Baron of Rais before and since, but the reasons he gave for his actions are, like those for burning Joan, characteristic of the times. Gilles wished, so he said, to replenish his fortune by magic; with the aid of the devil he sought to find gold.

As a young man he inherited wide lands in Brittany, which had once been a great feudal domain. His career started well; he joined the French king in the war against England. When Joan of Arc led the army to victory, he rode at her side and for his bravery was made a marshal of France. The war over, Gilles returned to Brittany and lived there in the most amazing splendor, lavishing his money on public feasts and entertainments for the people of the countryside. At last, when his fortune was nearly exhausted, he called to his aid the greatest alchemists and sorcerers of the day. Mysterious rites were performed in secret at his castle for the purpose of obtaining the philosophers' stone.

At the same time, in the country for miles around the castle, there occurred a series of mysterious disappearances. Small children, boys and girls of four and five and six and seven, left their homes to carry lunch to their fathers in the fields or to go on errands to neighboring farms and never returned. One such disappearance, even two or three, might have attracted no wide attention in a day when wolves and wild boars inhabited the thick forest; but when the number rose to dozens, scores, and even hundreds, sorrow gave way to excitement and horror. The country was bewitched. Children on the open road, in lane and lot, seemed to vanish into the air. One moment they were there; the next they were gone.

But one thing people noticed. Whenever a disappearance occurred, there had passed through the neighborhood at the time the mounted men of the Baron of Rais. Suspicion was aroused against the tall marshal with the blue-black beard. This was the fifteenth century; human lives were no longer sacrificed without protest at the mere word of a nobleman. The Baron was arrested. The bodies of some of the missing children, horribly mutilated, were discovered. Like savages, Gilles and his magicians had held blood orgies.

Gilles was tried before an ecclesiastical court for heresy and before a civil court for murder. He was found doubly guilty, excommunicated, and condemned to be hanged and burned. He did not fear death, but the penalty of excom-

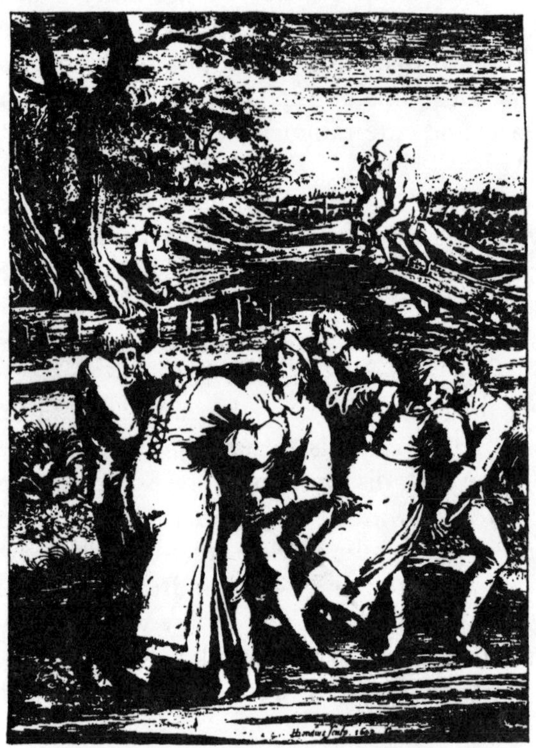

The Dancing Mania.

munication which carried with it the certainty of eternal damnation in hell terrified him.

When we told of the methods of scholarship of the thirteenth century, we said that fear of excommunication kept men from daring to risk the heresy of free thought. Here in the fifteenth century this warrior, sorcerer, and murderer broke down and begged in tears that he might die, but not be excommunicated. His prayer was granted; his confession was heard, and he was absolved of sin. He was simply hanged and burned.

Led to the gibbet, he climbed on a high stool; a rope was passed around his neck; the stool was pushed away. The faggots about his feet were lighted. The flames mounted over him and burned the rope. His body fell into the fire. At this sight the sentiment of the people, even of those who had lost their children, suddenly changed. A moment before they had been eager for revenge; now they were softened. Women from the crowd of spectators ran forward and rescued the body. It was given Christian burial. On the spot where Gilles died a shrine was erected. In time a legend grew about it; it was said to possess miraculous powers. Women flocked there to pray for abundance of milk that they might nurse their babies well!

The story of Gilles lived on, but changed in the telling and became confused with the tale of another monster of Brittany who lived in the sixth century, Comorre the Cursed. Gilles's blue-black beard stuck in men's memory. The garbled legend became the story of Bluebeard, written by the Frenchman Charles Perrault, who also told the stories of Cinderella and the Sleeping Beauty. What an ironical fate for the strong and terrible Baron of Rais—that the spot of his execution should become a magic shrine for mothers, and the story of his life a nursery tale to amuse children!

The ways of human nature and human behavior and belief are at times seemingly inexplicable. And if in the case of Gilles de Rais they seem strange, they were even stranger in the case of the Dancing Mania of the same century.

Perhaps the Black Death may give a clue to the origin of this strange phenomenon. The graves of the victims of that mortality were covered, but the memory of the horror remained; it haunted the survivors. A sense of insecurity, of panic, pervaded the people. The pent-up emotion broke out first in the town of Aix-la-Chapelle. There, one morning, the inhabitants awoke to find their city invaded by a strange band of people who had come from Germany. Silently, intent only on their own purposes, they walked through the

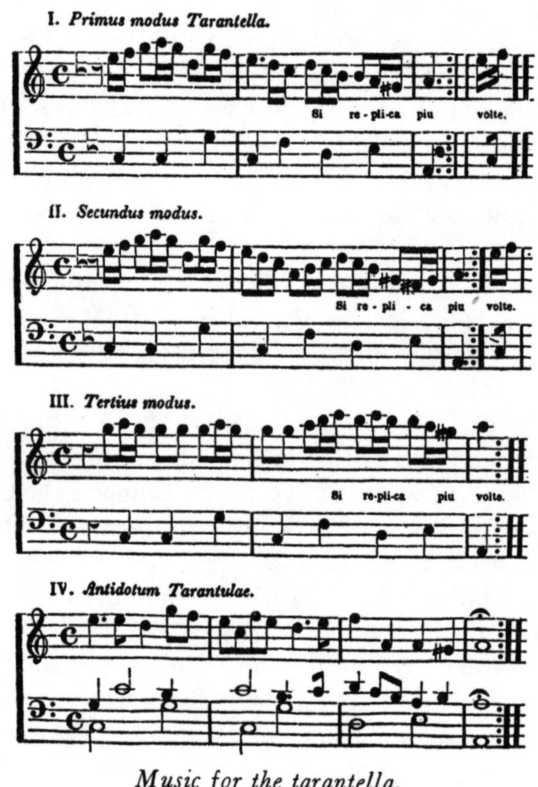

Music for the tarantella.

streets until they came to an open square. Then, forming in a circle, they began to dance. But it was such a dance as no one in the city had ever seen. Slowly at first and then faster and faster the dancers contorted their bodies, until finally they were writhing and jumping in a frenzy, screaming, their eyes fixed, foam dripping from their mouths. One by one they fell from exhaustion, but as they dropped their places were taken by the townspeople. The contagion of the Dancing Mania, a mental contagion, one of sympathy, of suggestion, was spread by the mere sight of the dancers.

Along country roads, from town to town, from city to city, went processions of the dancers. Shops were closed, farms neglected. Crowds followed in the wake of the dancers. Some were impelled by curiosity, but some were anxious parents seeking their children. And there were children crying pitifully as they crept among the hurrying feet of the spectators, seeking parents who had joined the dancers.

In 1418 the mental turmoil reached its climax in the city of Strasbourg. The priests of the church tried to comfort and soothe the victims of the mania. The sufferers took St. Vitus as their patron saint. They appealed to him to save them from their own wild outbreaks.

The Dancing Mania occurred five hundred years ago, but the term St. Vitus' dance still survives. It is applied now to a certain nervous disease called chorea in which there is twitching of the face and arms.

There is another word in the language that commemorates this wild outbreak that once spread over Europe. It is "tarantella," the name given to a lively form of Italian music which was originally played for those who were overcome by the Dancing Mania; music seemed to bring relief. Not knowing why they danced, people sought an explanation. They said that spiders bit them, tarantulas, and that the poison made them twist and squirm. The music of the tarantella healed them. This superstition lasted for three hundred years; to treat spider bites the village musicians were called to play on flute and oboe and Turkish drum the whirling music of the tarantella.

The strenuous exertion of the Dancing Mania was merely the physical expression of intense emotional excitement. Similar behavior has often been seen among people aroused to great religious enthusiasm; the zealous have shaken and trembled and even fallen unconscious. Some religious sects have been named after the queer behavior which marked their earlier days—especially the Shakers, the Jumpers, the Rollers, the Quakers, and the *Convulsionnaires*, not to mention the whirling dervishes.

Most of the mental epidemics, and there have been many before and since the Dancing Mania, have taken some form other than mere purposeless muscular activity. The Crusades to the Holy Lands, especially those incited by Peter the Hermit, and certainly the Children's Crusade, were the outcome of mental epidemics. So, also, years later, was the Tulip Mania that centered in Holland during which, in a frenzy of speculation, ordinarily sensible men paid out their entire fortunes for a few tulip bulbs.

A far sadder epidemic than the latter was the persecution of witches which started in the fifteenth century and lasted well into the eighteenth. Thousands of harmless old women were burned to death or drowned in the belief that they were witches. America was far from escaping the craze. There were men who made a business of witch-hunting, and sought out suspected people, looking for small projections on their bodies called "witch spots." Mob excitement waxed high over witchcraft. In solemn courts of law robed judges listened seriously to fantastic tales worthy of savage and primitive people, and condemned harmless old ladies to death. Many of those were poor insane people who had the misfortune to live in a day when the humane care of the mentally ill had not yet begun.

People in all ages who have lived in tribes or cities or nations have felt the influence of mental contagion. No germ causes it; the mania is not a disease; it is simply one of the manifestations of strange human nature and human behavior transmitted by imitation.

Why is it that one idea or the example of one man may influence a whole group of people and incite them to some peculiar course of action? Many years ago, in a nunnery in Europe, one of the sisters began to mew like a cat; soon another and another joined her until all of the inmates were

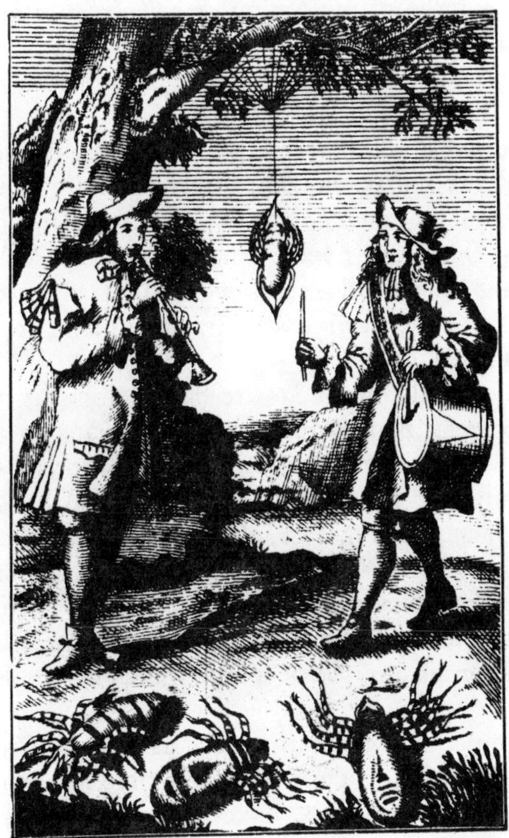

Killing tarantulas with music.

mewing industriously. Threats of punishment failed to stop them; they were whipped, but still they mewed on until the petty mania wore itself out and ceased. In a thousand other nunneries a sister might have mewed in vain—merely the butt of ridicule.

Why did the mewing spread in this one nunnery? Conditions, you say, were ripe for it; the mental attitude receptive. Such words mean little. But manias, small and great, are very real. You have seen the milder ones—the sudden success of a fashion in clothing or in cosmetics or in slang expressions, or a wave of enthusiasm for some new popular song which is sung and sung and sung and then dropped and forgotten.

War, perhaps, is the greatest of all the epidemic manias. A wave of excited patriotism, a mental contagion, spreads through a country; men go out to maim and kill their fellow men whom they have never seen. Then the war subsides as the Dancing Mania did; men lose their hatred for their erstwhile enemies; the survivors return once more to peace and international commerce.

Not all mental contagions are bad or foolish; not all of them deserve the name "mania," which means unreasonable excitement. Some mental contagions which spread by example and imitation are good and beneficial. Although contagion always suggests disease, there is no phrase but mental contagion to explain how in a short time the opinion, the attitude, even the guiding belief, of a great body of people may be completely altered. By means of mental contagion Peter the Hermit aroused people to march on the First Crusade.

Great humanitarian reforms, such as the Red Cross agreement to care for the wounded in war time, humane care of the insane and of animals, have been effected by the contagion of an idea, which has spread until it has become accepted and established in ways of living. We shall tell of these advances in their place, and you will see then that although they are good and helpful, they too, like the useless and harmful manias, bear a relation to the mental contagions.

Our present attitude toward the world had its beginnings in a fashion that arose in Italy in the fifteenth century. Near the end of the fourteenth century men for the first time discovered the beauty of the writings of classical antiquity. At first their attention was held by the Latin authors. But these authors themselves said so much about Greek literature that men were led to learn the language and discover the beauty of Homer, Plato, and the great Greek dramatists.

A wave of enthusiasm for the classics spread through Italy; classical literature and art became fashionable. To be a gentleman meant that a man was acquainted with scholarship and with the works of writers such as Plutarch, Isocrates, Virgil, Cicero, and Lucretius.

What is called a classical education had its beginnings then. In the colleges, the lecture rooms of the teachers of poetry and rhetoric were crowded. But the students did not attempt to follow deeply one single line of learning. Rather they learned a little of everything—a little medicine, a little philosophy, a little art—in order to develop the widest possible culture. They were not experts in anything.

In wealthy families, because of the new learning, tutors were employed to instruct boys in the works of poets and orators in order that they might quote them fluently in polished conversation and write prose and poetry in the ancient Latin style of Cicero.

With the discovery of the beauty of classical style came a wave of enthusiasm for the loveliness and grandeur of classical art and architecture. But men not only admired the technical beauty of style and the art of the ancients. They came for the first time to understand the Greek and Roman way of thinking about life. Greek influence was especially important. The Greeks had, as you recall, conceived life in the fullest sense of its possibilities and glories. Their art showed men and women ideally beautiful but still men and women. Their architecture was practical and direct; its beauty grew out of its very simplicity. The Greeks had looked at life face to face, and had tried to understand the real nature of man and the universe. The men of the Middle

Ages had shrouded all that was human with supernatural mystery; the Greeks had tried to make the supernatural less mysterious by making it more human.

The revival of ancient learning, carrying with it this point of view, opened the eyes of men to themselves and the world about them. Not only were the heavens good but so was the earth; man was good and nature was good; man was born

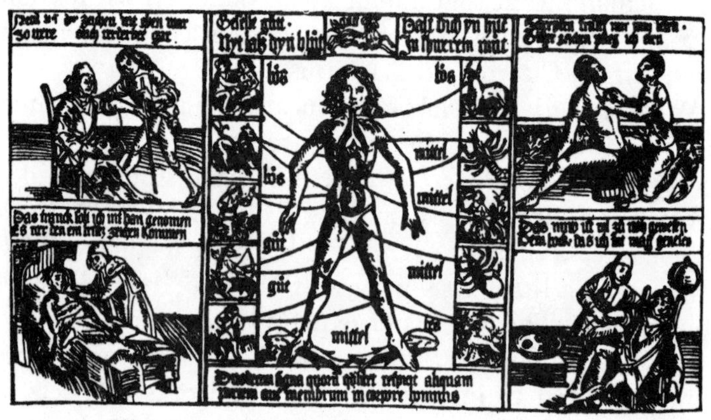

Illustration from a calendar printed in 1493.

with a right to use nature for his earthly benefit. These were ideas quite different from those held by medieval Christians.

From the intense emotional reaction of the Renaissance, there resulted in Italy some unpleasant social consequences. Men in a desire for earthly experience lost the restraint of piety which they had felt in the Middle Ages. The fear of excommunication which had frightened even the Baron of Rais no longer disturbed the Italian nobleman, who, yielding to the contagion of new ideals, yielded to the bad as well as the good. The somewhat refining experiences that we have gained since that time were lacking. There came a period when Italy was disgraced not only by political intrigue and dishonesty, but also by brutal assassinations and poisoning at the hands of cultured gentlemen and gentlewomen. It was a period of extreme sophistication, when people had no guiding principles of decency as we know them. Cesare and Lucrezia Borgia and Lorenzo de' Medici made the pages of history bloody with their deeds. But in one thing they differed from the terrible Gilles de Rais of Brittany. He gave way to temptations; he sinned and knew it; he was afraid; he repented. The murderous Italians of the Renaissance flouted religion; they knew no sin; they feared no spiritual vengeance. Their basic ideal was not very different from that of today in some schools for small children; it was to give way to complete self-expression in order to develop all the natural qualities of the personality. Following it, some of the Italians behaved like vicious, spoiled children.

Fortunately these unpleasant by-products of the Renaissance were largely limited to Italy. But the contagion of the spirit of learning, of free thinking, spread through Europe. It was tremendously accelerated after the invention of printing with movable type. Manuscripts copied by hand were inaccurate and expensive; printed books were more accurate and far cheaper. Printing unquestionably was the most important of all agents in spreading the new doctrines of the Renaissance.

Printing began in Germany soon after 1440, and in 1462 the sack of the town of Mainz by Adolph of Nassau drove the German printers to take refuge in the cities of other countries of Europe. Books were being issued from many presses and some of the earliest to be printed were medical works. In 1457 a purgation calendar was printed which told when the stars were propitious for taking a physic. In 1462 a similar astrological work on blood-letting appeared. The writings of Avicenna were printed in 1479 and a year later the first of many editions of the Sanitary Regimen of Salerno.

These were old and well-known books that were merely distributed more widely by printing; soon an entirely different kind of medical work was to appear from the new printing presses. The wave of enthusiasm which led men to collect and translate the manuscripts of pagan poetry and oratory led them also to the classical medical writings. The works of Galen and Hippocrates were translated directly from the original Greek and printed. Men began to see how the words of the masters had been garbled in passing through many translations at the hands of Romans, Syrians, Persians, Arabs, and Hebrews.

The fifteenth century was for medicine a period of the revival of ancient learning. The new ideals of freedom of thought and criticism, which characterized the Renaissance, affected art and literature and politics and religion more quickly than medicine. The physicians of the fifteenth century were busy translating, comparing, learning, and had as yet no desire to work out scientific methods, make observations, and perform experiments.

But in the closing days of the fifteenth century, a single year after the discovery of America by Columbus, a man was born who was destined to awaken the scientific spirit among physicians and to spread the contagion of the Renaissance to the field of medicine. In the one thousand years that have passed since the fall of Rome he is the first European doctor we have mentioned. His name was Aureolus Theophrastus Bombastus von Hohenheim. In those days it was the practice of learned men to take a Latin name, and so he called himself Paracelsus after the Roman physician Celsus, and it is by this name that we shall speak of him.

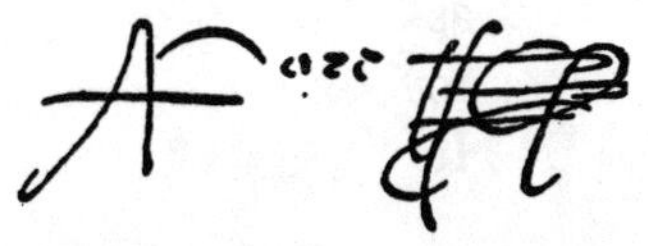

Part Six

PARACELSUS, THE CRITIC
VESALIUS, THE OBSERVER
PARÉ, THE EXPERIMENTER

CHAPTER XVI

Paracelsus, the Critic

EXPLORATION, trade, politics, war, religion, those ancient and dominating figures in the pageant of human history, stormed across the stage of the sixteenth century. And among their hulking shapes what a poor show the actors of medicine and science made; what a feeble voice they raised amid the din of loading ships, of rattling armor, of cries and shouts and exhortations! Medicine: one critic, one observer, and one experimenter. That strange character Paracelsus, moving across the stage with his crew of vagabond students; Vesalius, the courtier, glancing over his shoulder as he dissected in hiding a stolen body; and Paré, the barber, performing amazing feats of surgery on the battlefields of France.

And science? Gentle old Dr. Gilbert, who wrote his volume on that toy new to the West, the magnetic compass, and who was appointed physician to Queen Elizabeth, although he never treated her; she preferred the magic of the royal astronomer to the science of Gilbert. And Galileo, who climbed the leaning tower of Pisa to drop weights and so establish a law of physics and outrage the scholars of his day—for everyone knew that gentlemen settled matters of science by authority and argument, not by experiment.

Those whom we call heroes of medicine and science were humble men, pushed to one side, obscured in the onrush of exploration, trade, politics, war, religion. And why not? What indications were there then that these once lowly fellows of medicine and science would in time become leaders in the pageant of history?

Contrast them—one critic, one observer, one experimenter in medicine in a whole century—with the great men that history records for those years. There was Columbus, who died in the early years of the century, died without knowing that he had discovered a new continent. After him there trooped to the lands that he had found a procession of swash-buckling Spanish adventurers who tramped over the country, exploring, betraying, killing for the sake of the stream of gold that they sent back to Spain. And Portuguese crews, rotten with scurvy, disembarked from their tiny ships on these new lands. Spain, so the Pope decreed, should rule all the lands of America west of the 50th parallel, and Portugal all the rest. A mighty event, this serving up of a continent as though it was a pie to be divided with one stroke of the knife. That alone dwarfed to insignificance a wandering doctor, a dissector, an army surgeon, a man who played with compasses, and one who dropped stones from a building badly out of plumb.

And trade? What a scramble there was for naval supremacy and sea trade! On the outcome hinged the destiny of nations. Sea power was the key to the greatness of England, and the rise of the British Empire. The only advantage that this commerce held for medicine, a scant one at best, was that the articles dealt in were chiefly drugs. Medicaments were the lightest, safest, most valuable cargo a ship could carry. Two ducats worth of cloves from the Moluccas brought eight hundred ducats in London. And there was cinnamon to be had from Ceylon; aloes and pepper from Cochin China; ginger and benzoin from Sumatra; nutmeg and mace from Banda; camphor, musk, and rhubarb from China. Spices we call them now, but they were medicines then; they were the native herbs of the East that Rhazes and Avicenna had added to the medicaments of Dioscorides. But with them were powdered "mummy," odd stone-like concretions from the intestines of goats, and the horns of narwhals, to be used in treating disease. This was the drug trade. In the ships of the explorers came coffee and tea and tobacco and potatoes. Coffee and tea were used to treat "acidity," tobacco was a medicament of which many a sixteenth and seventeenth century physician wrote in highest praise; the potato sold for fabulous sums to cure disease and weakness. Gold and silver and drugs were the cargoes of that time—and human beings. The days of plantations were opening in the New World. The first African negroes were brought to the West Indies in 1502.

As for religion—this was the century in which Luther preached a Reformation, a century made bloody with religious strife. Men were exiled, tortured, slaughtered, not for the sake of Christianity, as they had been in Charlemagne's time, but for the sake of freedom of belief within the Christian religion.

In politics Machiavelian intrigue and war joined their bloody hands. Off to the East Suleiman the Magnificent ruled from Bagdad to Hungary. He besieged Vienna. But more important to the European kings and queens and princes and nobles than this outside enemy were their own intrigues. In England the much married Henry VIII held the throne, then the feeble and tuberculous Edward, next Bloody Mary, and finally Elizabeth. In France reigned Francis I, one of the few great kings ever captured and ransomed; next Henry II, who died in a tournament from a lance wound in his eye; then the feeble sons of the intriguing Florentine, Catherine de' Medici. In Spain and Germany there was that strange character whom no one understands very well, the Holy Roman Emperor Charles V, who ruled over nearly half of Europe and fought against the other half, whose troops sacked Rome to obtain their pay, and who as an old man finally turned over his kingdoms and his wars to his son Philip II in order that he might have leisure to eat like an epicure and worship like a monk. It was Philip's Armada that was sunk in the English channel.

Exploration, trade, politics, war, religion held the center of the stage. True there were in the background medical matters that now and again obtruded into the affairs of even kings and princes. There were four great pandemics of influenza, one wide outbreak of the plague and a dozen or more minor ones. Typhus appeared in the camps of the armies and broke out in the law courts, where it spread from the prisoners to the judges and jury and spectators and killed without regard for rank and dignity. These terms of court were afterwards called the Black Assizes. Diphtheria spread through Spain and the Rhinelands. More and more each year smallpox was branding the people with its pitted marks. And although men did not recognize the fact, the pneumonia that we have today was then starting its great increase.

Where were the doctors to hold in check not only these terrifying diseases, but the other invisible enemies, the common diseases, the croups, the consumptions, and all the infections that crept unceasingly across the baby's crib, through the schoolroom, the home, the church, the ship at sea, the camp of war—and crept unhindered?

The physician of the sixteenth century, though trained in a university, knew no more what a disease really was than did the savage. Theories he learned in books; some helpful treatment, some valuable remedies, some beneficial surgery he found there, but mingled with them always the false theories of the past. These were his guides—the theories of the four humors, of the planets that controlled the functions of the body, of plethora that led to treatment by bleeding, the theory of colors, and the theory of numbers.

Dignified and scholarly physicians sat in consultation rooms strewn with strange relics which would have delighted a befeathered medicine man—stuffed alligators, narwhal horns, and bizarre animals from the New World. Through the heavy leather-bound spectacles of the day they peered at yellowed manuscripts and drew astrological charts, made their diagnoses and prescribed a medicine of a hundred ingredients without perhaps ever having seen their patient.

The educated surgeon, dressed in his long robe, disdained to touch the wounded man. With his cane he pointed to the place where the barber surgeon should cut.

Such doctors as these were not for the common people. For them there were quacks and tinkers, bathhouse keepers, strolling mountebanks, and old women. Failing these, there were the holy shrines where hope and prayer and faith brought ease of mind and suffering as they had in the temples of Æsculapius. But the shrines stopped no disease; dis-

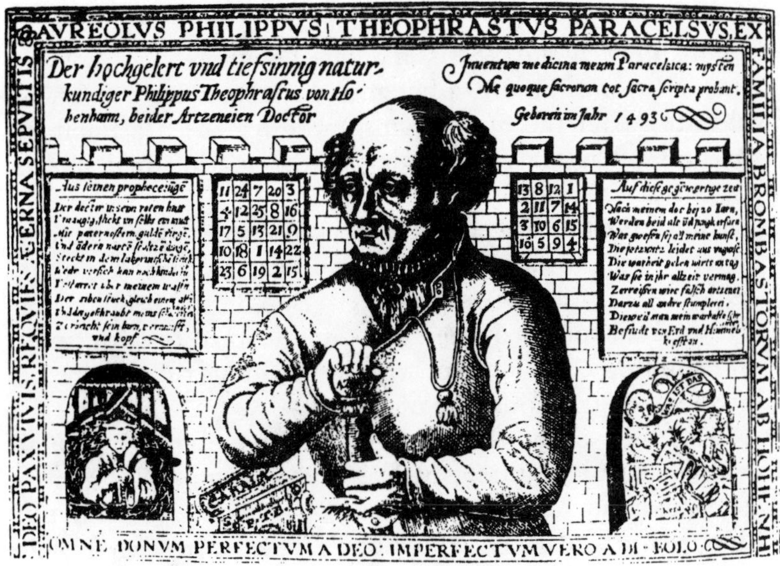

Paracelsus.

ease was most rampant when faith in shrines and holy relics was the greatest.

Neither physician nor surgeon nor quack knew the human structure; few had seen inside the body; none had studied it. None knew the simplest facts of physiology—how the blood circulates, why man breathes. None had heard of bacteria.

The physician of the sixteenth century lacked knowledge. But his greatest fault was his failure to seek knowledge.

Instead he was content with his cherished authorities, those newly translated volumes of Galen, written thirteen hundred years before. He had to break with the past before he could turn to the future, before he could advance. And to shake him from his reverence of the antiquated a critic was needed who would sow the seeds of dissatisfaction.

The man destined to this rôle, the idol breaker, was Paracelsus.

He was born in the rough mountains of Switzerland, of a German father and a Swiss mother. The father was a physician, a lover of nature, a botanist. He named his boy Theophrastus after the first botanist, who had been a pupil of Aristotle. The revived learning of the ancients had spread from Italy across the Alps.

When the boy Theophrastus was ten years old, the family moved to the town of Villach in Austria. This was a mining region where there were iron smelters. Young Theophrastus watched the miners at their work and learned the principles of metallurgy and of chemistry, just as in his Swiss home he had learned the principles of botany.

And then about the time that the popular Prince Hal was mounting the throne of England as Henry VIII, Theophrastus went to college to become a scholar. He made the slow journey to Italy, where at Ferrara the teacher Leoniceno had recently translated from the Greek some of the writings of Hippocrates.

Theophrastus was educated after the manner of all medical students of those days. He did not, as the modern student does, spend long hours in the dissecting room, in the laboratory, and at bedsides in the hospital. Instead, he studied from books of the ancients, of Hippocrates and Galen and Avicenna, and spoke, read, and wrote Latin. He read the classical orators, poets, and grammarians; the geographers, historians, and philosophers. He had a classical education, tinctured, but only tinctured, with medicine. When he had completed his training, he was well equipped to translate further works of the ancients and to dispute over their theories and their philosophies, but he was sadly equipped indeed to help his suffering fellow men as a physician or to contend hand to hand with the enemy disease.

However, in his short life Paracelsus was not destined to lead the sheltered and unreal existence of the scholar of medicine. Why was this so? We shall never know, but men have speculated as to the reason he became a critic; and it is a harmless speculation. Most investigators have concluded that his early training in Switzerland and his observations in the mines of Austria had made him too free and independent to be content with classrooms where there flitted only the ghosts of great men and of great observations. He wanted realities. These things are true no doubt, but there is more. The destinies of men are not shaped wholly by what men see and hear, but also by what is in them at birth.

Theophrastus was made of rebellious fiber. He was born to stand alone and lead, not follow. In war perhaps he would have been a doughty, impetuous, violent, and unruly hero. But he chose medicine. There was no battle to be waged there; all was submission to authority.

The schoolroom held him for a few years and then he was free. There was much to see in the world that the ancients had never dreamed of. He would see it. He threw away his scholarly costume and traveled far and wide as a simple wayfarer. Here then was a rarity, a trained scholar associating with common people, listening to them. Barber surgeons, bathhouse keepers, wise old women who treated the peasants, confided to him their funds of practical knowledge. These were things that the professors in the schoolrooms, getting their noses dusty in ancient tomes, had never heard. A mass of superstition, but mingled with it here and there sound knowledge made from observations by keen eyes unblinded by long reading of the old manuscripts.

Paracelsus had seen the miners break away the useless rocks from the rich ore. Like them he separated the useless from the valuable. He listened, he observed, he thought; and there grew on him the conviction that there was much error and much nonsense in the theories of the ancients. Hippocrates alone had been a true observer. The others had made theories. The students in the classrooms were being crammed with traditions which, for all the polished language they were written in, were as false as the superstitions of the garrulous peasants.

As Paracelsus' ideas changed during his travels, so did his manners and his speech. He found the rough native tongue better suited to his palate than the Latin of his school days, and the vulgar company of the tavern more to his liking than that of gentlemen. He was coarsened, roughened. He no longer disputed; now he fought to prove to the dandified scholars that the traditions of their medicine were false. He wrote not in Latin but in German, so that all his countrymen might learn what disease really was and how actual experience taught that it should be treated.

What he wrote seems to us now nearly as remote from the truth as were the theories of the ancients. Paracelsus for all his critical attitude was a product of the early sixteenth century. He believed in astrology and spirits (in fact he said he always carried one about in the hilt of his sword) and salamanders that walked through fire unscathed. He believed that nature had put on every plant the signature of the disease it would cure. He believed in weapon ointment, and here, perhaps, more clearly than anywhere else, we see his peculiar mixture of practical common sense, observation, and mystical nonsense. It was commonly believed that to cure a wound the healing ointment should be put not on the wound itself but on the blade of the weapon that caused the wound. The wound was left undisturbed or merely wrapped with linen. Paracelsus had observed that wounds actually healed better when treated this way—and he had observed correctly. But his ideas led him to find an explanation in a mysterious supernatural force which radiated from the weapon to the wound. His theory was wrong; his observation right. The ointments intended for wounds were made up of filthy ingredients, often bits of decayed animals and even dung. A wound healed better when the ointment was applied anywhere else than upon the wound.

The experience that Paracelsus had had in the mines of Villach led him to use mineral substances for medicines. Revolting against the herbs that Galen had employed, he prescribed iron, sulphur, mercury, and mineral waters. It did not disturb him in the least that the ancients gave no authority for this kind of treatment. He believed in many things, but he did not believe in authority.

Out of his writings on the use of simple mineral remedies there grew in the next century a great conflict in medical practice—the conflict between the doctors who believed in Galenical herbs and those who followed the lead of Paracelsus. The herbs were largely useless; they were also harmless. The mineral substances were often beneficial; but they might also be poisons and grave harm might, and often did, follow their excessive use.

It is not, however, the fact that Paracelsus introduced new methods of medical treatment that makes him a hero of medicine. His greatest contribution lies in his criticism of authority, his breaking with the past. Even his new remedies helped do that.

In his wanderings he had seen much, thought much, written much. It was time now to get his books published. With written words for his cudgel, he would beat the authorities into submission; bully them out of existence—all except Hippocrates. Hippocrates was a man after his own heart. The slavish nincompoops (Paracelsus would have used some such word, probably a less polite one) of medicine, those scholarly doctors who believed that truth was to be found only in the traditional doctrines, should see how a man of brains, a man who trusted his own senses and his own reason went about settling the problems of medicine.

Getting books published was no easy matter. But Paracelsus was lucky in this respect—for a little while. You will remember Galen's good fortune when he came to Rome and was called to treat Eudemus. Paracelsus stopped his wanderings and settled in Strasbourg, but his fame as a doctor who succeeded where others failed reached to the town of Basel. In Basel there was a wealthy printer by the name of Frobenius, who had for a long time suffered with a pain in his foot. His physician recommended that his leg be cut off.

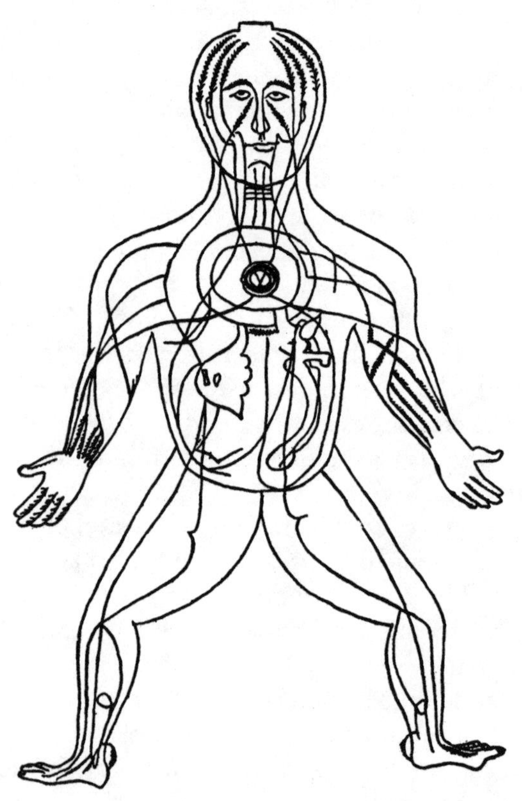

The nervous system as shown in a medieval manuscript.

Operations in those days, of course, were done without anæsthetics, without antiseptics, and without adequate means for controlling the hemorrhage. Frobenius decided that before he submitted to the operation he would consult the doctor of Strasbourg who boasted so boldly of his successes.

Paracelsus went to Basel. He treated the leg; to the joy of Frobenius the pain went away. This fellow Paracelsus for all his rough exterior was no mere braggart.

With an influential patron now, Paracelsus could not only get his books published, but, as seemed fitting for a man of his attainments, he could have the position of city physician and teach in the University as well.

Here at last was Paracelsus back in scholarship. Scholarship had not changed, but Paracelsus had. He would show these dry-as-dust delvers into books how medicine should be taught. He would tell them what he thought of them even before he started to teach. So he published a pamphlet not in scholarly Latin but in German, in order that all literate men might understand the great reform that he was going to bring about.

"Who is there who does not know," he wrote, "that doctors of today make frightful mistakes and greatly harm their patients? Who does not know that this is due to the fact that they cling firmly to the teachings of Galen, Avicenna, and such men?" I, Paracelsus, on the contrary "elucidate with industry and to the great advantage of all who will hear me, from books on the practice and the theory of medicine written by myself. I do not, like other medical authors, make these books up out of extracts from Hippocrates and Galen, but in never ending toil I create them anew upon the basis of experience, the supreme teacher of all things. If I want to prove anything, I do not try to do so by quoting authorities, but by observation and trial and reasoning. . . ."

This pamphlet was a bomb exploding in the scholarly precincts of the sedate University. There was no precedent in the ancient authorities prescribing how to deal with such behavior, but for once the professors needed no authority. They would throw out this bullying quack. He could not stay at their University.

But Paracelsus did stay—for a time at least. And what is more—a then unheard-of thing—he gave his lectures not in Latin but in German, the native tongue, the vernacular, as would be done today.

It is said that to impress his students with his contempt for authority he publicly burned the books of Galen and Avicenna.

In his lectures he told the students the practical and useful observations he had made; but he told them also his vague and mystical theories of disease. And, becoming excited, he challenged the authorities of antiquity and bullied his students. He, Paracelsus, alone of all men, knew medicine and the way to truth in medicine. The truth was not to be found in the teachings of the learned doctors of the universities. "All the universities," he declared, "have less experience than my beard; the down on my neck is more learned than my auditors." And on another occasion, he said, "You must follow in my footsteps; I shall not go in yours. Not one of you [the professors] will find a corner so well hidden but that the dogs will come and lift their legs to defile you. I shall become monarch; mine will be the monarchy over which I shall rule to make you gird up your loins. . . . You will eat dirt."

Vulgar, crude, egotistical—but mingled with his raillery there was profound wisdom.

During his short stay in the University his students failed to appreciate the real meaning and significance of his words. They laughed at him, ridiculed him, and finally lampooned him in a scurrilous poem posted on the door of the lecture room.

Paracelsus, the exponent of freedom, amazing as it may seem, turned to the city council for protection against his own students. But his bad manners counted against him. He treated the judges of the courts as contemptuously as he had the professors of the University. He was the great Paracelsus; they mere foolish, useless men of no consequence. He actually and sincerely believed this; it was his way of thinking.

In disgust at the treatment he received, Paracelsus left the University. If men would not listen to his words in lectures, they would read his words in books. He would write and demonstrate that the authorities themselves were men no greater than other men—certainly not as great as Paracelsus.

At the age of forty-eight he died. His enemies, and they were many, have said that he was killed in a drunken brawl, that he was deformed and physically abnormal; all that we really know is that he died, and we can be very sure that he died sadly misunderstood.

Who cared that in 1541 a vulgar man who boasted to his students and railed at his betters passed away? This was the century of great things—of exploration and trade, of kings, and princes, of wars and conquests; who cared that the first of the modern doctors died?—for Paracelsus was the first modern doctor. His ways were as different from those of the doctor of today as his times were from ours. But underneath his rough exterior he had the spirit of the modern doctor, the spirit of truth, progress, observation, independence, and self-reliance.

CHAPTER XVII

Vesalius, the Observer

IN 1514, when Paracelsus was twenty-one, a son was born to the Imperial Court apothecary of His Majesty the Emperor Charles V. The baby was christened Andreas. The father's family, though living now in Brussels, had come originally from Wesel and had taken as their name a Latinized form of this town—Vesalius. The boy, Andreas Vesalius, was destined to become the first critical observer in modern medicine, the father of anatomy.

How often the things we do in our youth affect our after life! Or is it that we do them because of something peculiar within ourselves, something in us that remains there all through our lives and shapes our actions in maturity as well as in youth? In the boy, can we see the man that is to come? I think so.

Young Vesalius, like most keen boys, had a hobby. It was a queer one, so it seemed in those days, but one that since then has fascinated many a budding young doctor. His hobby was dissection. Mice, and frogs, and even cats and dogs were his playthings; and he investigated them with that same irresistible desire to see what was inside that makes a modern boy take apart the mechanical toy and alarm clock. One can almost hear the voice of Andreas' nurse or tutor raised in protest—such nasty dirty things for a young gentleman to soil himself with—and always to be grubbing into the insides of rats and mice, and carrying them in his leather pouch!

Boys were not different then from now, nor were parents and nurses. And hobbies? Fortunately they existed then and still do—one of the most priceless things in any boy's life. Pity the poor mortal who has not some engrossing, soul-consuming interest!

Bloodthirsty, depraved, this hobby of dissection? Certainly not. What Vesalius saw in dissection was not blood and gore, but nature itself; his mind seethed with curiosity. The mangled rat, the half-skinned mouse to such a boy is a thing of beauty far beyond the flowers of the field. And it was in pursuit of his beloved study of anatomy that Vesalius went to Paris to the great school of medicine and to the greatest disappointment of his life.

In Paris in the year 1533 anatomy was taught, not by careful dissection, but instead as it had been in the Middle Ages by that old doctor of Bologna, Mondino de' Luzzi, who called himself Mundinus.

Before the opening of the Christian Era, the study of human anatomy died in Alexandria with Herophilus. Galen wrote a book of anatomy, an elaborate one, but he had not dissected the human body; there were religious reasons to prevent. Instead he used pigs and oxen and monkeys. But, being Galen and very sure that all God's creatures were created much alike, he did not admit that he had never dissected man himself. So when the Arabs translated his works, they stated positively that the things he described were all in man and had the shape and form he said they had. Galen described all the anatomy that any man need ever know—so thought the doctors of the past. But Mundinus held that a dissection, a demonstration now and then would make the facts stick better in the student's mind. And so early in the fourteenth century there began the first human dissections since Alexandrian days. The bodies used were those of condemned criminals, and at most only one or two were available to a medical school in a whole year.

The way in which the dissections were made was this: the professor of anatomy sat on a raised platform. Seated before him were the pupils. At his feet was the body and beside it a barber surgeon. The professor read aloud from Galen, and as he named a part of the body the barber surgeon pointed to it. In the days of Mundinus the affair—it would be absurd to call it a dissection—took up only four class periods. Today a medical student may spend on dissection four hours a day for a whole school year.

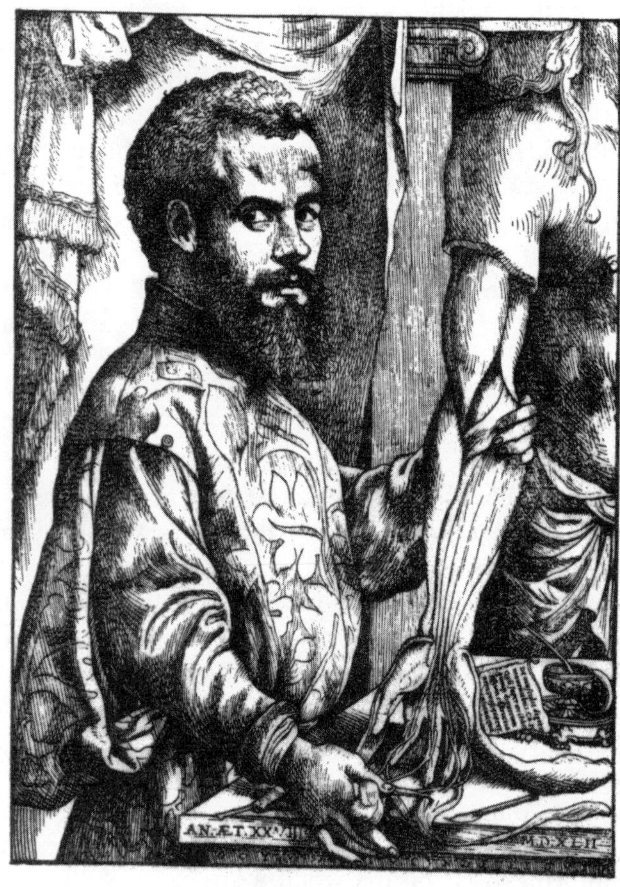

Andreas Vesalius.

The way that Mundinus had taught anatomy, more than a century before, was the way it was being taught when Vesalius came to Paris. In his disappointment he called the dissection he saw "an execrable rite." A careless barber surgeon mangled a body and an indifferent professor mumbled lines from Galen. It wasn't a dissection; it was a farce.

Vesalius was forced to study medicine as the other young men at the school did, but he wanted to study it differently. He wanted to do what no one in medicine had yet done. He wanted to specialize, give most of his time to one subject, anatomy, study it thoroughly, and become an expert. He made a vow that he would devote all his powers to the revival of anatomy and strive to reach a perfection of dissection, description, and understanding of the human body equal to that of the ancients.

From that very statement you see that Vesalius believed firmly that Galen's dissections and his descriptions were of human anatomy. This is a point to bear in mind, for his discovery later that Galen had not dissected human beings was the great turning point in his life.

As a young man in Paris Vesalius and a group of fellow students fired by his enthusiasm for anatomy searched through graveyards for bones—in those days coffins were of wood which rotted and the cemetery land was used century after century, so that sometimes a skull or a leg bone or an arm bone found its way to the surface; you will remember Hamlet and the skull over which he soliloquized. So thoroughly did Vesalius study the chance bones he found that he could identify each one by the mere sense of touch when he was blindfolded. But he had no such opportunity for studying the organs of the body or the muscles and nerves and blood vessels.

Twice he sat on the student benches and watched a barber surgeon hurriedly point to the main organs of the body while the professor recited snatches of Galen. On the third occasion—thanks to his zeal for anatomy—he was allowed to take the barber surgeon's place. But this was not dissection; this was merely a peep at those fascinating structures which he longed to study as he had studied the bones.

In 1536 war between France and Spain and Germany put

an end to Vesalius' schooling in Paris. His father, you will remember, was attached to the court of Emperor Charles V. Andreas went to Louvain to continue his studies. It was there that the most picturesque event of his life occurred.

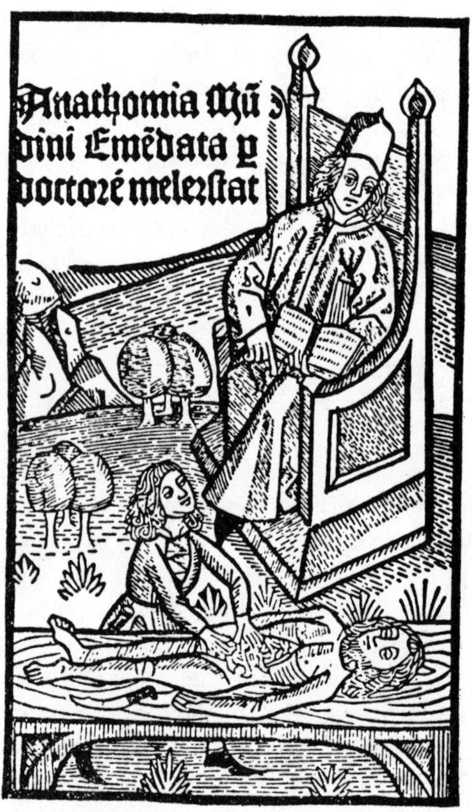

Title-page of the Anatomy *of Mundinus.*

In the dead of night he stole a skeleton from the gallows outside the city walls, the skeleton of a convict hanged in chains and left hanging, according to the custom, as a warning to all malefactors. If he had been caught in the act, he would no doubt have shared the same fate.

He spent a year in Louvain, and then went on to Venice. There he met a fellow countryman named Jan Calcar, a pupil of Titian, who could paint so adroitly that his work could hardly be told from that of his master. The two young men went on together to Padua. There at the University Vesalius completed his medical studies and received his doctor's degree. The day after he graduated he was made professor of surgery and anatomy. He was twenty-three years old.

In the following year, 1538, to aid his students, Vesalius published his first book of anatomy. It consisted of six large plates showing the skeleton, the blood vessels, and the organs of the body. His friend Calcar drew the pictures.

Now here is the peculiar thing about these pictures. The anatomy shown was exactly as Galen had described it. The breast bone of the skeleton had seven segments; the spleen was oblong in shape; the liver had five lobes. Vesalius had not seen the structures in this form in the human bodies he had examined, but who was he to compare his brief experience with the master, the great authority, Galen? Vesalius could be wrong—Galen never.

But as he conducted his dissections day after day in Padua, sometimes secretly on a body which he obtained we know not where, his wonder mounted, his perplexity grew. In all the bodies that he dissected the structures seemed the same, but they were not as Galen had described them.

And then one day in the year 1541 he found the answer to his dilemma. He was dissecting a monkey. On one of the vertebræ of its spine he noticed a small projection of the bone. That projection he had not been able to find in the vertebræ of human beings. Yet Galen had described it. Galen then had not dissected human beings, but only beasts. In all the centuries in between men had believed that it was human anatomy that Galen was describing. Instead of trusting their eyes they had been blinded by Galen's great authority.

It was preposterous! Here he had hoped to revive anatomy and make it as great as it was in Galen's day. And all the time he had known more anatomy, more human anatomy, than had Galen himself!

The enthusiasm that kept him at his work now had a new purpose. That purpose was to describe for the first time true human anatomy. His zeal redoubled. With Calcar at his side to draw and make the printing blocks of carved wood, he dissected, wrote, described. A year and a half of feverish activity and the great anatomy was ready for the press. Where should he publish it? Venice? No, at Basel, the very center of the printers' trade. Over the Alps went mules laden with the blocks for the pictures. Vesalius rode with them. He supervised each step of the printing. At last in June, 1543, there appeared complete the great book—*De Fabrica Humani Corporis.* It had 663 pages and more than 300 woodcuts.

Vesalius was twenty-eight years old. His work was done. In his twenty-one remaining years he did no more in anatomy. Henceforth there was to be no peace for him. He had dared to turn against the idol Galen. The scholarly physicians, the teachers of anatomy railed at him. If the anatomy of man was different from that described by Galen, then the anatomy of man had changed since Galen had described it! Strange, isn't it, how men will try to deny the facts? But that was not the worst. He was ostracized, his pupils left him, his fellows snubbed him, the authorities put difficulties in his way to embarrass him.

Vesalius in indignation burned his manuscripts. He left Padua, gave up anatomy, and became court physician to the Emperor Charles V. It would have been better had he borne the attacks against him and marked time until everything became quiet again. While Vesalius was buried at the court of Charles, men began timidly to look around to see if by chance he was right. They found that he was. Then forgetting Vesalius, so it seemed, they went on from where he had stopped. Soon Vesalius was only a name. A court physician in retirement, he was dead to medicine.

Perhaps his unmerited oblivion rankled in his mind and

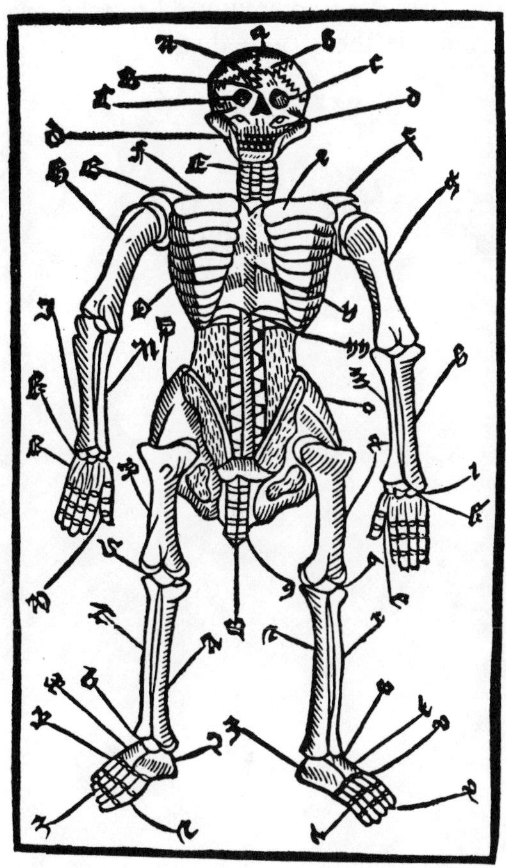

The skeleton according to Galen's description.

he longed to escape from the court, go back again and mingle with the men who were carrying on the work he loved. At any rate in 1563 he left the court and made his way to Venice. From this city twenty-six years before he had set out with Calcar, carefree, happy, on his way to Padua and fame. This time, we do not know why, he took a ship to Palestine.

In 1564 he made the return journey, hastened, some say, because he had received an invitation to take over his post at Padua again. On the way he died.

CHAPTER XVIII

Paré, the Experimenter

IN 1559 King Henry II of the Valois family had been on the throne of France twelve years; he was just forty years old. An interruption had come in the wars with Spain and Germany; one of the many treaties of peace had been agreed upon. And now to seal the peace the King's daughter Elizabeth was to marry the King of Spain and his sister the Duke of Savoy. June of that year, 1559, was a month of festivals, of balls, hunts, and jousts at the court. The King, to show his good fellowship to his officers and his athletic prowess to the ladies of the gallery, entered the lists. He called upon Gabriel, Comte de Montgomery, Seigneur de Lorges, Lieutenant in the Scottish Guard, to break a lance with him. Reluctantly allowing his armor to be put on, Montgomery mounted his horse. There was little for him to gain; if he lost, he would be ridiculed; if he won—well, royal favor and royal prejudice were fickle things, and many a brave if indiscreet man had lost his hold at court by winning from the King. But fate had more in store here than reputation and favors; two lives were at stake.

The joust was run. Montgomery's lance struck the King's helmet and broke and splintered. A fragment passed through the vizor, penetrated the King's eye, and passed on into his brain. The King fell to the ground and was borne away unconscious to his bedroom. He died. Montgomery fled to escape the vengeance of the Queen, Catherine de' Medici. Some years later he was captured, tortured, and executed.

Alexander Dumas, author of *The Three Musketeers*, describes this incident in his romantic tales of France. And he tells of the medical treatment that the King received. Ambroise Paré, the royal surgeon was summoned. He examined the wound. He knew too little of the anatomy of the head to dare attempt an operation in search of the splinter. So he sent for Andreas Vesalius. Loaned by the Spanish Court, the great anatomist rode night and day to reach Paris. After

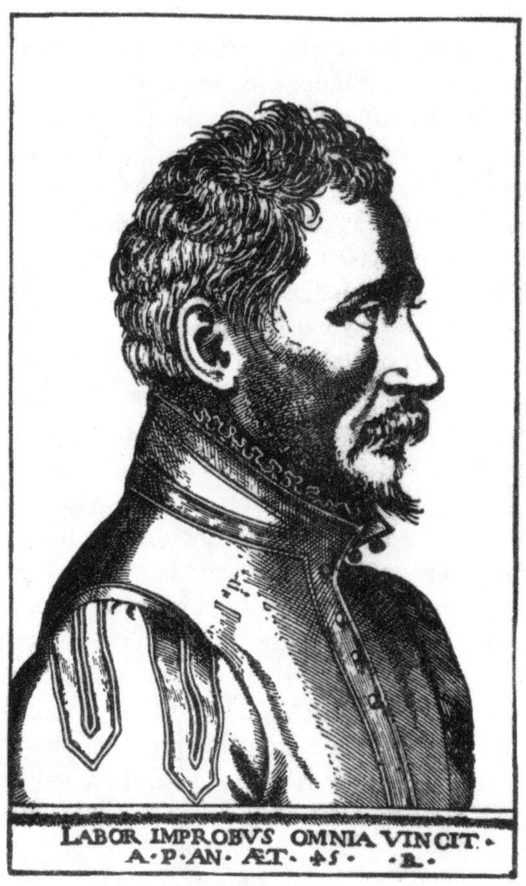

Ambroise Paré.

greeting Paré, he examined the King, and then ordered the heads of two executed criminals brought to him at once. There in the sick room he and Paré carried out their dissections to obtain the precise knowledge of anatomy necessary for the operation. But their efforts were in vain. The King died of an infection of the brain.

The tale of the meeting of Vesalius and Paré may be merely the invention of a romancer, but it has nevertheless a figurative significance. Paré's acquaintance with the anatomical knowledge of Vesalius resulted in a great advance in surgery. Paré applied to surgery the anatomy that Vesalius had described. He found surgery a degraded calling; he left it, if not a great profession, at least a dignified and competent branch of medicine. He was the first to start breaking down the attitude developed by the Arabs that the surgeon was a menial, far inferior to the physician.

Paré was quite a different kind of man from either of the other two medical heroes of the Renaissance with whom we have dealt. Paracelsus and Vesalius were well educated. The one had revolted against tradition and fought with all the violence of his personality against the theories of Galen; the other had painstakingly shown that Galen's facts were false. Ambroise Paré was not an educated man; he was a humble barber surgeon. The force that drove him on was not revolt, nor yet zeal for observation; it was love, the love arising from a deep compassion for those who suffer.

Paré was born about 1510. As a boy he was apprenticed to a barber. He was taught to clip hair and shave, and he learned the other duties of a barber of those days; to bleed, to pull teeth, to dress wounds. Surgery appealed to him, and so he went to Paris to work at the great hospital there, the Hôtel Dieu.

Being familiar with a modern hospital, you may have in mind an immaculately clean operating room, with tiled walls, an array of complicated, shiny instruments, and hallways where nurses move quickly and quietly in and out of rooms with neat white beds. But there were no such hospitals until late in the nineteenth century. The hospital that Paré went to, like all those of the time, was still a place of refuge. It was a great stone building, badly lighted by narrow, dusty windows opening into long rooms with rows of canopied beds. Sometimes two or three or even four or five patients were put in a bed, with no regard to the diseases they might have. In the halls on piles of straw lay others—men, women, and children, too. And for nurses there were only the Sisters of Charity, untrained for such work, who

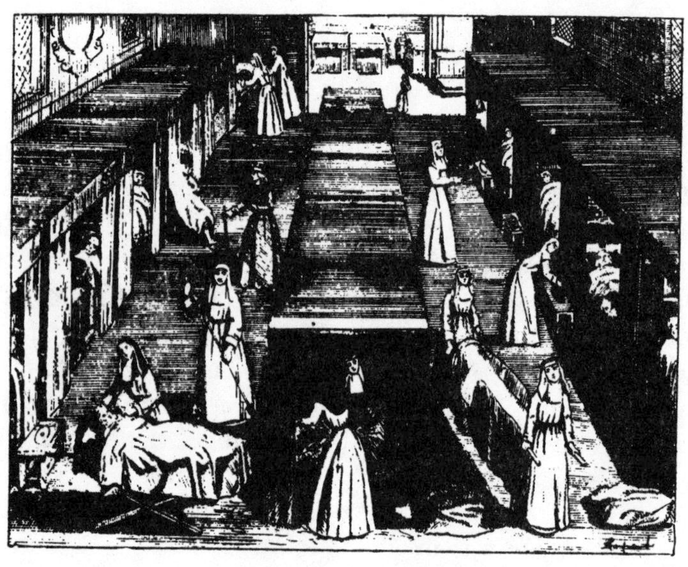

Scene in the Hôtel Dieu.

gave their services as a religious duty. The place was indescribably dirty; it was overrun with vermin; a vile smell of filth and disease and rotting flesh pervaded the building. The only operating room was a corner, a cubicle, or perhaps a dimly lighted vestibule.

In such a place Paré studied; there he learned to bandage wounds, put splints on broken limbs, and now and again to cut off a leg or an arm from some screaming fellow held down by strong men. Slim chance indeed did such patients have for recovery. Infection usually killed them in spite of all his efforts.

In 1536 the war that drove Vesalius from Paris called Paré into the army. The forces of the French crossed the Alps and laid siege to Turin. Paré accompanied Marshal Montejan as regimental surgeon.

It was a new life for the young surgeon. He was, as he said, a greenhorn not yet hardened to the cruelties of war; this is the tale he tells of his first experience:

"We thronged at the city and passed over the dead bodies and some that were not yet dead, hearing them cry under the feet of our horses, which made a great pity in my heart, and truly I repented that I had gone forth from Paris to see so pitiful a spectacle. Being in the city, I entered a stable, thinking to lodge my horse, where I found four dead soldiers and two others who were not yet dead propped against the wall, their faces wholly disfigured, and they neither saw, nor heard, nor spoke, and their clothes yet flamed with the gunpowder which had burnt them. Beholding them with pity, there came an old soldier who asked me if there was any means of curing them. I told him no. At once he approached them and cut their throats gently and without anger. Seeing the great cruelty, I said to him that he was an evil man. He answered me that he prayed God that when he should be in such a case, he might find some one who would do the same for him, to the end that he might not languish miserably."

During this campaign Paré made the first of his great innovations in surgery; it concerned the treatment of gunshot wounds, which were a new feature of warfare. The muzzle-loading arquebus, shooting a ball as large as a walnut, inflicted horrible wounds. The sword, the lance, and the battle-ax made clean open wounds, usually only slightly infected. But the gunshot wound was deep and narrow, and bits of clothes and filth were carried into it. Such wounds became badly infected.

The leading scholarly writer on the surgery of the century was Giovanni di Vigo, who was physician to Pope Julius II. He had stated that gunshot wounds were poisoned with gunpowder. It was an ancient doctrine of Arabian surgery that "diseases not curable by iron were curable by fire." That is, if the surgeon could not give relief with his knife, he should use cautery. Since gunshot wounds, then, were thought to be poisoned burns (it was a century later that men discovered that bullets were not hot enough to burn the

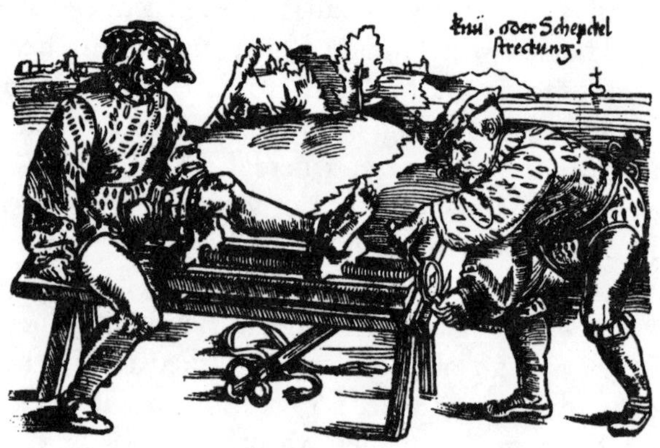

Setting a broken leg on the battlefield.

flesh), they were to be treated at the first dressing by pouring into them oil boiling hot. Good logic, but from a false premise!

Here is Paré's first experience in treating wounds by the method then in vogue: "Now all the soldiers at the Chateau, seeing our men coming with great fury, did all they could to defend themselves and killed and wounded a great number of our soldiers with pikes, arquebuses, and stones, whereupon the surgeons had much work cut out for them. Now I was at that time an untried soldier; I had not yet seen wounds made by gunshot at the first dressing. It is true that I had read in Jean di Vigo that wounds made by firearms were poisoned wounds, because of the powder, and for their cure he commands to cauterize them with oil of elder, scalding hot, in which should be mixed a little theriac; and in order not to err before using the oil, knowing that such a thing would bring great pain to the patient, I wished to know first, how the other surgeons did for the first dressing, which was to pour oil as hot as possible into the wounds, of whom I took courage to do as they did. At last my oil lacked and I was constrained to apply in its place a digestive made of the yolks of eggs, oil of roses, and turpentine. That night I could not sleep at my ease, fearing that by lack of cauterization I should find the wounded upon whom I had failed to put the oil dead or poisoned, which made me rise early to visit them, where beyond my hope I found those upon whom I had not put the oil feeling little pain, their wounds without inflammation or swelling, having rested fairly well throughout the night; the others, to whom I had applied the boiling oil, I found feverish, with great pain and swelling about their wounds. Then I resolved with myself never more to burn thus cruelly poor men wounded with gunshot."

Ambroise Paré was, you see, a rare surgeon for his day. He could do what so few men then could do; he could trust and follow his own intelligence and reasoning regardless of authority. He cared not what the noble Giovanni di Vigo, the Pope's physician, said. Paré saw with his own eyes—he never more would "burn thus cruelly poor men wounded with gunshot."

It was this same keenness and compassion that led Paré on to develop many other valuable methods for surgery. It was he who introduced, or rather reintroduced, for it had been used centuries before by the Romans, the ligature for stopping hemorrhage. In his day surgeons staunched the flow of blood with red-hot irons which seared the flesh and made a painful wound slow to heal. Paré used pieces of twine, ligatures, to tie shut the ends of the bleeding vessels. The surgeon of today uses the method he introduced.

A multitude of ingenious operations, artificial eyes, greatly improved artificial arms and legs, massage, and implanted teeth, are some of the things Paré gave to surgery. But the most important contribution he made was to anatomy. It

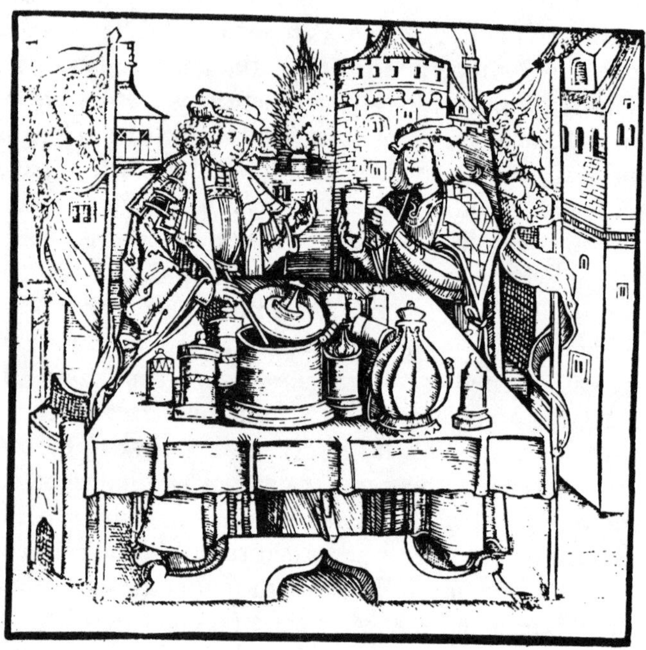

Making theriac.

was he who popularized for surgeons the anatomy that Vesalius had described.

It is unthinkable now for a surgeon to attempt an operation without knowing in exact detail the structure of the body. But in the days before Paré, the surgeon learned as craftsman a few simple operations; the trick of doing them was handed on from surgeon to surgeon by apprenticeship. The operations could not be varied to suit the needs of the patient; nor could new operations be developed. But with knowledge of anatomy a whole new field was opened to the surgeon; his operations no longer needed to be merely the tricks of a trade; with a knowledge of what lay beneath his knife he could now plan operations intelligently and vary them to suit the occasion.

Paré, as we have said, made surgery a skilled craft. It remained as he left it for two hundred years, and we shall therefore have little to say of it until we come to the medical heroes of the eighteenth and nineteenth centuries—to the Scotchman, John Hunter, who made a science of surgery, and the Englishman, Joseph Lister, who introduced antiseptics to prevent infection, and the Americans, Long and Wells and Morton who gave us the blessing of anesthesia to abolish the pain of operation.

Before we tell more of Paré and his work, there are two terms that we have used that deserve explanation. One is theriac. You will remember that when Paré wrote of Di Vigo's treatment for gunshot wounds he said, "cauterize them with oil of elder, scalding hot, in which should be mixed a little theriac." This word theriac takes us back some sixteen centuries before the days of Paré. We mentioned Mithridates, King of Pontus, and his private herb doctor Crateuas. Mithridates was a dabbler in medicine; he wished to make himself immune to all poisons (a very useful state for a king of those days) by taking small but gradually increasing doses of the poisons. He was reputed to have discovered a universal antidote—a theriac. The theriac that Paré mentions was supposed to be made after the original formula; it contained vipers' flesh and some sixty-three other ingredients, none of which had any beneficial medicinal effect. Theriac was a most popular remedy until well into the eighteenth century.

The other term concerns an operation which we said Paré introduced: the implantation of teeth. The only dentists in Paré's time—if we exclude the bathhouse keepers, peddlers, and old women—were the barber surgeons. Dentistry at their hands was merely the pulling of aching teeth. The extraction was performed with formidable instruments called pelicans and keys, which seized on the suffering tooth, and often one or two sound ones as well, as a pipe wrench seizes on a pipe. It was a brutal form of dentistry, but there was no other. In order to cover up the gap made by missirg teeth,

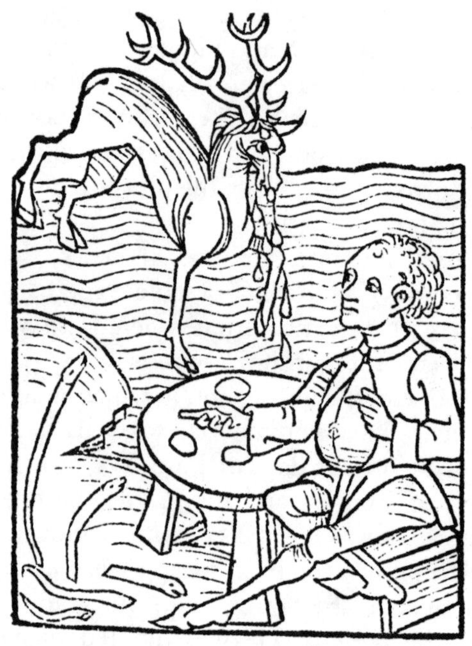

The legend of the bezoar stone.

artificial teeth carved from bone or ivory were sometimes wired in place. Paré's method of implantation was to pull the aching tooth and then insert into the wound in the jaw a sound tooth extracted from the mouth of some poor chap willing to sell a tooth. The tooth thus stuck in grew firmly to the bone and often lasted several years. Of course no one in those days dreamed of infection of the teeth or its consequences, nor were such things known until late in the nineteenth century. It was only then that modern dentistry began.

We have said that Paré raised surgery from a trade followed by menials to a skilled craft carried out by trained men. After his time instruction in surgery became more and more a part of medical education. The distinction between the surgeons of the long robe and those of the short robe was gradually broken down. Surgery became respectable.

It is hard to turn from Paré to the other medical heroes who await us in the centuries ahead. If you ever read the tales Paré wrote, you will know why. In reading them you see the man; you know and love him. To part with him is to leave a friend.

Paré was a man at home equally in the strife of the battlefield, the turmoil of the camp, and in the intrigue of a polished court. He lived beloved by the common soldiers, respected by kings. His unvarying purpose in life was the one that has moved all truly great doctors: the desire to help, to heal, to relieve the suffering of their fellow men. It was love—not maudlin sentiment, or the compassion of those who shrink from the sight of suffering—but the aggressive warfare of men who for love of their fellows devote their lives to the fight against the enemy disease.

Paré was a fighter of tough fiber, and yet he was not ashamed to show gentleness and humility. Nowhere is his gentle character more clearly seen than in the words with which he closed his descriptions of the cases he treated. They were: "I dressed his wounds; God healed him."

There remains yet one more thing to be said of Paré. He was one of the first men in modern medicine to perform experiments. Moreover, he used what is now called the method of the control experiment. Here is an instance.

In one of his army experiences he was called to treat a man who had been badly burned. He went to the supply tent to get a healing ointment but on the way he met an old woman among the camp followers of the army. She told him that the best way to treat a burn (remember this is the sixteenth century and not today) was to put on the wound chopped-up onion. Paré never ignored suggestions. He tried the onion. The man's face healed well. The treatment seemed of benefit. A lesser man than Paré, one who did not possess that blessed thing called skepticism, would have

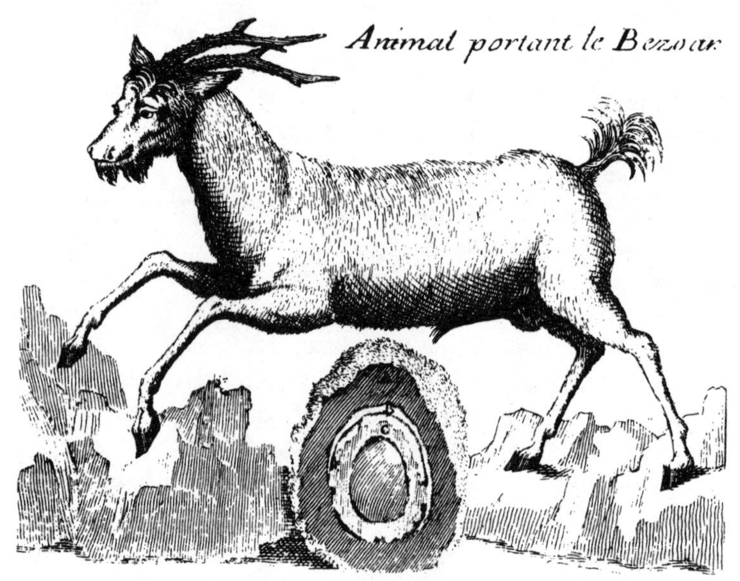

A bezoar stone and the animal from which it really came.

said, "the onion healed the burn." Because of that kind of uncritical reasoning, medicine since primitive times has been encumbered with its multitude of useless remedies and treatments. But Paré asked a question, the question that made him a scientist. It was: "Might not the burn have healed as quickly as it did even if the onion had not been put upon it? Did the onion help the healing or did the burn heal in spite of the onion?"

To answer that question he tried an experiment. Soon a

soldier came to him with his face burned on both sides. To one cheek Paré applied his chopped-up onion; but on the other he put nothing. The untreated cheek was his control, his standard of comparison. He found that the side treated with onion healed more quickly than the side untreated. Thus by sound experimental evidence he proved that the treatment was of benefit.

And here is another of Paré's experiments that gives an idea of the kind of remedies then in use. There were four medicaments in which the physicians of those times had great confidence. Theriac, of course, was one; then there were powdered "mummy" from Egypt to heal wounds, unicorns' horns to detect poison in wines, and bezoar stones as antidotes against poison. Paré wrote a scathing condemnation of "mummy"; as chief surgeon and counselor to the King he told His Majesty that the unicorn's horn which was dipped in the royal wine by the poison tester was useless; and he proved that the bezoar stone was not an antidote against poison. It is with the incident of the bezoar stone that we are concerned here. A bezoar was, so legend said, a crystallized tear from the eye of a deer bitten by a snake; it was in reality a concretion, a sort of gallstone, found in the stomachs and intestines of goats and similar animals. It had, of course, no medicinal value. But it was firmly believed that if one was poisoned, all he need do was swallow the stone and the poison would have no effect. A great many people who thought they were poisoned had swallowed stones and had recovered. But Paré raised the question: "Were they really poisoned, or did they merely think they were?"

King Charles IX, who, by the way, had been marked by smallpox so badly that his nose was split in two, possessed a valuable bezoar stone, one that he prized highly. Paré suggested an experiment that would prove or disprove its value as an antidote—try the stone on a condemned criminal given poison. The King sent for his provost and asked if there was such a criminal in the prisons. He was told that there was a poor cook who had stolen two silver plates from his master and who in accord with the pitiless custom of the time was to be hanged and strangled. "The King," said Paré, "told the provost that he wished to experiment with a stone which they said was good against all poisons, and

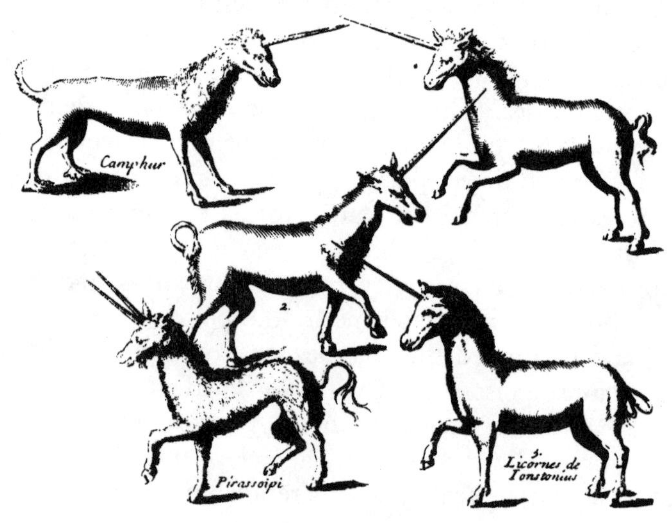

A variety of unicorns.

that he should ask the cook if he would take a certain poison, and that they would at once give him an antidote; to which the cook very willingly agreed, saying that he liked much better to die of poison in the prison than to be strangled in view of the people." (Apparently the cook did not share the King's faith in the bezoar stone.)

The prisoner was given the poison and the bezoar. He died seven hours later. The stone was returned to the King. He is said to have thrown it in the fire.

The method of the control experiment which Paré used is the one, although without the human subjects, by which the medicaments and treatments used by modern physicians have been proved to be effective. Needless to say there are far fewer remedies in use today than there were in the sixteenth century or even the seventeenth and eighteenth.

It took many years for the experimental method to come into wide use in medicine. It would perhaps never have been used if such great doctors as Ambroise Paré and Paracelsus and Vesalius had not carried into medicine the spirit of independent observation, of criticism, and of progress which grew out of the Renaissance. But for the spirit and the practical results that have grown from it, you and I today would be dosed with horrid and useless concoctions, would read our fate in the stars, would scream in pain while we were mangled by the barber surgeons who knew no anatomy, have our teeth extracted by peddlers, and go to hospitals that were filthy and reeking with infection. But worst of all by far—we should be defenseless against disease, as defenseless as men were when the Black Death threatened to wipe out the human race.

Little more than three centuries lie ahead of us in our story, a mere moment in the vast expanse of time through which we have traced medicine. In these few years medicine and surgery and dentistry have grown from what they were in Paré's time to the highly developed sciences we know today.

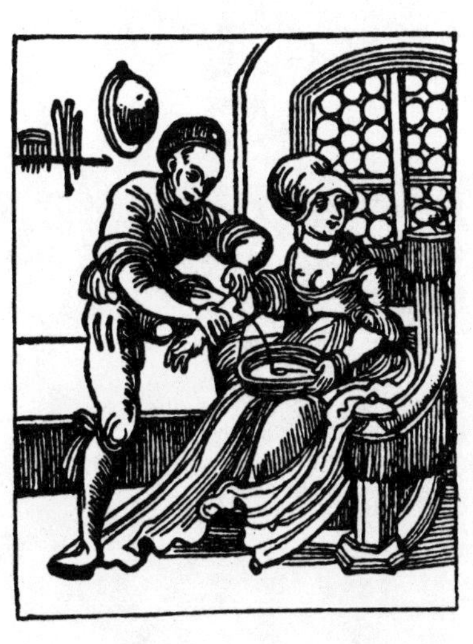

Part Seven

THE SCIENCE OF MEDICINE

THE SUPERSTITIONS OF MEDICINE

THE PRACTICE OF MEDICINE

CHAPTER XIX

The Science of Medicine

MANY, many years ago when men believed in the philosophers' stone that changed base metals into gold, there was a formula, said to be infallible, for obtaining the stone. Its sly author, though he lacked in science, was wise in understanding the contradictions of human ways. Go to a mountain top, said the directions, and mix together certain ingredients—their names are unimportant—and then sit for half an hour without once thinking of the word hippopotamus. That was the important thing, not to let that word hippopotamus slip into your mind; if it did, as it always did, the formula failed.

To Galileo the fateful and forbidden word was not hippopotamus but mathematics. You will remember Galileo, whom we have mentioned as dropping weights from the leaning tower to prove a law of physics. It was in 1581 that his father sent him as a boy of seventeen to the medical school of Pisa where he was to study to become a doctor.

The father, fearing that mathematics—then a most flourishing science—would catch and hold the boy's attention and take his interest from medicine, had kept him from studying the subject and warned him not to think of it when he went to college.

Galileo, dutiful and devout, sat one day in the cathedral of Pisa. He must not think of mathematics. But swinging enticingly before his eyes was a lamp hung on a chain from the ceiling. Back and forth like a pendulum it moved. One, two, three, four; its swing grew less; five, six, seven, eight; his finger strayed to the artery pulsing in his wrist; nine, ten, eleven, twelve; he could count the pulse and the pendulum together, so many swings, so many beats, so many swings, so many beats. The forbidden mathematics! But after all it was important to know that there were always the same number of swings to the same number of beats, even though the distance of the swings grew less and less. No one had ever known before that the rate of the pendulum was largely independent of the range of its swing.

Galileo kept on with medicine; but again the forbidden mathematics intruded. He chanced to hear part of a lecture

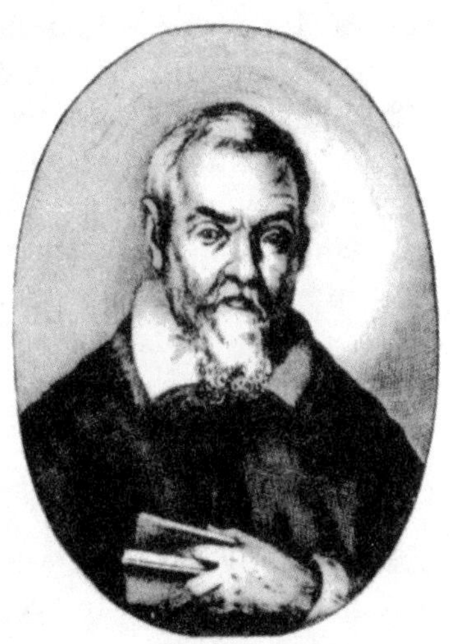

Sanctorius.

on geometry. This was a fascinating subject; there were facts to be proved by mathematics, and things to be measured exactly. Compared to mathematics, medicine, the treating of disease, was a blundering, uncertain sort of business. Reluctantly the father yielded to the son's enthusiasm, and gave his permission; Galileo left medicine and took up instead the study of mathematics. And from this change science was to benefit. It owes to Galileo many principles of physics, the law of the swing of the pendulum, of falling bodies, of the movement of projectiles. It owes to him also great improvements in the telescope, and the invention of the microscope and the thermometer. But most of all it owes to him a method of study. It is the method of making measurements to determine the facts of nature, of using mathematical proof to replace vague guesses and often wrong guesses.

It is indeed rare that we can count medicine as fortunate when a great man leaves its ranks; but that was true in Galileo's case. The physician of today, when he takes the temperature of his patient, counts his pulse and rate of breathing, determines the pressure of the blood in his arteries, weighs him, carries out any of the precise measurements that make modern medicine so vastly more exact than the medicine of the past, is following the method of Galileo. But what is more, the nature of the very bodily functions to which he applies his tests was found out in part at least by Galileo's method.

Medical science as we have traced it so far in our story has followed two methods only. Vesalius was using one when in his dissections he observed and described. Paré, when he experimented with remedies by trial and comparison, was using the second. And now in the seventeenth century there came into use a third, the method of Galileo, of measurement and mathematical proof.

The first man to apply the new method of science to the problems of medicine was a physician named Santorio Santorio; he is usually called by his Latinized name, Sanctorius. Graduated in 1582 from the famous School of Padua, he led a varied career; he was physician to the court of Poland, then a professor at Padua, and finally a private citizen of Venice, where he practiced medicine and carried on the scientific studies which so aroused his enthusiasm.

Men, for centuries before Sanctorius, had observed the fact that in illness there is fever, but no one had ever measured the rise in temperature nor was it certain that the body had a normally constant temperature. Sanctorius was the first physician to use a thermometer to measure body temperature. His thermometer was vastly different from the one that the doctor of today draws from his pocket. It was a long twisted tube with a bulb nearly as large as an egg at the top; the open end at the bottom was placed in water. The patient held the bulb in his mouth; the air in it, becoming warmed, expanded and escaped through the water. When no more air leaked out, the bulb was taken from the mouth; on cooling, the air contracted and water rose in the tube. The height to which it rose was a measure of the air expelled and hence of the temperature that had been about the bulb—the patient's temperature.

For centuries, physicians had felt the pulse at the wrist; they had judged the nature of disease from the quality of the pulse, its firmness, its regularity. But no one had counted it to see how rapid it was. Galileo, some say, counted his pulse with the pendulum; but what he really did was to time a pendulum with his pulse. It was Sanctorius who counted the pulse. He did not use a watch, for a very good reason. Watches had been invented in 1510 but in the early years of the seventeenth century they had no second hand or even minute hand. Sanctorius used a pendulum and varied the length until the rate of the pendulum corresponded to that of the pulse. The rate of the pulse was recorded not in so many beats per minute, as we record it now, but as so many inches of pendulum length. I paused for a moment in writing these lines to measure my pulse: it beat twenty-six inches; my watch said seventy-two beats to the minute.

Sanctorius carried out many experiments in measurement. One of the most famous concerns the weight of the body. He had attached to the ceiling of his dining room a steelyard to which his chair was hung. He weighed himself while he ate and recorded his loss of weight hour after hour from insensible perspiration.

The methods that Sanctorius used are by modern standards crude indeed, but the principle of these methods is the same as that used by the physicians of today in the most refined procedures of modern science, the principle of measurement, of expressing facts in numbers—expressing them objectively.

During the seventeenth century this method was used to yield one of the greatest of all discoveries in medicine. It was the discovery of the function of the heart. The English physician William Harvey demonstrated that the heart

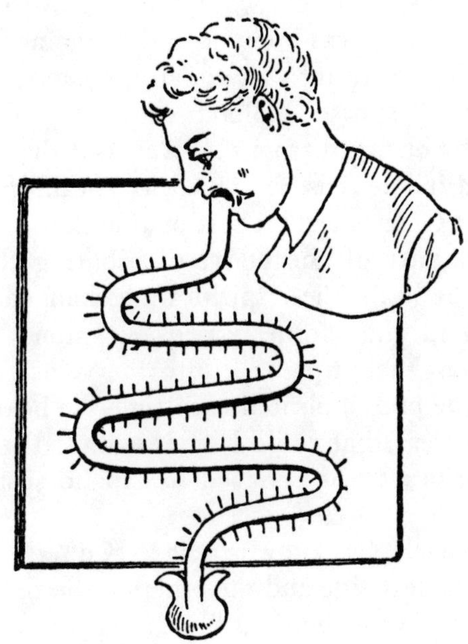

The thermometer of Sanctorius.

pumps blood and that the blood circulates in the blood vessels. He discovered these facts by observation, he demonstrated them experimentally, and he proved them mathematically—the three great methods of science.

We have said little so far concerning the function of any organ of the body; but that does not mean that much had not been said by the physicians and the philosophers in every age. There was indeed a theory to explain every known function of every known organ. But there was little fact in most of these theories. True, Galen had actually performed experiments to show the function of nerves and muscles. But he had performed none to show the function of the heart, and yet he gave an explanation of its action in an elaborate theory. It was the one held by every physician at the beginning of the seventeenth century.

The liver, so said Galen, was the center of the blood system. The food eaten was brought to the liver and changed in some mysterious way into an equally mysterious substance called "natural spirits." Blood containing the "natural spirits" flowed outward from the liver. But the word "flow" was not used in the sense in which we speak of the flow of blood; rather Galen meant a sort of tide that moved slowly out to every part of the body, distributing the "natural spirits." In the brain these spirits were changed to "animal spirits" and in that form passed out along the nerves, emptying from their tips back into the veins. The arteries throughout the body pulsated each time the heart beat. But in giving the beat that could be felt against the ribs on the left side, the heart was believed to expand just as did the arteries.

The heart itself was known to have two sets of chambers, one pair on the left side and the other on the right. To those on the right the veins holding bluish-black blood were connected and to those on the left the arteries holding bright vermilion blood. Between the two sides of the heart, so said Galen, there were minute pores through which the blue blood and the red blood mingled.

It had not occurred to Galen that the heart was a pump; instead, like Aristotle, he thought of it as a churn and a furnace. It heated the blood and stirred into it something called "vital spirits." The lungs were fans that cooled the blood.

Galen's theory gave support to the old idea that bleeding, the drawing off of blood, was beneficial in the treatment of disease. That belief arose, as we have told, among primitive people; it was promoted by the false theories of ancient physicians; it was widely practiced by the physicians of the fifteenth, sixteenth, seventeenth and, sad to say, even of the eighteenth and early nineteenth centuries. Believing Galen's theory, men were unaware of the fact that there was only a small quantity of blood in the body, perhaps a gallon, rapidly circulated. They thought rather that it was continually formed and stagnated. To bleed relieved the body of "bad blood"; and new and good blood was made to take its place. Sometimes there was too much blood, so they thought, on one side of the body, and in order to establish a balance some was drawn off.

Bleeding at one time was the physician's chief method of treating disease. Read the story of *Gil Blas*, as we have suggested in an earlier chapter, and you will see to what excesses bleeding was carried by the famous character, Dr. Sangrado, "the tall, withered, wan executioner of the sisters three." The story is fiction, of course, but it is based on fact. In Paris in the seventeenth century a prominent physician named Guy Patin wrote that he bled himself seven times for a head cold, and his son twenty times in the course of a few days. His procedure was not exceptional.

The story of the discovery of the circulation of the blood takes us first to Padua—the Padua of Vesalius and of Sanctorius. The English boy, William Harvey, came there to study medicine after his graduation from Cambridge University. In 1602—the same year that Shakespeare's *Hamlet* was first played—Harvey received his doctor's degree from the University of Padua. But Padua gave him something in addition that no other school of that time could have given him, a love for anatomical observation. True to the memory of the great Vesalius, it was the leading school of anatomy.

While he was there Harvey may have read the famous lines that Vesalius wrote when he looked for the tiny pores through which Galen had said the blue blood and the red blood were supposed to mingle—and did not find them: "We are driven to wonder at the handiwork of the Almighty, by means of which the blood sweats from the right into the

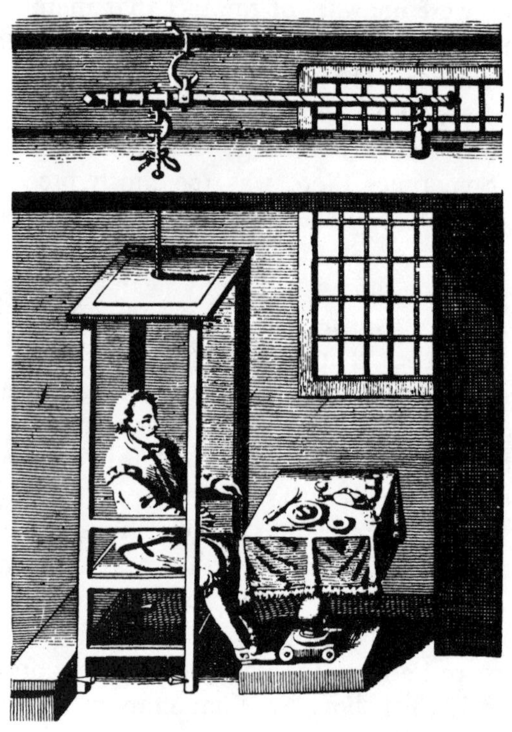

Sanctorius on the steelyard.

left ventricle through passages which escape human vision."

Perhaps Vesalius suspected even more than he implied. But his was a dangerous time in which to hint that ancient theories of how the organs of the body worked might be wrong. Such things were still closely linked to religious beliefs. Men could be burned for upsetting established views.

Another man, Miguel Serveto or Servetus, less prudent

than Vesalius, published his discovery that the blood passed from the right side to the left of the heart, not through the partition but through the lungs. And of all places he chose to print it in a book pointing out what he thought were errors in religion. Galen's mistake was one of the errors he enumerated. Servetus was burned to death in 1553.

Servetus' discovery did not by any means settle the problem of what the heart does. That was left for Harvey. This young man, newly made a doctor, was back in London practicing medicine.

The London of his day had a population of less than a quarter of a million. And it was a plague-ridden place; one outbreak after another tortured the people, until the greatest and last of all in 1665, a year before the fire that burned a large section of the city.

Between treating his patients, Harvey carried on the study of anatomy that he had begun at Padua. His interest centered on the heart. What was the meaning of its movement? He could see it move in fishes, in turtles, in frogs. And as he watched the living heart pulsate, he pondered. Here was something different from the descriptions of Galen and of Aristotle. Had they looked as carefully as he? They had said the heart expanded when they felt it beat against the ribs, when the pulse could be felt in the arteries. Instead he saw the heart contract. It was pushing out—squeezing out—the blood it held. The pulse in the artery was caused by the rhythmic onrush of the blood.

Then came a question. If the heart pushes out the blood, does the blood run back into the heart when it relaxes? An experiment was needed. He tied a cord about the forearm of a man. The cord pressed hard enough to shut off the flow of blood in the veins but not in the arteries. With each beat of the heart blood flowed into the arm; the veins of the hand were distended, the arm swollen. The veins above the band were collapsed. Clearly the experiment showed that the blood flowed from the heart through the arteries but did not flow back through them when the heart relaxed. Instead it flowed from the arteries into the veins. This was science by the method of observation and experiment, but it alone did not supply the answers to the questions Harvey raised.

Where did the blood in the veins go? And, if the heart kept pumping blood where did the blood come from? Was it possible that it was the same blood being pumped round and round? Measurements, mathematics would supply the answers.

Harvey calculated that each time the heart squeezed down and emptied out its blood two ounces of blood went into the arteries. The heart of a man at rest beat some seventy-two times a minute. Seventy-two beats, 72 x 2 ounces, 144 ounces a minute; 540 pounds an hour; more than 16 tons in 24 hours! Absurd to think that the body produced that much blood. There could be only one answer; the blood circulated. It went from the left side of the heart into the arteries, from the arteries to the veins, from the veins to the right side of the heart and from the right side of the heart—as Servetus had shown—through the lungs and back to the starting point. The heart was a pump; the blood circulated.

In 1618 William Harvey had learned these facts. Ten years later, when he was certain beyond question of a doubt, he published them. His book, *Exercitatio anatomica de motu cordis et sanguinis in animalibus*, is one of the great landmarks of medicine.

We need hardly say that a storm of opposition met Harvey's statements. He had dared to doubt Galen. The repetition of that cry "You deny Galen?" may have become a bit tiresome even to the men of that time. Eighty-five years had passed since Vesalius had been driven from his post at Padua. Harvey lost some patients; he heard some uncomplimentary things about himself; but the storm soon passed. He stayed on in his post as royal physician to His Majesty King Charles I and lived to see his discoveries accepted.

And the man himself? Those who knew him said that he

was rather quick of temper when crossed in an argument, given to fingering the handle of the dagger he wore at his belt, and that "in person he was not tall but of the lowest stature; round-faced, olivaster complexion, little eyes, round, very black, full of spirit, his hair black as a raven,

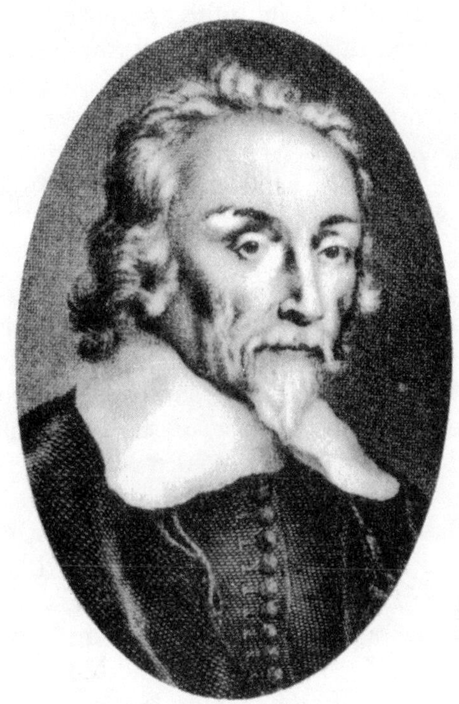

William Harvey.

but quite white twenty years before he died." He died in 1657—four years too soon to know the answer to the question that must have puzzled him all his days. How did the blood flow from the arteries to the veins; how did it flow through the lungs?

It was the Italian physician Marcello Malpighi who solved the riddle. He used the method of observation but he had at hand a new instrument—the microscope that Galileo had invented.

Under the lens of even the crude microscope of those days a whole new field of study was opened up by the physician. The tissues of the body had definite and important structures invisible to the unaided eye.

In the year 1661 Malpighi, then professor of anatomy at Bologna, reported that he had seen in the lungs and about the intestines of frogs, minute blood vessels, far too small to be visible to the naked eye, connecting the arteries and veins. In the flesh of a living animal he saw blood move through these capillary vessels, saw it flow from artery to vein.

Harvey, Servetus, and Malpighi supplied all the main facts concerning the circulation of the blood. Since their time only details have been added. But in spite of their knowledge, none of these men knew what functions the blood served in the body. The microscope showed it a clear, faintly yellow fluid in which were suspended many minute red disks; Malpighi had thought them drops of red fat. But what did the fluid do in the body; why was it circulated? Again theories. Since earliest times blood had been looked upon as a fluid denoting the very essence of life. It was the ingredient passed on in heredity to carry the family traits—witness, "blood relations." Men were distinguished temperamentally as "hot blooded" or "cold blooded." When in the seventeenth century the first crude transfusions of blood, the drawing of blood from the veins of one man and putting it into the veins of another, were performed, there was much speculation as to what would happen to the character of the recipient. Would a sheep bark when transfused with the blood of a dog; how would an English bishop behave if he were transfused with the blood of a Quaker?

Nowhere has modern science dealt more unkindly with old beliefs than with those concerning blood; to the modern physician blood is simply the least alive of all the tissues of the body; it has nothing to do with temperament; notions that one hears even today of disease due to "bad blood" the physician knows are absurd. The one peculiarity of blood lies in the fact that it is a liquid and can escape when the body is wounded. The body needs its blood to carry oxygen

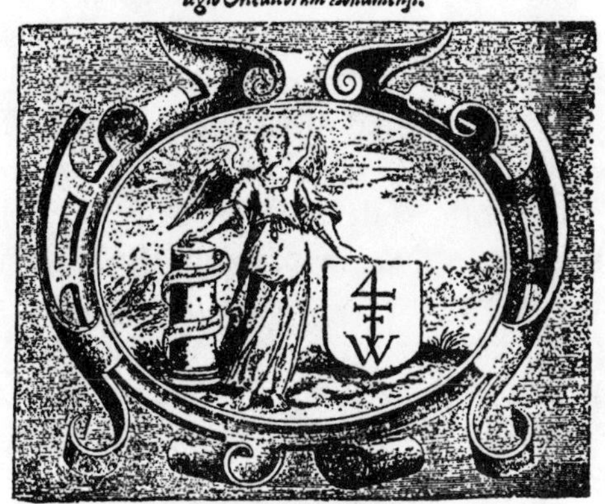

EXERCITATIO.
ANATOMICA DE
MOTV CORDIS ET SAN-
GVINIS IN ANIMALI-
BVS,
GVILIELMI HARVEI ANGLI,
Medici Regii, & Professoris Anatomiæ in Col-
legio Medicorum Londinensi.

FRANCOFVRTI,
Sumptibus GVILIELMI FITZERI.

ANNO M. DC. XXVIII.

Title-page of De Motu Cordis.

and food and waste materials from one part of the system to another. Blood is merely a vehicle.

It was not until the nineteenth century that these facts were known fully, but in the seventeenth century the first step was taken toward finding them out. An Englishman from Cornwall, named John Mayow, showed that the bluish blood found in veins turned red in passing through the lungs because it took something from the air. What that something was he did not know. He called it nitro-aërial—spirit of air; we call it oxygen, but oxygen had not been discovered in his day.

In reading here of Galileo, Sanctorius, Servetus, Harvey, Malpighi, and Mayow, you may have noticed a fact that in a way makes their work different from that of the medical heroes of the sixteenth century. Paracelsus, Vesalius, and Paré were reformers; they revolted against the medical beliefs of their time; they attempted to change the course of medicine; their achievements depended largely upon their peculiar personalities.

In the seventeenth century medical science was still in the hands of independent workers but there were the beginnings of close coöperation. Thus Harvey, following the anatomy of Vesalius and the method of Galileo, went on from where Servetus had left off and was able to demonstrate the circulation of blood; both Malpighi and Mayow followed with their contributions to this one problem. Individual contributions were becoming merely a part of a united whole that each year grew, and still grows, more nearly completed. From now on our story of medical science will deal less with the lives of men; their work, their contributions to the unfolding scheme of things, and not their personalities, become the dominating theme. Personality and chance shape the destiny of each great man; but the work that has come before likewise shapes his work. We are to find fewer reformers but many new contributors.

In recognition of this coöperation, this interdependence, the scientists of the seventeenth century were founding societies in which they might exchange ideas to their mutual benefit. Scientific journals were appearing; one of the greatest of them was the *Philosophical Transactions* of the Royal Society of London. The society itself was formed in 1645 and given a charter by Charles II in 1662; the *Transactions* first appeared in 1664. In this journal a few years after its founding, a discovery was reported, the importance of which was not realized until almost two centuries had passed. A man named Leeuwenhoek of Delft had written a letter to the editor of the *Transactions*. He was not a physician but

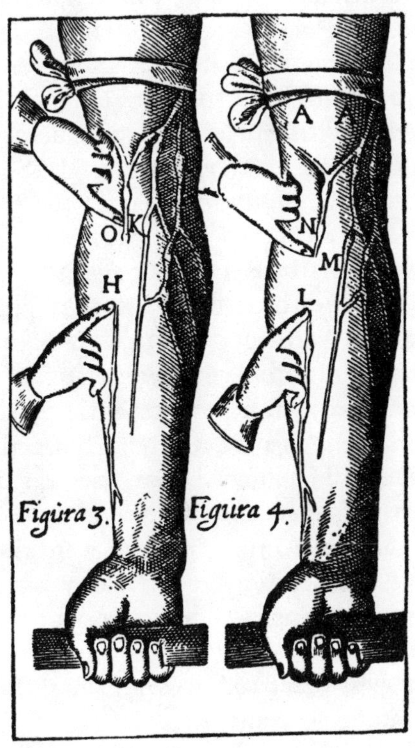

An illustration from De Motu Cordis.

the janitor of the city hall. He had, however, a profitable hobby, the microscope. He ground his own lenses, made his own microscopes, and turned them on everything he could find.

In 1683 he wrote that in scrapings from a tooth he had

seen what we call bacteria. He described them accurately. Bacteria were of no interest at all except as curiosities to physicians of those days. Leeuwenhoek's was an isolated fact of observation.

While Leeuwenhoek peered through his microscope, off in Italy another naturalist was studying flies, making his isolated contribution of a fact. Francesco Redi by experiment disproved a theory held strongly in his day—that maggots develop spontaneously in filth and rotting things. He placed some meat in jars; some of the jars he left open; others he covered with gauze. The meat decayed. Attracted by the smell, flies buzzed about the vessels. Soon there were maggots in the meat of the open jars; there were none in the meat of the jars covered with gauze. But on top of the gauze where eggs had been laid maggots appeared. Flies, not something in the rotten meat, were responsible for the maggots. Maggots were not generated spontaneously.

These observations of Leeuwenhoek and of Redi lay isolated for nearly two hundred years. Then in the nineteenth century the French chemist Pasteur built them into the scheme of science. He showed that bacteria, like maggots, did not arise spontaneously, but were produced by other bacteria; and he proved that bacteria were the cause of infectious disease. This was a revolutionary advance of medicine, but it had its beginnings in the work of scientists of the seventeenth century: Galileo who invented the microscope, Leeuwenhoek who described bacteria, and Redi who first disproved spontaneous generation.

This chapter which we have entitled "science" is really one act in the drama of medicine. The other two acts could be named, as we have named the next two chapters, "superstition" and "practice." The stage is set here for the seventeenth century; it could as well have been set for the eighteenth, nineteenth, or twentieth. We have chosen the seventeenth because then the contrasts between science, superstition, and practice were greatest.

The science of medicine is knowledge concerning the body in health and disease, knowledge proved by experiment and reduced to rules, precise, exact, unvarying.

The superstitions of medicine are the false beliefs concerning disease and its treatment that linger in the minds of many people.

Science and superstition are conflicting forces. One makes for progress; the other retards it.

The practice of medicine concerns all the ways in which the doctor deals not only with disease but also with the people who have disease. Behind him, supplying him with new facts, weapons with which to fight disease, is science. But science has not even yet told him all, far from it. The doctor must know not only science but men as well, with all their fears, their false beliefs, their superstitions.

A time may come perhaps, though not in your day or mine, when medicine will be a single thing—science. Superstitions will have died, and science will have reduced to rules not only the knowledge of how the body works and how disease can be prevented and cured but also how human beings behave.

In the seventeenth century little use was made in medical practice of the science that we have described in this chapter, vastly important though it was for later events.

CHAPTER XX

The Superstitions of Medicine

AN automobile mired in the unpaved streets of London in the seventeenth century; an aëroplane soaring over the modest homes of the Pilgrim fathers of New England, or those homes lighted with electricity—these things would be anachronisms.

But it is just as much an anachronism to bring forward in time something old and out of date as it is to move something back in time. A primitive medicine man in the surroundings of the Royal Court of England would be an anachronism. Standing there, his nakedness barely covered with bits of fur, he would be out of place among ladies dressed in the flowing gowns of the seventeenth century and gentlemen with tight satin breeches, velvet coats, and powdered wigs. In the decorous surroundings of civilization the medicine man shouting, gesticulating, carrying out his rites and incantations, would most certainly appear absurd. But suppose that we were to dress this medicine man in the costume of the times and change his rites and ceremonies, not in principle but only in form, so that they no longer seemed grotesque; then he would not appear as an absurdity but he still would be an anachronism. He would represent something old brought forward in time, misplaced.

With this idea in mind let us read from the diary of an English writer of the seventeenth century—John Evelyn, a cultured gentleman and friend of King Charles II. Here is what he said concerning an incident he witnessed on July 6, 1660:

"His Majesty began to touch for the Evil according to custom, thus: His Majesty sitting under his state in the banqueting house, the chirurgeons cause the sick to be brought, or led, up to the throne, where they kneel; the King strokes their faces or cheeks with both hands at once, at which instance a chaplain in his formality says, 'He put his hands upon them, and he healed them.' . . . When they have been all touched, they come up again in the same order, and the other chaplain kneeling, and having angel gold strung on white ribbon on his arm, delivers them one by one to His Majesty, who puts them about the necks of the touched as they pass, while the chaplain repeats, 'That is the true light who come into the world.' Then follows an epistle with liturgy, prayers for the sick, lastly blessings; and then the Lord Chamberlain and the Comptroller of the Household bring a basin, ewer, and towel, for His Majesty to wash."

The same ceremony as described by Shakespeare in *Macbeth*, Act IV, Scene 3, reads:

> *—strangely-visited people,*
> *All swoln and ulcerous, pitiful to the eye;*
> *The mere despair of surgery, he cures;*
> *Hanging a golden stamp about their necks,*
> *Put on with holy prayers.*

These are faithful descriptions of the ceremony of the Royal Touch for the disease of the King's Evil. If it were carried out in some forest glade by a shouting, sweating savage, if the gold pieces were perforated shells on a grass string, the primitive nature of the ceremony would be apparent. In principle it was the same in the court of England in the days of the seventeenth century; for all its regal surroundings it was primitive, savage, superstitious medicine.

The King of England played the rôle of a primitive medicine man. He was only one in an unbroken succession that has carried the medical beliefs of the savage through all ages even to our day. In guise ever changed to suit the times but with principle unaltered, we shall meet these "primitive medicine men" again and again in the centuries that remain before us in our story. They are the ignorant healers, the leaders of healing cults, the great quacks.

The Royal Touch for the King's Evil was merely one of many superstitions in the seventeenth century, but it was perhaps the most striking. The disease, the King's Evil, was scrofula; and scrofula, as we know now, is tuberculosis of the glands of the neck.

The belief in the power of the laying on of hands is an ancient one. The primitive medicine man stretched out his hand, touched the ailing place, and bade the tormenting spirit leave. In early civilization the priest was an emissary of the gods, sharing their healing powers; often he wrought cures by touch. Later when kings, so it was believed, ruled by divine right, they too had healing power. Why their virtues were limited to one disease, scrofula, we cannot say, but the fact remains that Edward the Confessor in England touched for this disease in the eleventh century.

From the time of Henry VII in 1465 to William of Orange in 1689 the Royal Touch was an accepted court ceremony. William, far from superstitious in this matter, touched only once and then greatly against his will. He laid his hands on the sick person and said, "May God give you better health; and more sense." In the eighteenth century, however, Queen Anne revived the practice. Dr. Johnson was one of the last persons she touched: it was done in his infancy; he retained his scrofula all his life.

The French kings from Clovis to Louis XVI also touched for the evil. In 1775 Louis XVI, the last king before the Revolution, touched 2400 sick persons on the day of his coronation. But men were becoming openly skeptical of the ancient practice. An investigation was made of the 2400 cases. In only five were there any signs whatever of improvement. In spite of skepticism the practice was revived in 1824 at the coronation of Charles X; he touched 121 sick people.

The Royal Touch has not been used now for more than a century, that is, not used by royalty; but the laying on of hands is still performed as manipulation of the feet or spine by men who have a following for their primitive, superstitious medicine quite as great as was the king's in the past.

For a time in the seventeenth century there was no king on the English throne. The head of Charles I had fallen under the ax of the public executioner. Cromwell was in

KINGS-EVIL.

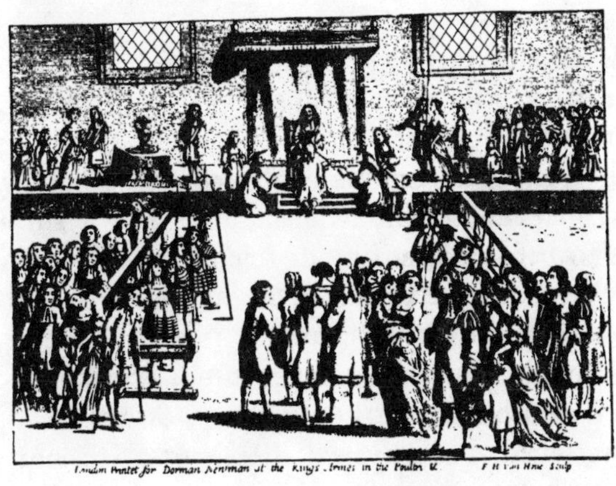

A broadside printed in 1697 showing King Charles touching for the evil.

power, but he refused to attempt the touch for the evil. And so the public turned to one of those odd characters who in every century, even the present, have carried on the healing of the primitive medicine man. It was Valentine Greatrakes, one of Cromwell's soldiers, who, so he said, was told in a dream that he possessed healing powers over the evil. He began to practice his art and was quite as successful as the kings had been. That is to say, he satisfied the people. By successive dreams it was revealed that his healing powers covered almost every disease. Thousands of people flocked to him; he obligingly touched them; they were "cured." Many prominent men, even Robert Boyle, the "father of modern chemistry," spoke in praise of Greatrakes.

There in the countryside of England was an ignorant man practicing in his quiet way the principle of healing that had been used by the medicine men of primitive people, by the magicians of Egypt, the priests of Æsculapius, and the sorcerers of Syria. The principle is the same regardless of the way it is applied; the medicine man shouted and danced; the magician drew his magic circles; the priest of Æsculapius commanded sleep and dreams; the kings of France and England, and Greatrakes touched. After their times men were to turn to still other means, to mesmerism, to electricity, to manipulation of joints, and even to healing philosophies. The principle remains unaltered; the primitive medicine man in ever-changing guise stalks down through the centuries to become in a day of science an anachronism.

Whatever form the principle takes, the result is the same. As we have said in earlier chapters, primitive medicine acts largely through its effect upon the mind. If confidence is obtained and fear banished, the symptoms of disease may for a time be relieved, but physical disease itself is not altered. But the important thing here is the fact that the cure used by the kings and Greatrakes and all of the superstitious healers in all ages was applied to physical as well as mental disturbances; no distinction was made. Only in the momentary wave of their enthusiasm did the physically ill feel better and then, as their diseases progressed, they became worse than they had been before they were treated.

Valentine Greatrakes for a few months was a tremendous success; and then his prestige began to wane. The pains and aches and infirmities which had yielded to confidence returned. His fame diminished; the crowds no longer sought him.

Another of the medical superstitions of the seventeenth century was the amazing powder of sympathy that was exploited by Sir Kenelm Digby. Digby was at various times a student at Oxford, an English ambassador, a Commissioner of the Navy, a follower of Cromwell, and a courtier of

Plants.
Sym: Powder.
his Cookery
Rec: in Physick &c
Sr K Digby of Bodyes
The truly Learned and Honoble
Sr. Kenelme Digby Kt. Chancellor
to the Q: Mother
Aged 62.
Cross sculpsit

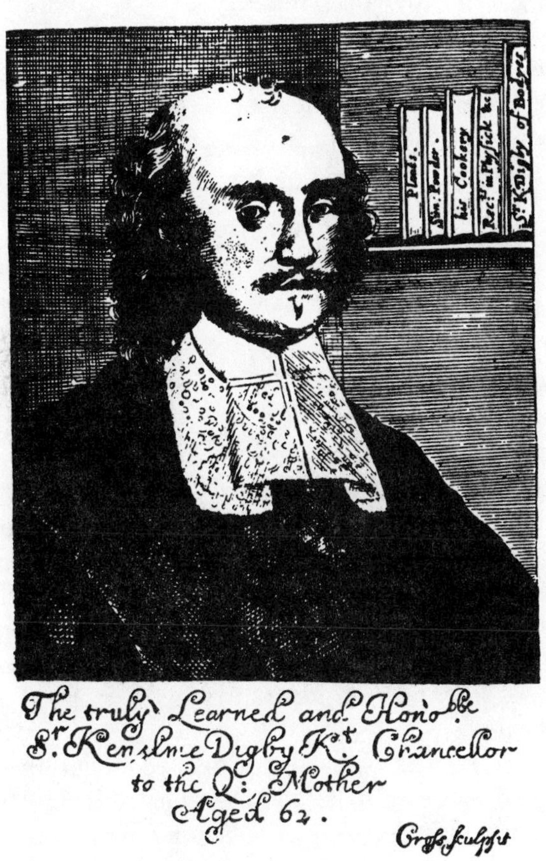

Sir Kenelm Digby who used the powder of sympathy.

James I, Charles I, and Charles II. Quite a checkered career. He was energetic, he had wild schemes which he could present with amazing conviction. It is said that he hastened the death of his sorely abused consumptive wife by trying out on her a remedy made of vipers' flesh, intended to beautify her.

After he had traveled for some time on the continent he had returned to the court of King James with his amazing remedy, the powder of sympathy. It was a variant of the weapon ointment of which we have spoken in connection with Paracelsus. You will find mention of weapon ointment in Sir Walter Scott's "The Lay of the Last Minstrel," in the episode in which Lady Margaret finds William of Deloraine wounded:

She drew the splinter from the wound,
And with a charm she stanched the blood.
She bade the gash be cleansed and bound:
No longer by his couch she stood;
But she has ta'en the broken lance,
And washed it from the clotted gore,
And salved the splinter o'er and o'er.

Now sometimes, as you may well imagine, it was difficult to obtain the weapon that caused the wound. The enemy might escape with his sword or dagger. It was in just such instances that the sympathetic powder of Sir Kenelm came in so helpfully. It was applied not to the weapon but to blood-stained clothing. Scraps of cloth were soaked in a solution of the powder; instantly pain stopped and the wound healed.

King James was particularly excited about the remedy and begged to be told its composition. Reluctantly Digby divulged it. This mysterious substance was iron sulphate, green vitriol.

Kings of those days had their personal medical superstitions. Henry VIII was interested especially in "cramp rings," rings to be worn to prevent stomach ache. But we can forgive him any superstitions he may have had in view of his one great gift to medicine. It was he who first decreed that births and deaths should be carefully recorded; later, causes of death were added, and the way thus opened for medical statistics. Queen Elizabeth wore a magic locket about her neck that kept her free from infection; William of Orange used the dried ground-up eyes of crabs for a medicament (he had consumption); and Queen Anne's medical superstitions aside from the Royal Touch led to her making tailors and tinkers into eye specialists to treat her failing sight.

The most striking of Charles II's many connections with medical superstitions occurred while he was unconscious. We shall come to it soon when we talk of popular remedies; first, let us see some of the more common medical superstitions of the people at large. We could go on endlessly recounting local superstitions that prevailed in one region or another—a spider in a bag to cure fits; a horse chestnut carried in the pocket to prevent rheumatism; a cleft in a tree through which a child could be pushed to cure rickets; coral to drive off malarial fever and keep dogs from going mad; cobwebs to stop hemorrhage; a black snake put around the neck to cure goiter; the blood of a black hen killed in the dark of the moon to cure a variety of diseases; and so on and so on. There were literally thousands, yes, hundreds of thousands of these remarkable remedies. Many of them persist today.

There were, however, in the seventeenth century, three superstitions that were thoroughly believed in as influencing matters of health and disease. These were palmistry, astrology, and witchcraft.

Palmistry is one of the most ancient arts of divination. From the shape of the hands, from the swellings and depressions, and from the creases, the health of the individual, his character, and his future could be determined—so it had been believed from prehistoric times. The life line, the crease at the base of the thumb; the liver line across the wrist; and the heart line ending near the index finger were the most important in determining health, although perhaps the heart line was studied more often in relation to the tender emotion supposed to be centered in this organ than in relation to diseases. Of course, the creases in the hands are simply places where the skin is firmly tied down to the

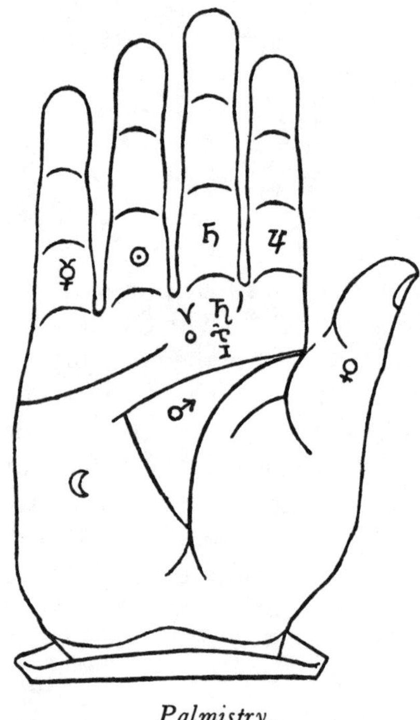

Palmistry.

underlying flesh; the lines are no more indicative of states of health than are finger prints.

In the seventeenth century astrology bulked large in medical superstitions. It was to hold its place until the eventful year 1758. Halley, the astronomer, calculated that the comet which now bears his name would appear in that year. It did. And men realized then that comets were not the gods' token of disease but instead were themselves under the rule of mathematics.

We mentioned astrology, the so-called science of the influence of the heavenly bodies on human life and health, when we talked about Arabian medicine. But astrology was older than the Arabian civilization; it probably arose among the Babylonians or Chaldeans. About the fourth century B.C. it spread to Greece and under Greek influence was woven into every phase of art and science and indeed every act of daily life. From Greece, astrology followed the stream of knowledge; it went into Egypt in a new form with the Ptolemies; it reached Rome shortly before the opening of the Christian Era; it spread to the Moslem Empire; it was carried into Western Europe and throve there from the thirteenth to the seventeenth centuries. Among ignorant people it still flourishes even in America of today. The almanacs of patent medicines still occasionally show the typical picture of a man surrounded by the constellations of the zodiac, from each of which a line extends to the organ that the particular constellation controls. Again in the columns of newspapers and magazines and over the radio, astrological advice is given concerning the indications of the stars for lucky days and ventures. Fortune tellers, in spite of laws prohibiting their practice, still for a fee draw horoscopes showing the fate of the individual as predicted from the position of the constellation at the moment of birth.

The absurdity of astrology is apparent to any moderately well educated and intelligent person of today; but three hundred years ago astrology was an accepted and serious part of medicine. The time for bleeding, the time for taking medicines, indeed, even the form of treatment used, as well as the kind of disease present, were often determined from the stars. The royal astrologer was a very important man at court.

In 1621 the scholar Robert Burton published an amazing book called the *Anatomy of Melancholy*. In it was his horoscope showing that his death would occur in 1640. He died on the twenty-fifth of January, 1640—some say at his own hands so that his horoscope would come out correctly. Cromwell is said to have had his "lucky days," and the great astronomer Kepler occasionally drew horoscopes. But in the seventeenth century many people were becoming skeptical of astrology; astronomical discoveries were yielding a new conception of the stars and planets. It was just after the close of the seventeenth century that Jonathan Swift, the author of *Gulliver's Travels*, perpetrated a hoax on astrology that by ridicule hastened the discarding of the practice in England. Swift, as you know, wielded a satirical pen that could drive home his points by astute exaggeration. Thus in his paper *Modest Proposal for Preventing the Children of Poor People from being a Burden to their Parents or the Country*, he ridiculed the futile schemes of impractical writers on social problems. His suggestion was to fatten the children and eat them.

His astrological hoax was in the form of an announcement that on March 29, 1708, a certain Mr. Partridge would die. Instead of his own name on the announcement, Swift signed that of Isaac Bickerstaff. Mr. Partridge was a famous almanac maker and predictor of events. On March 30 Mr. Bickerstaff published a notice that his prediction was correct and that Partridge was dead. Partridge at once protested that he was alive; Bickerstaff denied it. The silliness of the controversy between the indignant Partridge and the sarcastic and insistent Bickerstaff amused the public. When a thing is ridiculed and parodied it is difficult ever again to view it seriously. Astrology declined rapidly.

But our language, which is in itself a record of the past, still keeps words derived from astrology. Lunatic is one of them—from luna, the moon that shone on men in their sleep and made them insane.

More pernicious by far than astrology was the superstitious belief, still existent in the seventeenth century, in witchcraft. By witchcraft, so it was thought, a spell could be cast upon some victim and disease and misfortune produced.

This, as you will recognize, was a belief that had persisted from the time of primitive people when the medicine man was supposed to be able to do black magic. There were many efforts made by men and women of the sixteenth and seventeenth centuries to dispose of their enemies or their rivals by using black magic. Sometimes little images were shaped in wax and needles stuck with proper ceremony in the part where the disease was to strike, or the image was melted to cause death. Needless to say no ill effects came from these

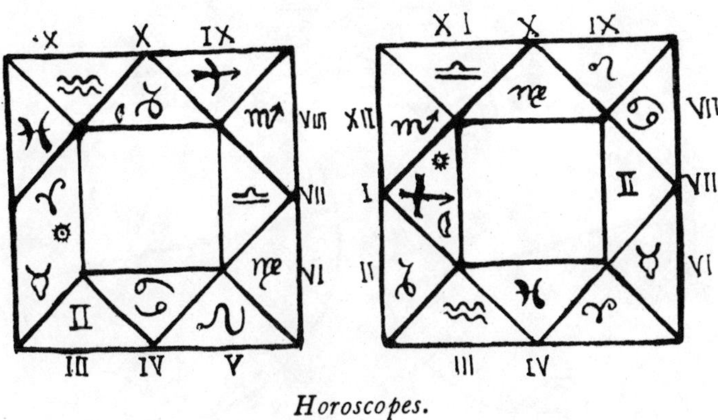

Horoscopes.

vindictive if harmless practices. But there was another aspect which was far from harmless. Sometimes when people had misfortunes or disease they believed them caused by black magic and accordingly sought to find the enemy who was attacking them. As like as not they hit on some poor wretch who was insane, who lived alone, was queer in her actions, and muttered meaningless words. She was accused of being a witch, and was drowned or burned.

Superstition in the seventeenth century still prevented men from realizing that the insane were really sick people. The savage superstition of possession by evil demons persisted in the midst of the elaborate civilizations of France, England, Germany, and Italy. Little kindness was shown to the insane; they were often taken to be witches or else possessed. But some institutions had arisen for the care of the more violent and incurable cases. The most famous of all was the hospital of St. Mary's of Bethlehem in London. With the English genius for such things, the name was shortened to Bedlam; the word has come down to our time to signify a place of discord and turmoil—a lasting commentary on the conditions of this institution. It was super-

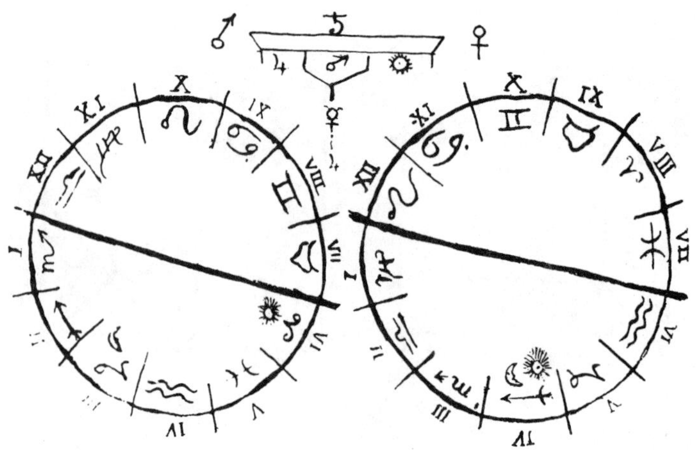

Horoscope in geometrical form.

stition, ancient savage beliefs, that prevented people from realizing that the insane man was a sick man, as deserving of care and sympathy as the man who was physically ill. Shakespeare had spoken of insanity as "a mind diseased," but three centuries were to pass—three centuries of stupid brutality—before this knowledge was to become widespread and the insane were to receive humane care. In the sixteenth century Bedlam, with its imprisoned, tortured inmates, was a sort of zoo where of a Sunday afternoon the curious could for a penny see the mad men. It was one of the sights of London.

When we spoke in passing of some of the minor personal superstitions of the kings and queens of the period—the cramp rings of Henry and the charmed locket of Elizabeth—we said that we would tell of the medical ritual in which Charles II was involved. It was a superstitious proceeding at the hands of his physician. Remember nearly a century had passed since the days when gentle old Ambroise Paré showed Charles IX how to test the bezoar stone by the method of control experiment. Here, on the other hand, are the remedies that the royal physicians applied to a dying king in the year 1685.

The records tell us that at eight o'clock on the morning of February second, King Charles fell unconscious while shaving in his bedroom. His physician, on being summoned, bled the King to the extent of a pint from his right arm. Next he drew eight ounces of blood from the left shoulder (Harvey had described the circulation of the blood fifty-seven years before), gave an emetic to make the King vomit, two physics and an enema containing antimony, rock salt, marsh-mallow leaves, violets, beet root, camomile flowers, fennel seed, linseed, cardamom seed, cinnamon, saffron, cochineal, and aloes. The King's head was then shaved and a blister raised on his scalp. A sneezing powder of hellebore root was given to purge his brain and a powder of cowslip administered to strengthen it, for it was the belief in those days that the nasal secretion came from the brain. The emetics were continued at frequent intervals and meanwhile a soothing drink given, composed of barley water, licorice, and sweet almonds, light wine, oil of wormwood, anise, thistle leaves, mint, rose, and angelica. A plaster of pitch and pigeon dung was put on the King's feet. Next there was more bleeding followed by the administration of melon seeds, manna, slippery elm, black cherry water, extract of lily of the valley, peony, lavender, pearls dissolved in vinegar, gentian root, nutmeg, and cloves. To this mixture were added forty drops of the extract of human skull. Finally in desperation a bezoar stone was tried. The King died.

Hardly a single one of the medicines given the King had, as we know now, any effect upon the body whatever. The mixture of drugs sounds more like something prepared in a nightmare than in a drugstore.

We should call these remedies superstitious ones today; they were not then. A superstition, as we said many chapters earlier, is a belief inconsistent with generally prevailing knowledge. As we shall see in the next chapter the medicaments used on poor King Charles were unfortunately consistent with the knowledge of the time.

Few of the scientists of those days—such men as Harvey, Sanctorius, and Malpighi—had turned their attention to the treatment of disease. They were interested in finding out how the body worked rather than how to treat the sick man. The remedies of the seventeenth century, barring only a few, were nearly as unscientific as those that the savage used.

In 1618, the first *London Pharmacopœia* appeared. A pharmacopœia is a book listing the remedies used in treating disease and giving the recipes for their preparation. There were nearly two thousand remedies described in this book, the vast majority of which were herb medicaments. A few of the remedies were valuable beyond question and are in use today: there was quinine, the great medical discovery of the seventeenth century, and mercury salts, the potent mineral medicament that Paracelsus had advocated, and "steel" tonics for the treatment of anæmia. But with these few there were many showing only too clearly that five thousand years and more of civilization had not changed the beliefs of ignorant people. That the great inventions of movable type and ink and paper should be used to record such remedies was itself an anachronism. There were pills made of viper flesh, the dried lungs of foxes for shortness of breath, ground up jewels, oil squeezed from bricks, bear grease to grow hair, and snake oil to limber muscles, moss scraped from the skull of a convict hanged in chains (a popular remedy), crabs' eyes, hoofs of animals, fly specks, the dung of many different kinds of animals (crocodile dung was especially beneficial), human sweat, saliva, spider's webs, snake skins, lice, oil of puppies boiled with earthworms, and cat-fat ointment! The very witches' caldron was brewed in the pharmacopœia of the seventeenth century.

CHAPTER XXI

The Practice of Medicine

IN the seventeenth century medicine as it was practiced was out of date. The satires of the great French dramatist Molière held the doctors up to ridicule before an amused public. It is said that Molière had a personal grievance against physicians; they were unable to cure him of the consumption from which he was dying; they had failed to save the life of his son, and of his dearest friend. Whatever his motive may have been, his keen satire dissected medical practice and laid bare its greatest fault. Medicine was out of date.

The doctors of the seventeenth century were trained as doctors had been trained in the Middle Ages. Disputation, hair-splitting argument over the authoritative statements of Galen and the Arabian physicians was still the essence of medical education. The great medical school of Paris allowed no student to read or discuss the works of Paracelsus. Medical practice was what it had been in the fourteenth, fifteenth, and sixteenth centuries. The doctors were educated, but they were not educated to treat diseases. They were the same scholarly and pompous gentlemen against whom a century before Paracelsus had directed his shafts.

In one scene of Molière's play, *L'Amour Médecin*, five physicians in their best professional manner bring all their powers of subtle disputation to bear upon the momentous subject of whether it fits their dignity better to ride to their patients on a horse or a mule. And that argument had truly as much importance as many upon which the doctors wasted their energies.

The last play written by Molière was *Le Malade Imaginaire;* it had to do with a man sick only in his imagination, a hypochondriac, who took all sorts of patent medicines and consulted many doctors. The part that satirized medical practice dealt with the elaborate ceremony of graduation from a medical school, a form of ceremony that had sur-

Semeiotica Uranica:
OR, AN
ASTROLOGICAL
JUDGEMENT
OF
DISEASES
From the Decumbiture of the ſick
much Enlarged.
1. *From* Aven Ezra *by way of Introduction.*
2. *From* Noel Duret *by way of Direction.*
Wherein is laid down,
The way and manner of finding out the
Cauſe, Change, and End of the diſeaſe. Alſo
whether the ſick be likely to live or die; and the time
when Recovery or Death is to be expected.
With the Signs of Life or Death by the body of the Sick
party, according to the judgment of *Hippocrates.*
Whereunto is added,
A Table of Logiſticall Logarithmes, to find the exact
time of the Criſis *Hermes Triſmegiſtus* upon the firſt Decumbiture of the ſick: ſhewing the ſigns & conjectures
of the diſeaſe, and of life and death, by the good or evil
poſition of the Moon at the time of the Patients lying
down, or demanding the queſtion: Infallible ſigns to
know of what complexion any perſon is whatſoever:
With a compendious Treatiſe of Urine.

By NICHOLAS CULPEPER *Gent.*
Student in Phyſick and Aſtrologie.

Diſce, ſed ira cadat naſo, rugoſaque ſanna. Perſius.

London, Printed for *Nath. Brookes* at the Golden Angel on *Cornhil*, neer the *Exchange*, 1658.

Diagnosis of disease from the stars.

vived from the Middle Ages. It actually took a week or more of banqueting, arguing, speech making, and parading before the student was pronounced a doctor. In Moliere's play the graduation disputation is burlesqued by a ballet singing in a sort of "pig Latin." Latin was still the language of medicine, in spite of the efforts of Paracelsus to break down the tradition.

It was in the fourth performance of *Le Malade Imaginaire* that Molière, while playing his part, became weak and faint; he covered his hesitation with a forced laugh. After the play he was carried home; he died that night.

The seventeenth century was a period of scientific progress. There, for all to see, was an amazing contrast: on the one hand, science that flourished in the work of Vesalius, Sanctorius, Harvey, Malpighi; and, on the other, a practice of medicine that remained unchanged.

But the truth is, science did not help the doctor. It was of no assistance to him to learn that the blood circulated, for he did not know what function the blood served in the body; the knowledge of the circulation merely cast doubt on his cherished practice of bleeding. The measurements that Sanctorius had made did not help the doctor in the treatment of disease, for no one yet knew the significance of these measurements. The anatomy of Vesalius helped the surgeons, it is true, but not the physicians; there was as yet no connection between anatomy and disease except in the case of diseases curable with the knife.

The doctors were bewildered. The whole structure upon which they depended was being torn down about them. Galen was wrong; Arabian medicine was little better than superstition. The scientists told them that, but gave them nothing to replace the things they took away. Paracelsus said study Nature; the philosopher Descartes said the body was a machine to be studied as a machine; Van Helmont said it was a chemical reaction. The scientists could not even agree among themselves except in saying that Galen was wrong and the Arabs were wrong.

Science did no more for medicine than did the satire of

Molière. Both simply showed that medicine had not kept pace with the progress of the time. But the scientists themselves, when they practiced medicine, discarded their science and dealt with disease as Galen had directed. We have described the treatment given King Charles II; it was carried out in the same royal court in which half a century before Harvey himself had been physician.

This was the unfortunate situation when there entered upon the scene a man destined to start medical practice on the path of progress. What Hippocrates had done for the medicine of the fifth century B.C., Thomas Sydenham did for the medicine of the seventeenth century. He gave to medicine the form it holds today, he made it a discipline to which experimental science and mathematical science could make their contributions.

Sydenham was an English practitioner of medicine. He disclaimed the use of all science but nevertheless he was a scientist. He did not use the principle of experiment, he did not use mathematical proof, but he did observe and describe. He dealt with the practice of medicine in the same way that Vesalius had dealt with anatomy.

Sydenham was born in 1624, four years after the Pilgrims landed at Plymouth Rock. These were troublesome times for men of the Puritan faith; and Thomas had been brought up a Puritan. The year he entered Oxford University the Great Rebellion broke out. Leaving school he joined the forces against the king. Four years later the army disbanded, but Sydenham, then twenty-two, felt too old to start again in college. At a loss for a career, he decided to take up medicine. He entered the medical school of Oxford but he learned little there, for in the years that he had been campaigning he had forgotten his Latin. After two years of struggle with books and lectures, he was granted, largely through political influence, so it is said, the degree of bachelor of medicine. That was in the year 1648.

Almost at once war broke out again and Sydenham turned from medicine, with some relief we may suspect, to serve in the army, not as a surgeon, but as a captain of cavalry.

Events moved fast. In 1649 Charles I was beheaded; his son Charles II, then a refugee in Paris, took ship and landed first in Jersey and then in Scotland, where in 1651 he was crowned King of the Scots. The same year he was defeated by the army of Cromwell, and after many adventures he again escaped to France. In 1653 Oliver Cromwell became Lord Protector and Thomas Sydenham reluctantly settled down to practice medicine in Westminster. Politics still held his attention and he obtained an official position. But that was lost, and with it all hope of a political career, when in 1660 King Charles II was restored to the throne.

It looked very much as if Sydenham would have to practice medicine after all. He must have thought so himself, for he went for a year to the Medical School of Montpellier to make up some of the deficiencies of his education. Sydenham was thirty-nine when he passed his examination permitting him to practice medicine in London; he was fifty-two before he obtained his degree of doctor of medicine.

In his career with its many interruptions Sydenham had no opportunity to learn the science of the time, to study the anatomy of Vesalius, ponder over the discovery of Harvey, try the measurements of Sanctorius, or discuss the theories of Descartes. He was above all else a practical man, a soldier turned doctor. He approached the problem of medical practice with an open mind. The fact is that he had not had enough medical education to be spoiled by having drilled into him with all their weight the beliefs that the practitioners of medicine then held.

Education colors our views, determines the way we see and interpret the facts before us. If the views are false then we are actually blinded to realities; we cannot see them in their true importance and true relation. Instead, we see them only through the tinted and distorting glasses which bad education has put before our eyes. Primitive man, trained to believe in spirits, interpreted every fact of nature as a manifestation of spirits; the doctors of the seventeenth century, trained in the beliefs of Galen and of the Arabian physicians, saw in sickness only what these men had pointed out.

Paracelsus, you will remember, with all the strength of his egotistical personality, revolted against this kind of education. He wanted to use his own eyes and to see clearly. He came near seeing what Sydenham saw, but he expressed himself in a fashion far too mystical for other physicians of his time to understand.

There was nothing mystical about Sydenham. It was his practical army training rather than his medical training that seemed to influence his views and determine the way he would attack the problem of disease.

From earliest times, men had looked upon disease as one common thing with many different manifestations in the body. What physicians, philosophers, scientists had sought for was the cause of disease; they wished to solve the problem of disease as a whole.

Sydenham saw the problem differently. He knew that a good general does not plan his attack against enemies as a whole, but against each enemy separately. In warfare the general finds out first all there is to be learned about the enemy he is facing. He must study his position, numbers, armament. Then only when he has obtained all necessary information about the particular enemy can he plan and execute a successful attack.

Sydenham recognized that the same principle applied to diseases. He said in effect: the human mind is far too limited in its ability and knowledge to settle the great problems of what disease is and why there should be disease. While we debate such questions there are sick men who need help and for whom we as physicians are "answerable to God." The place to study disease is at the bedside of the sick man; by observation and experience we can learn the nature of diseases.

Hippocrates might have spoken these words. But there was one great difference between the method of Hippocrates

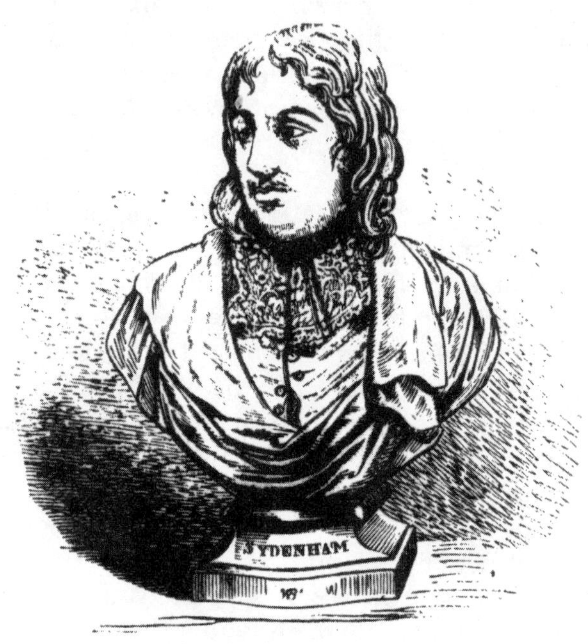

Sydenham.

and that of Sydenham. Hippocrates had studied the appearance and behavior of men who suffered from disease; he described how they looked and acted. From observation and experience he learned that when certain symptoms appeared the illness followed one course; with other symptoms it followed another course. He could thus judge, prognosticate, the probable outcome of the illness.

Sydenham on the contrary studied diseases. He believed that there was not one general illness with many different forms but that there were many different diseases. Each one was as definite and separate as were the different species of plants and animals. By careful study the physician could recognize the particular disease that affected the man just as a biologist could recognize a plant or animal.

According to Sydenham the particular disease attacks the body; the body in turn resists the disease and tries to overcome it by its inherent healing powers. The symptoms of disease result from the struggle between the body and the disease. These symptoms—the pain, the fever, the weakness—are not the disease itself, they are merely signs of the struggle that is going on, they are part of the body's effort to overcome the disease. With each kind of disease the struggle made by the body is different; therefore the symptoms are different. By studying the course of the illness carefully from the appearance of the first symptoms to the disappearance of the last, it should be possible, so Sydenham thought, to write a description of the disease itself—to write, as it were, the natural history of each disease.

It was to this task that he set himself. In 1675 he gave the first full and accurate account of scarlet fever and measles. He described smallpox, malaria, and dysentery. His masterpiece, published in 1683, was a description of gout, a disease from which he himself suffered.

Sydenham based his treatment on the idea that the physician should attempt to assist the natural healing powers of the body, to help it overcome the particular disease that affected it, not merely to overcome the symptoms—the signs of the struggle. He had no use whatever for the vast array of herbs and vile concoctions with which the pharmacopœia of his day supplied the doctor. He used only the few remedies which observation and experience showed him to be definitely beneficial—iron for anæmia, quinine for malaria, and sedatives to give rest and sleep and so to restore strength. Instead of using many medicines, as was the common procedure in medical practice then—you will recall those used on poor King Charles—he turned to other forms of treatment designed to build up the inherent self-healing powers of the body. He introduced such innovations as fresh air in the sick room, horseback riding for consumption, and cooling drinks for smallpox. Instead of attempting to adjust the disordered humors of the body or drive out disease with foul medicines, he tried to help the body heal itself.

The work of Sydenham brought system and order into medical practice to replace confusion. Since his time physicians have continued to describe diseases in the way that he did—separately.

If you look at an old textbook of medicine you will find it mainly a discussion of symptoms. One large section is devoted to fevers of all kinds, simple fevers, intermittent fevers, malignant fevers, fevers with eruptions, and so on. If then you turn to the pages of a modern text on the practice of medicine, you will find, thanks to Sydenham, not symptoms as the headings, but diseases, named, classified, and described so that they can be recognized.

Look under smallpox. You will find that smallpox is in brief an acute infection developing nine to fifteen days after exposure; that it begins with a chill, headache, pain in the back, and often vomiting followed by a rise in temperature and rapid pulse. Usually on the fourth day bright red spots appear, first on the face and arms and legs. The temperature falls. On the fifth or sixth day the red spots change to small blisters. About the eighth day pus appears in the blisters and the temperature again rises. In favorable cases the eruption subsides, the sores heal, often leaving scars, and normal health slowly returns. You will find much more detail, of course, for recognizing a disease even when it is fully described is sometimes difficult.

After reading a full description of smallpox and carefully examining many people with the disease, the physician has in mind a clear conception of the disease itself; he knows its natural history and its behavior and probable outcome. He can differentiate and treat each disease separately and not waste his efforts trying to treat diseases in general. But to do so he must study each patient thoroughly.

This conception was new in medicine. Hippocrates had urged physicians to study the sick man; Paracelsus had told them to turn from books and theories to the study of the disease state. But it was Sydenham who told them what to look for, how to describe disease, how to classify it. Here then was something concrete and practical for the physician to deal with—the natural history of separate diseases.

Following the method of Sydenham, many physicians began to study their patients carefully, began the work of compiling the description of individual diseases.

In making the study every possible clue that would lead to a more thorough description of the disease was followed. It was here that the contributions of mathematical science had their place. In smallpox the pulse was rapid; there was fever. These were clues. The pulse must be counted, the temperature taken in all diseases and comparison made so that these clues could be used to help distinguish one disease from another. New methods of diagnosis made the separation of the diseases easier and more certain. In the centuries between the time of Sydenham and our own we shall see in our story the rise and development of means of diagnosis, the stethoscope, the art of percussion, the X-ray, the serum tests and all the array of precise methods at the command of the modern physician.

In the scheme of diseases that Sydenham presented there was another place for science; it was to determine what changes occurred in the organs and tissues of the body in the separate diseases. It was here that the anatomy of Vesalius and the microscope of Galileo were to play their parts. In the centuries ahead of us we shall see the rise of a new study in medicine called pathology, the study of the changes in the flesh caused by diseases, the changes from which the symptoms of disease arise. Into the same scheme fitted the work of Harvey and all other scientists who were to study the functions of organs. How was the action of the heart affected by one disease or another; what was the significance of its altered action; what symptoms, what changes, what diseases even, arose from the disturbed function of the various organs? First the scientist must tell the physician what the organs did in the body, must describe their physiology.

And finally we shall come to still another study, of the cause of each separate disease, the thing which acts to produce the changes in the flesh and in the function. In that field, as we shall see, lies one of the greatest discoveries of modern science, the discovery of the bacterial cause of infectious diseases.

The great practical triumphs of modern medicine have been achieved in the years which lie between Sydenham's time and ours. For the majority of diseases there are precise descriptions, exact methods of diagnosis, an understanding of the changes within the body, and knowledge of means for prevention or treatment. It was Sydenham who pointed the way for the progress of medicine, who made it possible for medicine to keep up with science. Perhaps if Sydenham had not shown us how to attack the enemy disease, we today, in spite of science, might be as ignorant about diseases, as unhealthy, as short lived, as were the people of the seventeenth century.

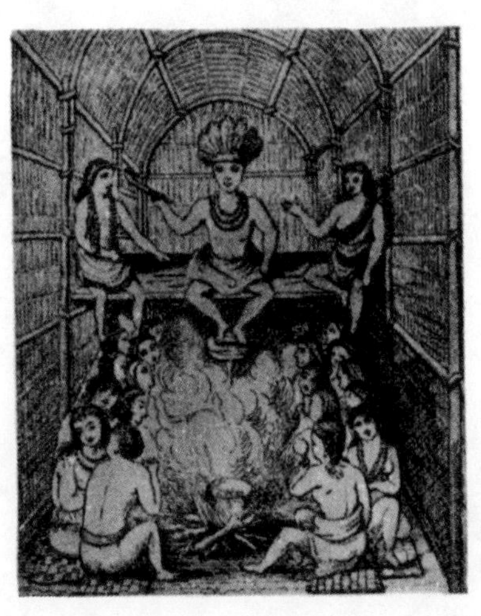

Part Eight

EUROPEAN MEDICINE COMES TO AMERICA

A CENTURY IN AMERICA

DOCTORS IN LACES AND FRILLS

CHAPTER XXII

European Medicine Comes to America

IN early chapters we saw the stream of medical knowledge emerge from the spirit-infested swamp in which primitive man lived, and flow turbid, muddy with false beliefs, into the earliest civilizations. We followed it from Egypt to Greece where it was freshened and widened by new sources. From Greece we traced it westward with Alexander and still farther westward with the Roman conquests. And then with the fall of the Empire we saw it recede eastward, through Byzantium, Syria, and into the Arabian Empire. In the days of the Crusades we again followed it westward into Italy, Germany, France, and England, sluggish and slow, but gradually gaining impetus. Finally in the seventeenth century we saw it abruptly widen and quicken, still carrying some of the flotsam and jetsam of the past, some superstitions, but flowing broader and deeper and more swiftly than it ever had before.

In the seventeenth century it again turned westward. English settlers bore their medical knowledge to the eastern shores of the New World. And there on plain and in forest, wherever settler met Indian, a curious contrast could be found. Medical knowledge accumulated through five thousand years and more of progress was brought face to face with the source from which it sprang. The medicine of the Indian was the medicine of primitive peoples, unchanged in one hundred and fifty centuries. The medicine of the settlers was that of Europe in the seventeenth century.

In the opening years of the century both settler and Indian were confronted with conditions new to them. The Spanish explorers, earlier comers to the New World than the settlers of Virginia and Plymouth, had brought to the continent infectious diseases from which the Indians had never before suffered. In great waves epidemics swept over the tribes, threatening to exterminate them.

What the disease or diseases were we do not know for sure; but it is certain that if the Indians had not been stricken they would have opposed more strongly than they did the landing of the colonists. Quite naturally, but rather uncharitably, the Pilgrims looked upon the affliction of the Indians as a special blessing sent by God to aid in the establishment upon these shores, as they said, of "a better stock."

The descriptions that eye-witnesses have left of the "prodigious pestilence" of the Indians are too meager and too biased to afford certain recognition. Some physicians of later date thought it smallpox, but that hardly seems likely, for the settlers were not affected at the time by the disease of the Indians, although in later years smallpox became a sore trial to them. Others have thought it bubonic plague, but certainly immigrants from plague-ridden London would have recognized that disease. And still others have believed it yellow fever, although it could not have been this disease, for yellow fever is carried only by a mosquito and the outbreaks occurred in the winter when there are no mosquitoes.

It seems very probable that the epidemic may have been measles. This is a disease that we consider one of the less important illnesses of childhood, but it can be very serious. There is a common belief among doctors that when a large part of the population of any country has suffered generation after generation from some disease, a partial resistance to it develops. The disease becomes as mild as measles is with us. But when this apparently mild disease is introduced to a people who have never had it, and hence are completely unresistant to it, it again becomes virulent and mortal.

In quite modern times an outbreak similar to that among the Indians occurred in the Fiji Islands. The King of Fiji, his family, and a number of his followers went aboard a British warship and were exposed to measles. The disease, which none of the natives had ever had, spread throughout the Islands. Within a few months nearly a third of the population had died. But the question has been raised: did they die because this disease became for a time more deadly among them or from lack of care? In civilized surroundings measles attacks a majority of the population, but only a few are sick at any one time and these are mostly children cared for by parents who years before have had measles and become immune. There in the Fiji Islands, however, nearly all the natives fell sick at the same time. There was no one left to care for them. Many, too ill to provide for their own wants, actually died of starvation.

Whatever the pestilence of the American Indians may have been, it afflicted them severely; all writers of the times agree on that. Daniel Gookin in his account of the Indian tribes says of the outbreak among the Pawkunnawkutts: "This people were a potent nation in former times, and could raise . . . about three thousand men . . . a very great number of them were swept away by an epidemic and unwonted sickness, An. 1612 and 1613. [It was in reality 1616 and 1617.] Thereby divine providence made way for the quiet and peaceable settlement of the English in those nations."

Of the Pawtuckets he says: "They were also a considerable people heretofore, about three thousand men. . . . But they also were almost completely destroyed by the great sickness . . . ; so that at this day they are not above two hundred and fifty men, besides women and children."

Of the way in which the Indians treated infectious diseases we have a description in the writings of an English traveler, John Josselyn, who visited the early settlements. He writes: "Their physicians are the Powaws or Indian Priests who cure sometimes by charms or medicines, but in general infections they seldom come amongst them, therefore they use their own remedies, which is sweating, etc. Their manner is when they have the plague as smallpox amongst them to cover their Wigwams with Bark so close that no Air can enter in . . . and making a great fire till they are in top sweat, and then run out in the Sea or River, and presently after they come into their Hutts again; they either recover or give up the Ghost."

John Lawson, who at the close of the century was surveyor-general of North Carolina, has left us an account of Indian surgery, although in this instance it is of a form hardly more beneficial than the common practice of scalping. He describes the way in which the Seneca Indians prevented prisoners from escaping:

"The Indian that put us in our path, had been a prisoner among the Sinnegars [Seneca Indians] but had outrun them, although they had cut his toes and half his feet away, which is a practice common amongst them. They first raise the skin, then cut away half the feet, and so wrap the skin over the stump and make a present cure of the wounds. This commonly disables them from making their escape, they being not so good travellers as before, and the impression of their half feet makes it easy to trace them."

Of the actual ministrations of the medicine man Lawson gives this account: "As soon as the doctor comes into the cabin, the sick person is set on a mat or skin stark naked, except some trifle. . . . In this manner the patient lies when the conjurer appears, and the King of that nation comes to attend him with a rattle made of a gourd with peas in it. This the King delivers into the doctor's hand whilst another brings a bowl of water and sets it down. Then the doctor begins and utters some few words very softly; afterwards he smells the patient's navel and belly; and sometimes scarifies him a little with a flint, or an instrument made of rattlesnake teeth for this purpose; then he sucks the patient and gets out a mouthful of blood and serum . . . which he spits in the bowl of water. Then he begins to mutter and talk apace, and at last to cut capers and clap his hands on his breech and sides, till he gets into a sweat, so that a stranger would think that he was running mad, now and then sucking the patient . . . still continuing his grimaces and antic postures, which are not to be matched in Bedlam. At last you will see the doctor all over of a dropping sweat, and scarcely able to utter one word, having quite spent himself; and then he will cease for awhile, and so begin again till he comes in the same pitch of raving and seeming madness as

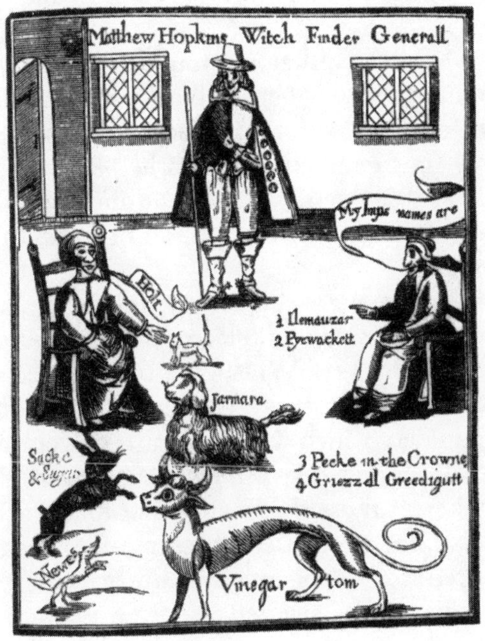

Matthew Hopkins, the famous "witch-finder."

before; all this time the sick body never so much as moves, although doubtless the lancing and sucking must be a great punishment to them. . . . At last the conjurer makes an end, and tells the patient's friends whether the patient will live or die; and then one that waits at this ceremony takes the blood away . . . and buries it in the ground in a place unknown to anyone but he that inters it."

Certainly the most famous example of the actual meeting

of primitive medicine and seventeenth-century medicine on the shores of America was the treatment of the Indian chief Massasoit. Word came to Plymouth that Massasoit, who had befriended the colonists, was dying. Edward Winslow, later Governor of the Plymouth Colony, and John Hamden went to offer sympathy and help to the chief. Governor Winslow in his *Good News from New England* tells of the incident:

"When we came thither we found the house so full of men as we could scarcely get in; though they used their best diligence to make way for us. They were in the midst of their charms for him making such a hellish noise, as to distemper us that were well. . . . About him were six or eight women, who chafed his arms, legs, and thighs, to keep heat in him."

Winslow finally made his way through the milling Indians to the chief's side and offered help. Massasoit nodded his consent. "And," says Winslow, "having a confection of many comfortable conserves, etc.; on the point of my knife I gave him some; which I could scarcely get through his teeth. When it was dissolved in his mouth, he swallowed the juice of it whereat those that were about him much rejoiced, saying, he had not swallowed anything in two days before. I then desired to see his mouth which was exceedingly furred; and his tongue swelled in such a manner, as it was not possible for him to eat such meat as they had, his [throat] being stopped up. Then I washed his mouth and scraped his tongue; and got abundance of corruption out of the same. . . . Then he desired to drink; I dissolved some of it [the confection] in water and gave him thereof. Within half an hour, this wrought a great alteration in him, in the eyes of all that beheld him." Next Winslow sent back to the colony for a chicken for broth and "such physic as the Surgeon durst administer."

While waiting the return of the messenger, Massasoit asked Winslow to go among the Indians, "requesting me to wash their mouths also and give to each of them some of the same I gave him. . . . This pains I took with willingness; though it were much offensive to me, not being accustomed to such poisonous savours."

The cure of Massasoit, as you will remember, had a most fortunate outcome for the colonists. In gratitude the chief revealed to Winslow the details of a conspiracy among the Indians to murder the English.

Winslow was not a doctor, but in those early days every man in the colonies of necessity learned something of practical medicine, just as he learned carpentry, farming, fishing, and hunting.

In the early years of the century, while the Indians suffered from the epidemics, the settlers themselves were having a tragic time learning to live under the conditions which they found in America. The voyage across the sea was long and there was sickness on the boats, especially scurvy from the lack of fresh food. When Francis Blackwell sailed from Amsterdam in 1618, only 50 out of 180 of the crew and passengers reached Virginia. That was of course an exceptionally high mortality, but even after more fortunate passages the survivors were weak and ill-nourished—and, one cannot doubt, frightfully homesick. Nor did their troubles end with the voyage; far from it; privation and sickness were awaiting them.

The colonists who landed at Cape Henry, Virginia, on April 26, 1607, and settled at Jamestown, had made a voyage of some ninety-six days. They disembarked on a fair day when the land was fresh with the flowers and grass of spring. William Strachey, secretary and recorder of the colony, described the new country in glowing terms. It seems to have been a failing of the early colonists to write home to friends and relatives of the comforts and prosperity they were enjoying in America, when in reality they were suffering and dying. Perhaps they were whistling to keep up their flagging courage, for George Percy, brother of the Earl of

Northumberland and one of the first settlers in Jamestown, has left quite a different account of conditions in the colony. He wrote: "Our men are destroyed with cruel disease, as swellings, flixes, burning fevers, and by wars and some departed suddenly. But for the most part they died of mere famine. There were never Englishmen left in a foreign country in such misery as we were, in this newly discovered Virginia. We watched every three nights lying on the bare, cold ground, what weather soever came; working all the next day which brought our men to be most feeble wretches. Our food was but a small can of barley sod in water to five men a day; our drink cold water taken out of the river, which was at flood very salty, at a low tide full of slime and filth . . . our men night and day groaned in every corner of the fort most pitiful to hear. If there were any conscience in men it would make their hearts bleed to hear the pitiful murmurings and outcries of our sick men, without relief every night and day for the space of six weeks; some departed out of the world, many times three or four in a night, in the morning their bodies trailed out of their cabins like dogs to be buried."

It has been estimated that 4170 immigrants landed in Virginia between 1607 and 1621. In 1624 the actual population was 1800.

Out of the hundred Pilgrims who landed at Plymouth in December, 1620, only fifty were alive in March. The immigrants who settled at Charlestown, although they arrived in the summer, suffered nearly as badly. They became ill when they ate berries in the fields and forests; they became ill again when they tried to live on the salt meat they had brought with them. The country was far hotter than any climate they had experienced. Sickness spread through the camp.

The Plymouth colony, more fortunate in having a man who acted as physician, Samuel Fuller, loaned their medical man to the inhabitants of Charlestown. He was unable to handle the situation there and wrote back, "Many are sick, and many are dead, the Lord in mercy look upon them." The immigrants, wholly ignorant of how a camp should be run, had allowed the grounds of their settlement to become filthy with decaying refuse. It was unfit for human habitation. The people deserted it and settled in what is now Boston.

Dr. Fuller of the Mayflower was not the first English physician to come to America; in fact he really held no medical degree. There is said to have been a doctor among the colonists of Jamestown. However he left soon and was replaced the following year by another who accompanied Captain John Smith on some of his voyages of exploration. After a few months his place was taken by still another doctor. None of these physicians appears to have remained long in the settlement. Perhaps they were merely recent medical graduates in search of experience. In those times it was common for such men to join a ship's company. In any event Captain Smith, when wounded in 1609 by an explosion of gunpowder, was forced to return to London for treatment, since at that date there were no physicians in the colony. Dr. John Pott was the first physician to live permanently in Virginia; he became governor in 1628.

With the growth of towns and harvesting of crops, the most trying days for the colonists were over. Immigrants came in ever increasing numbers and among them were a few trained physicians. Of these certainly the most famous was Dr. John Winthrop, Jr., first Governor of Connecticut and one of the early members of the Royal Society of England. Some of these early doctors were preachers as well; there was a strong tendency to combine the two callings. This situation may account at least in part for the fact that during epidemics of disease there were often proclaimed days for fasting and prayers of deliverance, to be followed by a feast of thanksgiving when the outbreak had passed. These spiritual appeals had something in common with what we call public health. Today, however, with public health, we turn to quarantine, sewage disposal, and water purification instead of fast days.

The earliest of the fast days proclaimed against disease was July 3, 1644; the records do not state what the disease was, but merely that "there was much sickness in the land." In the course of an epidemic of "chin-cough"—whooping cough—in the Plymouth colony about the year 1649, a number of fast days were held.

One after another the more common infectious diseases found their way to America; some in the seventeenth century and some not until the eighteenth. Influenza was epidemic in 1647, and in the same year yellow fever appeared in Massachusetts; in the next century it was to decimate the inhabitants of Philadelphia. Yellow fever was then prevalent in the Barbados, and to prevent its further spread to the mainland the first quarantine regulation in America was put into effect. In 1665 this quarantine was extended to all boats coming from England, for that was the year of the last great epidemic of bubonic plague in London. Diphtheria first appeared in 1659, in Kingston, New Hampshire, so it is said, and spread from there through the colonies, causing a frightful mortality among children. Scarlet fever was first observed in 1783.

The most important date in the history of American epidemics is 1663. That year virulent smallpox appeared in the Dutch settlement of New Netherlands. Fast days were proclaimed in rapid succession as the disease spread from town to town. We shall follow the history of smallpox in America in the next chapter, for the most important developments connected with it occurred in the eighteenth century; it was then that inoculation was first used in America to control it, and then also that vaccination was discovered in England. Smallpox in the seventeenth century in the colonies is, however, connected with one event of at least historical importance. The wide interest in the disease occasioned by the recurring epidemics led to the publication of the first medical book in America, the only one published here in the seventeenth century. It was written by a doctor-preacher of Boston named Thomas Thacher, and was called *Brief Rule to guide the Common People of New-England how to order themselves and theirs in the Small Pocks or Measels.* It consisted of a single page.

The first physicians who came to this country came before Sydenham's innovations had had any influence on medical education. They were trained in the theories of Galen; perhaps they knew something of the remedies of Paracelsus, and the anatomy of Vesalius, and the surgery of Paré. Oliver Wendell Holmes described a typical colonial physician:

"His pharmacopœia consisted mainly of simples, . . . St. John's wort and Clown's All-heal, with Spurge and Fennel, Saffron and Parsley, Elder and Snakeroot, with opium in some form, and roasted rhubarb and the Four Great Cold Seeds, and the two Resins . . . with the more familiar Scammony and Jalap and Black Hellebore. . . . He would order Iron now and then and possibly an occasional dose of Antimony. He would perhaps have had a rheumatic patient wrapped in the skin of a wolf or wild cat, and in case of a malignant fever with 'purples' . . . or of an obstinate king's evil he might have prescribed a certain black powder, which had been made by calcining toads in an earthen pot. . . . Sydenham had not yet cleansed the Pharmacopœia of its perilous stuff, but there is no doubt that the more sensible doctors of that day knew well enough that a good honest herb-tea which amused the patient and his nurse was all that was required to carry him through all common disorders."

Dr. Holmes used the words "sensible doctors," and certainly that applies to most of those who came to the colonies. Indeed there was about American medicine a practicality that distinguished it from European medicine, which in these years Molière was satirizing with his barbed pen. There was no appreciable audience for medical theorizers in the colonies; life was very hard and very serious for people there. Doctors must help and struggle as everyone helped and struggled.

There were no medical schools in America until well into the eighteenth century; the immigrant doctors were far too few to care for the population. Some of the young men went back to England for medical training, but many more obtained it by apprenticeship. The boy who intended to devote his life to medicine became a doctor's assistant. He lived in the doctor's home; took care of the doctor's horse and carriage, and rolled pills and mixed powders. In his spare moments he read in the doctor's library and learned the theories of medicine. But his real training was gained when he accompanied the doctor on visits to his patients. There at the bedside the older man pointed out to him the symptoms of disease and the treatment. As they walked or rode on to the home of the next patient, they discussed the case. This was a far different kind of education from that which young men were receiving in Europe where they learned largely from books. The apprenticeship of colonial days was essentially the same as the training given in the hospitals of the modern medical school. It is what is known as clinical instruction, one of the greatest advances in medical education. In colonial days the young doctors learned their medicine in the great school of practical experience.

CHAPTER XXIII

A Century in America

COTTON MATHER, the Puritan preacher of Boston, and Benjamin Franklin, the printer, diplomat, and philosopher, both played prominent parts in the medicine of the colonies in the early eighteenth century. Neither of them was a doctor.

Cotton Mather was a son of the President of Harvard College, Increase Mather. He was hot-headed and energetic and although he was primarily concerned with religion, he turned his restless attention to every event of the day. He wrote on witchcraft, in which he believed firmly, and he was implicated in the Salem witchcraft trials of 1692; he dabbled in politics with no success, he wrote on religion, science, history, and he tried his hand at treating his parishioners' physical as well as spiritual ailments. It is said that his favorite remedy was "sow-bugs" drowned in wine, a remedy quite in line with many then in the pharmacopœia of London. His fame, not as a doctor, but as a scholar, became international, but in 1713 he was elected to the Royal Society of London.

That was the first of a train of events leading to the establishing of his medical importance. As a member of the Society he received copies of the *Transactions*. Some time in the spring of 1721 he read in that august journal two descriptions of how the people of Turkey "buy the smallpox." Now smallpox in those days both in America and Europe, had become a frightfully prevalent disease, a terrifying specter in every home where there were children. Few indeed escaped the infection; millions died—in Europe alone in the eighteenth century sixty million—and many millions more were left marked and deformed for life. According to the article in the *Transactions*, the people of Turkey avoided the unpleasant consequences of the disease by a process called inoculation. Inoculation is not vaccination. The discovery of vaccination, the event with which we shall close the next chapter, came in 1798.

For an inoculation some of the pus was taken from the sores of a man actually sick with smallpox. A drop of this matter was then put in a scratch on the skin of a man who had not yet had smallpox. From this infection he soon developed the disease. But here is the important point: If he were to acquire smallpox by the usual means of infection, which seems to be connected with the salivary and nasal secretions, his illness would be severe indeed; of those who had smallpox, ten to seventy-five in every hundred died and those who survived were usually pockmarked. But when smallpox was given by inoculation the illness was mild; of those inoculated only one to three in every hundred died, and those who survived were not pockmarked. After smallpox by inoculation, as after smallpox by infection, there was immunity to the disease, that is, it was very rare for anyone to have a second attack. Inoculation was used by the people of Asia just as we now use vaccination—as a means of obtaining immunity to smallpox. There was, however, one great drawback to it. The people who "bought" the mild disease could spread the severe disease just as could those who acquired it by the usual mode of infection. Unless everyone were inoculated when very young, the practice tended to spread smallpox.

The description of inoculation that Cotton Mather read in the *Transactions* excited him immensely; here was a heaven-sent method for controlling a disease that at that moment was scourging the people of Boston. He would have them inoculated. But the procedure was beyond the medical skill of the enthusiastic Puritan—or perhaps for once in his life he did not want to take so great a responsibility. In any event he succeeded in obtaining the aid of a prominent Boston doctor, Zabdiel Boylston. Dr. Boylston, before he would risk it on any of his patients, tried it first on his only son, a boy of thirteen, and two negro servants. That was on June 26, 1721. The young men inoculated suffered no ill effects nor did they take the smallpox when a few weeks later Dr. Boylston took them to the pesthouse and exposed them freely to the patients with the disease.

Quite unknown to the colonists, the same experiment had been tried in April of the same year in England. Lady Mary

INOCULATION.

THE ſubſcriber reſpectfully informs the public that he has lately opened an Inoculation, at the pleaſantly ſituated hoſpital in Glaſtenbury; Gentlemen and Ladies who wiſh to have the Small-Pox by this ſafe and eaſy method, may be boarded, and have faithful attendance paid them, by their obedient,

ASAPH COLEMAN.

March 23, 1797.

EIGHT months is allowed by the Court of Probate for the diſtrict of Hartford, for the creditors of the eſtate of Col SAMUEL TALCOTT, late of Hartford deceaſed;

An advertisement of an "inoculation farm."

Wortley Montagu, wife of the Ambassador to Turkey, had her son inoculated while the family was still in Turkey. Returning to England, she attempted to interest the doctors of London in the advantages of inoculation. She had little better success in her efforts than did Cotton Mather and Dr. Boylston in the colonies.

During the epidemic of 1721 and 1722, Dr. Boylston inoculated 247 people in Boston; 39 were inoculated by other physicians. Six died. During the same period, 5759 citizens (more than half the population of Boston) acquired the disease by infection. Of these, 844 died. Many of those who recovered were disfigured with scars and broken in health.

Scarcely had the epidemic subsided when a violent controversy arose over inoculation. The physicians themselves turned against Dr. Boylston. The preachers from their pulpits and editors through their newspapers hurled invectives against inoculation. If a patient died, they said, the doctor who performed the inoculation should be hanged. Admittedly six patients had died. A bomb was thrown into Cotton Mather's home; Dr. Boylston was attacked on the streets; his house was set on fire, and a bomb was thrown into the parlor where his wife was sitting. The Massachusetts House of Representatives passed a bill to prohibit inoculation; but before it became a law, popular feeling had turned in favor of inoculation. Other epidemics of smallpox threatened.

Among the bitterest opponents of inoculation were the Franklin brothers, James and Benjamin, who in August of 1721 had established a paper called the *New England Courant*. The editorials in the journal were sensational for those days, and the denunciation of inoculation was particularly unsparing. Benjamin was then only sixteen years of age; as he grew older his views about inoculation changed. He had a son of his own who died of smallpox in 1736. In his famous *Autobiography* Franklin wrote: "A fine boy of four years old, by the smallpox, taken in the common way. I long regretted bitterly, and still regret I had not given it to him by inoculation. This I mention for the sake of parents who omit that operation, on the supposition that they should never forgive themselves, if a child died under it, my example showing that the regret may be the same either way, and therefore that the safer should be chosen."

Benjamin Franklin became one of the strongest supporters of inoculation; he urged the adoption of the practice in Philadelphia, where he set up his own printing press after leaving his brother James. The practice spread slowly, especially among those whom Franklin called "the common people of America." But opposition was not confined to them, for in 1747 Governor Clinton of New York issued a proclamation in which it was "strictly prohibited and forbidden all and every of the Doctors, Physicians, Surgeons and Practitioners of Physick . . . to inoculate for the smallpox any person or persons within the City and County of New York, on pain of being prosecuted to the utmost rigour of the law."

In equally stringent terms the practice is forbidden by law today, but for an entirely different reason. The modern laws were passed when at the close of the eighteenth century vaccination replaced inoculation. Smallpox cannot be spread by the person vaccinated, as it can by someone who has been inoculated.

In spite of Governor Clinton's proclamation the practice of inoculation grew, especially in Massachusetts, Connecticut, and Pennsylvania. In September, 1774, when the Continental Congress was in session, the physicians of Philadelphia agreed to inoculate no one during the time the visiting congressmen were there "as several of the Northern and Southern delegates are understood not to have had that disorder [smallpox]." It was feared that they might become infected from inoculated cases.

In Connecticut especially, judging from the advertisements in the papers, danger of infection was avoided by establishing "inoculation farms" out in the country, where "Ladies and Gentlemen who wish to have the smallpox by this safe and easy method may be boarded and have faithful attendance paid them."

George Washington was a strong advocate of inoculation and during the Revolutionary War ordered that all recruits to the Continental Army who had not already had smallpox should be inoculated. Martha Washington took the disease in this manner. In spite of the growing tolerance toward inoculation, it was by no means universally used; the epidemics of smallpox continued with frightful mortality among the uninoculated.

It was largely through the efforts of Benjamin Franklin that the first hospital was erected in the American colonies.

Franklin had come to Philadelphia in 1726 as an almost penniless young man. Twenty-five years later, wealthy and influential, he found time from his printing ventures to indulge in his many interests—politics, literature, philosophy,

To the Honorable
The Congress of the United-States
of America,

And to every Friend and Well-Wisher
To the Rights and Liberties of Mankind,

The following
VINDICATION
of his Public Character.

In the Station of Director-General
Of the Military Hospitals,

And Physician in Chief
To the American Army,

is,
With all deference to Rank and Authority,
And with all becoming Freedom,

Chearfully submitted
by
Their most Respectful
and most obedient
humble Servant,
JOHN MORGAN

Title-page of Dr. Morgan's Vindication.

medicine, and science. He became known abroad for his demonstration that lightning was electricity and his invention of the lightning rod, and was recognized as America's leading citizen.

In 1751 the idea was suggested to him by a friend, Dr.

Thomas Bond, that Philadelphia, the metropolis of the colonies, needed a hospital. In Franklin's masterly hands the idea soon grew into a reality. The hospital was opened in 1752 in a rented building. A few years later it was moved to a building erected for the purpose which stands today and is called the Pennsylvania Hospital.

In this hospital—and this is strange for the eighteenth century—insane people were taken as patients. The antics of the insane seem to have attracted many idle people who gathered about the windows and teased the inmates. The board of managers had a fence built; but the crowd clamored outside for admission. A gate was put in the fence and a notice posted that "persons who came out of curiosity to visit the house should pay a sum of money, a Groat at least, for admission."

Although people ill with all sorts of disease were admitted to the hospital, it was the insane, caged in the cellar, who aroused the most interest. One incident connected with a patient named Polly shows the rather informal hospital care of the times and incidentally casts some light on the amusements of the residents of Philadelphia. The records kept by one of the managers are full of the exploits of Polly. Here is one anecdote:

". . . I was walking on the Commons and heard a great noise. Where it came from I could not tell, but list'ning Attentively, I discovered it was from the blue house, and directing my course there, I found it to be the shouting of a great number of people. They were assembled to a Bull baiting. . . . The Animal appeared to be in a great rage, tho' much exhausted by the Dogs, before I reached the Scene of Action. Soon after I got there, a Small Mastiff was sett on, which he threw about ten feet high, and fell to the ground with his upper Jaw broke and Every tooth Out.

"A short rest was now again given to the Bull, when a presumptious little Man, to shew what he could do, ran towards the Animal, but returned faster than he went, for the creature took him under his breeches and tossed him about twelve feet from the end of the Rope.

"A new pack of dogs being procured to renew the fight, every Eye was turned to the Onset.

"At this moment Polly scaled the high fence, thro' the Crack of which she saw the battle and pitying the Bull, she pierced unseen thro' the Circle and ran up directly to the Ring; and without Shoes or Stockings; with her neck bare and her beautiful Ringlets wildly dangling over her Shoulders—her other Cloathing was her Shift only and a white petty coat; so that she appear'd more like a Ghost than a human Creature. When she reached the Bull (tho' almost before, he was in a Rage) she Accosted him—'Poor Bully! have they hurt you? they shall not hurt you any more,' and stroking his forehead and face she repeated 'they shall not, they shall not hurt thee.' This was indeed wonderful; but the Animal's behavior was not less so, for he no sooner saw her approach him, than he dropt his Head and became Mild and Gentle. As tho' he knew she was sent to deliver him.

"The whole Concourse of spectators saw it, and were Struck with Astonishment—not one of whom dared to enter into the Ring to save her; but stood trembling for Polly's life, afraid to stir a step and even to follow her on the Return, thro' the Midst of the dumb Struck Company, like an Arrow from the Bow Over the high fence again to the Hospital from which she eloped."

When this incident occurred, Philadelphia was the largest city in the colonies. Its population was about forty thousand; that of New York about thirty thousand; and that of the entire country less than four million.

It was in Philadelphia that the first medical school of the colonies was founded. Several of the more prominent physicians of Philadelphia had gone to Europe for their medical education, but many young men could not afford this expense. It was in their interest that Dr. John Morgan, on his return to Philadelphia from Europe, urged the founding of a medical school. There was in the city the college that later became the University of Pennsylvania; in 1765 in response to Dr. Morgan's urging, it opened a department for instruction in medicine. In this first medical school the doctors who were soon to become prominent in the Revolutionary War

EXTRACTS from LETTERS to the AUTHOR of the METALLIC DISCOVERY,

PIERPONT EDWARDS, Efq. Diftrict Attorney for the State of Connecticut.

DEAR SIR, *New-Haven, October 7, 1796.*

I SHOULD have written you laft week, had I then been able to afcertain certain facts, the rumor of which I had heard. A Mrs. Beers, a near neighbor to me, the wife of Eber Beers, and daughter of Capt. Samuel Huggins, of this town, had been, for fourteen weeks, exceedingly diftreffed with the Rheumatifm, to fuch a degree that for the fourteen weeks, previous to the 29th of laft month, fhe had not been able to walk acrofs her room even with crutches, fave only once, when fhe made out with the affiftance of crutches, to hobble part of the way acrofs her room.—On the 29th of September laft, fhe procured a fet of your Metallic Subftances, and in lefs than an hour after fhe had begun to ufe them, in the manner directed by you, fhe rofe from her chair, and walked about her houfe, and on the next day fhe went abroad to her neighbors, having thrown afide her crutches. I have this day

A testimonial for Perkins' tractors.

acted as teachers. They were Dr. Morgan, Dr. William Shippen, Jr., and Dr. Benjamin Rush.

The beginning of the war, as you know, found the colonies in a state of unpreparedness. There was little military organization, and there was no medical organization to care for the sick and wounded, and no time to build hospitals or to make surgical instruments. Each district sent out with its fighting men such doctors as were available; some were good and some were useless; some had surgical and medical supplies and some had none.

The first step toward organizing a medical department of the Continental Army was made in July, 1775, when the Continental Congress passed a resolution creating such a department with a director-general and chief physician at its head. Dr. Benjamin Church of Boston was appointed to this office. In October of the same year he was tried for treason and found guilty. Probably the grounds for the accusation were not well founded, for those were chaotic times when a breath of suspicion was enough to damn a man as a Tory. Dr. Church was put in prison, but obtained permission to sail to the West Indies. His boat was wrecked and all aboard were drowned.

Dr. Morgan became the next director-general. He, too, was soon dismissed. His vigorous efforts to establish a really effective medical service aroused the animosity of many of the less efficient doctors. Through political intrigue they succeeded in having Congress deprive him of his post. Dr. William Shippen, Jr., was appointed to succeed him. Benjamin Rush served under Shippen as surgeon-general of the Middle Division.

In spite of the work of Morgan, Shippen, and Rush, medical care during the Revolution was pitifully inadequate. The hospitals improvised in public buildings and private houses were hotbeds of infectious disease. There was an almost complete lack of surgical instruments and all the men capable of making these were manufacturing guns. The sick and wounded suffered frightfully from lack of food and bedding and nursing.

There were heroic doctors in the Revolution, but they were hopelessly handicapped by the conditions under which they were forced to work. However, if patients profited little from the doctors, the doctors profited a good deal from the war. It was the first time that men trained in medicine by apprenticeship in small towns were brought in contact with physicians educated in Europe. Ideas were exchanged, new interests aroused, and wider experience gained. American medicine grew up during the Revolution. In spirit at least the physicians were no longer colonial doctors of the backwoods; they were now doctors of a new country, the United States, and as such, they turned with a new vigor, a new feeling of union, to meet the scientific advances of the nineteenth century.

But before we come to that greatest of all centuries in medicine, there remains to be told the medical progress of Europe in the eighteenth century. We have dealt so far only with America. And there is also the story of America's first great contribution to medical quackery.

Science in America in the eighteenth century consisted of Benjamin Franklin's discoveries in electricity and some half dozen descriptions of diseases by American doctors after the manner of Sydenham. America aroused Europe's greatest interest with the amazing medical fad of Dr. Elisha Perkins. This was perhaps not extraordinary in view of the fact that medical superstition was more vigorous in Europe than in the colonies.

Elisha Perkins was graduated from Yale College late in the eighteenth century. He took up medicine, but in 1798 he developed a device that did away—so it seemed—with all further need for doctors. He invented the Perkins' tractor. The tractor consisted of a compass-like device of two rods, one sharp pointed and the other blunt. They were made of combinations of different kinds of metal, copper and zinc, gold and iron, or platinum and silver.

The tractor was stroked over the skin above the ailing place and the pain disappeared. The bimetallic rod suggested strongly a discovery that Luigi Galvani of Bologna had made in 1786; he observed that the legs of a dead frog twitched when brought in contact with two different metals. In 1792 the famous Alessandro Volta of Pavia, inventor of the electric battery, had written on animal electricity; and in America Franklin had brought electricity out of the clouds. Electricity was the subject of much popular discussion and much speculation; there was as yet little knowledge about its properties. But people were willing to credit miracles to this mysterious thing; and they were willing to believe in Perkins' tractors.

Of course, after going this far in our story you know that almost any remedy or medical procedure that catches and holds interest will drive pain away and make many people think for a time that they are cured of disease. Perkins with his tractors was practicing the same kind of medicine that the medicine man of primitive people, and Valentine Greatrakes and all such healers had used. Dr. Perkins was entirely sincere in his belief in the benefit to be derived from the tractors, and so were many thousands of people who bought and used them and gave testimonials.

The fad spread to Europe. An Institute of Perkinism was erected in London. The Perkins' tractor was the sensation of the day.

But in Europe there had been a whole century of progress since the days of the Touch for the King's Evil. Some men were learning to be skeptical in matters of science and to test remedies.

A Dr. John Haygarth of England tested the tractors. He used a method that Ambroise Paré might have and that a modern doctor certainly would have used—the control experiment. He made a pair of tractors out of wood and painted them to resemble metal. When he applied these to ailing people, their pain disappeared and they recovered just as quickly as when the real bimetallic tractors were used. He, too, collected testimonials. And then he disclosed his deception. At once the enthusiasm for Perkins' tractors collapsed. People were willing to be impressed by something that suggested electricity, but they knew that a chip of wood scratched over the skin cured no disease.

CHAPTER XXIV

Doctors in Laces and Frills

IN the seventeenth century Molière ridiculed the doctors of Europe as pompous asses. But in that same century Harvey and Sydenham did their work. If Molière had lived and written in the eighteenth century, he certainly would have characterized the doctors as fashionable fops; and he would have found rich fields for his satire in the charlatans and their patent medicines, for this was the "golden age" of quacks. And yet this century gave us the great French scientist Lavoisier who supplied the answer to the question of why men breathe; Morgagni who showed the changes in the body due to diseases; and Jenner who provided the race with one of its great boons, vaccination against smallpox.

In manners and customs the eighteenth was a century of artificiality, of strong class distinction, of powdered wigs and lace ruffs, of elaborate etiquette and poverty and brutality. It was not with pen and ink that the revolt against the injustices of the times was written but with steel and blood—the pike and guillotine of the French Revolution, the sword and musket of the American Revolution.

The fashionable doctor of England dressed as became an aristocrat; he wore a red coat, satin breeches, silk stockings, buckled shoes, a powdered wig and a three-cornered hat; he carried a goldheaded cane and often a fur muff to protect the delicacy of his hands. Perhaps behind him as he walked, which he rarely did, there followed at a respectful distance a footman bearing his gloves and satchel. More often he rode in a fashionable carriage drawn by elegantly equipped horses. Many doctors, so it is said, made it part of their business to gallop about London for the admiration of the people and to create the impression that they had very large practices.

Now when doctors pretended to the foppery of fashion it was easy for quacks to ape them, because what the public saw and admired in the doctor was not his skill in science but his polished behavior. All that the charlatan needed was an equal ostentation, an equal snobbery, an equal effrontery,

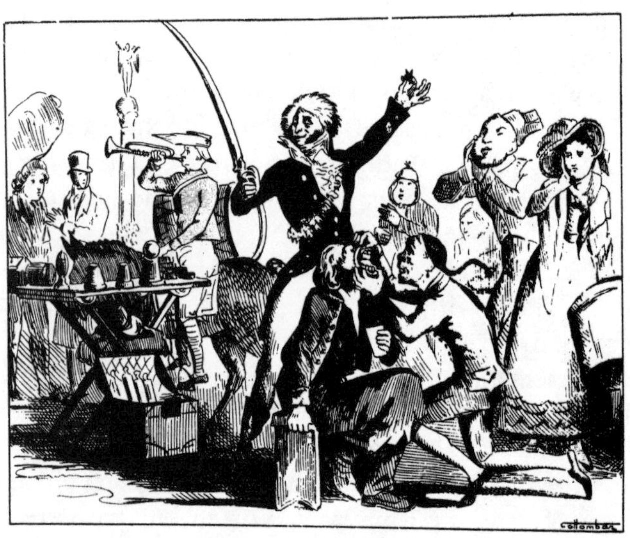

A mountebank dentist.

and he, as judged by the standards of the time, was likewise a great doctor. Many were the quacks who followed this device and made their fortunes.

The artist Hogarth in a satirical engraving has given us with others the likenesses of three of the greatest quacks of the century—"Spot" Ward, Chevalier Taylor, and Sally Mapp. The engraving is designed in heraldic fashion and is called the "Undertaker's Arms."

Joshua Ward, nicknamed "Spot" because of a birthmark on his face, took up medicine, but his preparation for it was slight. He had failed first as a drysalter and then as politician. He invented a variety of medicaments which had great popularity. Among his "patients" were Lord Chesterfield, Horace Walpole, and Edward Gibbon, the historian. He had the very good luck to cure by a sudden pull a dislocation of the thumb of King George II. After that his fortune was made. He was given a room at Whitehall; he asked that he might be buried in Westminster Abbey. His greatest claim to lasting distinction is that the poet Pope, and the lexicographer Johnson, deigned to notice him. Pope wrote of him:

Of late, without the least pretence to skill,
Ward's grown a famed physician by a pill.

And Johnson said: "Taylor was the most ignorant man I ever knew, but sprightly; Ward the dullest."

Taylor was the Chevalier Taylor of Hogarth's engraving. He was an apothecary's assistant; but he set himself up as an eye specialist. In this he did badly at first but he became a success as a traveling mountebank, dressed in the height of fashion, lecturing to the people from his carriage in inverted sentences to create, as he said, the impression that he spoke like Cicero. Among his patients was Gibbon, who seemed to have a failing for quacks, and Handel, the great German composer. Taylor was appointed oculist to King George II.

Taylor and Ward are shown in Hogarth's engraving holding goldheaded canes; Mrs. Mapp is brandishing a bone. Her claim to medical distinction lay in what is called "bonesetting." Bonesetting in turn arose from the idea that pain and illness result from bones slipping from their proper places. The bonesetter manipulates the leg, or foot, or arm, or spine, corrects the misplacement, and health is presumed to follow. The whole procedure is a "laying on of hands" but done with impressive force. Mrs. Mapp made a small fortune out of such manipulation and rivaled the fashionable physician with the magnificence of her dress and carriage and footmen.

Probably the greatest medical absurdity of the eighteenth century was perpetrated by another English woman, Joanna Stevens. She had, so she claimed, a remedy that was a certain cure for stone in the bladder, a complaint common in those times. Being a public-spirited lady she consented to part with the secret for $25,000. The amazing thing is that the money was actually given to her in the interest of the public by Act of Parliament. When published in 1739 in the *London Gazette*, her "cure" turned out to be a mixture of eggshells, soap, snails, together with an assortment of weeds and herbs.

It was to the same public that hoped to benefit from her medicine that Perkins' tractors made so strong an appeal. But unfortunately for the American, he appeared late on the scene; by the end of the eighteenth century physicians at least were not quite as gullible as they were in the more fashionable days before the Revolution.

The medical troubles of the eighteenth century went deeper than the mere foibles of fashionable medical practice and quackery; they extended even into the theories of medicine. Some physicians, to the profit of medical progress, patiently followed the rigorous method that Sydenham had pointed out—studying disease at the bedside of the patient. But many more, carried away by the tendencies around them, turned to making systems and building up classifications of disease quite as artificial as the manners of the times.

The fashion for classification was set by a physician who is known best as a botanist, Carl von Linné or Linnæus. His interest in medicine was romantic rather than scientific. He fell in love with the daughter of a wealthy physician; and the father would only consent to her marrying a physician. Linnæus thereupon studied medicine, and then, duly wed, returned to botany and zoölogy. He gave us the best classification of plants and animals that had been made up to that time; one that though modified is still in use. It was he who

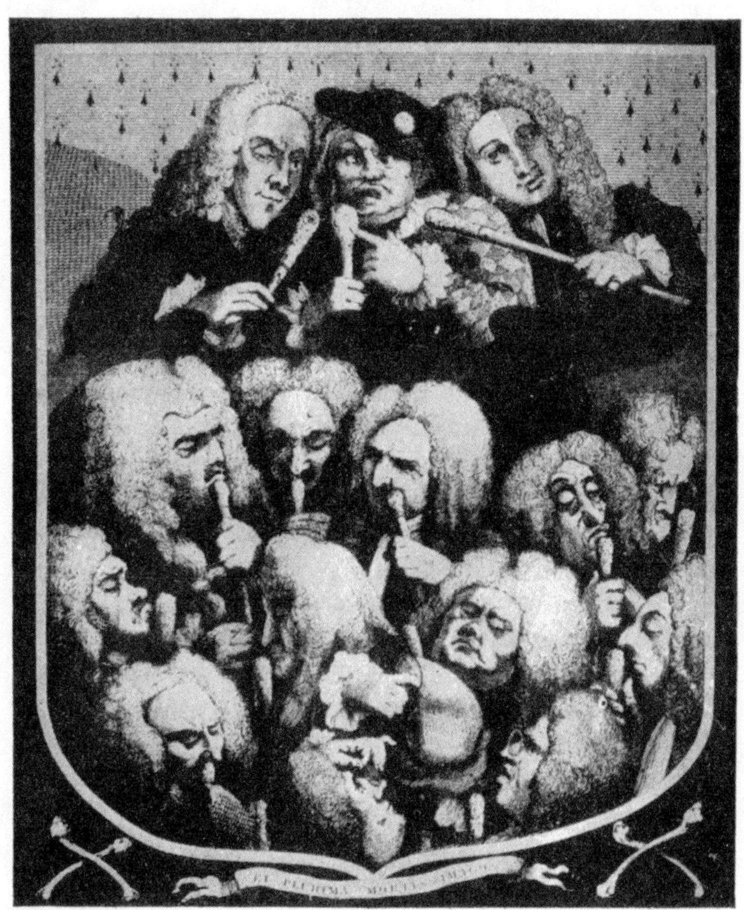

The "Undertaker's Arms."

classified man as an animal in the order of Primates and called him *Homo sapiens*—intelligent man.

Now man, for all of his intelligence, allows himself to be led easily from the arduous paths of search for facts. He finds it simpler to pause and speculate, and systematize. The great usefulness of the system of classifications made by Linnæus served as an excuse for physicians to attempt similar classifications of diseases and their symptoms and indeed of all aspects of life itself. Medicine was advanced little by these attempts at systematizing on which men wasted their energies and over which they engaged in violent controversies.

Certainly the most silly and at the same time the most popular of all the systems was one devised by Dr. John Brown of England. It had a tremendous influence on medical thought. As late as 1802 the argument between the Brunonian and non-Brunonian medical students of the University of Göttingen became so violent that it broke into a riot which was quelled only by the militia. The Brunonian system had at least the advantage of simplicity. According to it the essential of life was excitability; in disease there was either too much or too little "excitement." The remedy was to reëstablish the proper degree of excitability. To do this Dr. Brown used mainly two medicaments, opium and alcohol. He died of an overdose of his favorite remedies.

In the seventeenth century the greatest advance made in physiology had been allied to mechanics—the discovery of the circulation of the blood by the physician Harvey. In the eighteenth century there was an equally important advance, but it came this time from the new and rapidly growing field of chemistry—the discovery of the significance of breathing.

The chemists of the eighteenth century were particularly interested in air. Here was a thing that had always been taken for granted, but only in its physical aspects—its movements. The winds drove the boats across the water and, blowing over the land, turned windmills. And it was known that man must have air to live; but the belief again concerned the physical properties: the lungs were bellows which moved the air, and the resulting breeze cooled the blood. It was in the seventeenth and especially the eighteenth centuries that scientists began to realize that air had important chemical as well as physical properties. They were interested in the airlike substances to which the physician Van Helmont had given the name gases.

Robert Boyle, the English chemist, who took many but

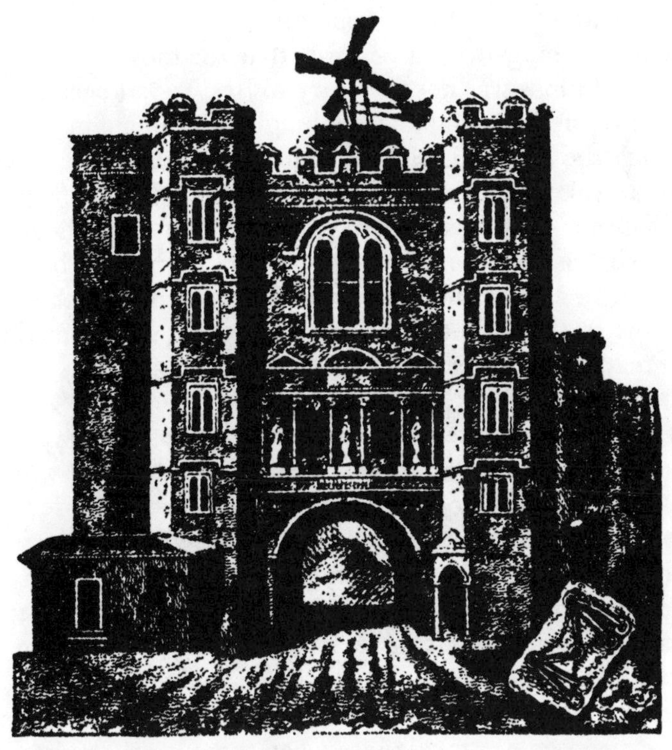

Stephen Hales's windmill ventilator on Newgate Prison.

not all of the useless and unpleasant medicaments out of the pharmacopœia in the seventeenth century, performed an experiment to show that an animal could not live or a flame burn in a vacuum. It was more than a hundred and fifty years later that the French scientist Antoine Laurent Lavoisier showed that man and the flame needed air for the same reason—because the process of living is one of combustion in which food is burned.

In the intervening years, clue after clue had been revealed to show the secret of breathing. Many of the more common gases had been discovered: those that we now call hydrogen, nitrogen, carbon dioxide and oxygen. It had been shown that an animal could be kept alive when air was blown through its lungs with a bellows, that the movement of the chest and lungs was not necessary to life. It had been shown also that the blood takes something from the air in passing through the lungs, and its color changes from purple to vermilion. Likewise men had learned that when a flame is burned in a closed vessel something is taken from the air so that what is left is no longer good for animals to breathe. In breathing, men and animals and fire not only took something from the air but they added something to it, something that made lime water turn white and turbid—the gas carbon dioxide.

Lavoisier took these separate observations and systematized them. He showed that nearly four-fifths of the volume of air is a gas, nitrogen, which will not support life; and one-fifth is a gas which he called oxygen, which is necessary to maintain life. It is the oxygen that combines with the blood in the lungs and changes its color. When a man breathes air into his lungs, part of the oxygen is taken up by his blood and in return another gas, carbon dioxide, is given off and breathed out. Lavosier showed that exactly this same exchange takes place when carbon such as charcoal is burned in air—oxygen from the air is used up and carbon dioxide formed.

Combustion, a burning of food, takes place then in the living body. The energy of the combustion appears as the heat that keeps the body warm, and as the work that the muscles perform. Air is necessary to life because oxygen is needed for the vital combustion. We breathe—not to cool the blood—but to obtain oxygen and to throw off carbon dioxide. Although it is the mechanical part of breathing that is most apparent, it is the chemical part that is the essential.

Physicians had small part indeed in the great discovery of why men breathe. But they had at least a connection—an unfortunate one—with the discoverer. Lavoisier was condemned to death by one doctor and executed on a machine invented by another.

Lavoisier was wealthy, he was an aristocrat, he dabbled in politics, and he lived in France during the closing years of the eighteenth century. An unpleasant combination for those days when common men were revolting in violence against social injustices.

Jean Paul Marat, the firebrand of the French Revolution, was a physician, and it was he who brought against Lavoisier the charge that as farmer-general he had oppressed the people. Lavoisier was condemned to death. He died under the guillotine invented by Dr. Joseph Ignace Guillotin.

Physicians had not even this much connection with another discovery in physiology made in the eighteenth century. It is to an English preacher, Stephen Hales that medicine owes the first attempt to measure the pressure of blood in the arteries—the blood pressure. Hales diversified his religious duties with scientific investigation; he invented artificial ventilation. A law had been passed putting a tax on windows; and to avoid payment the windows of tenements and prisons, which were then operated as concessions by private individuals, were boarded up. An epidemic of typhus fever broke out. The typhus of course was attributed to "bad air" and unpleasant smells. Hales attempted to purify the air in Newgate Prison by erecting on its tower a large fan wheel driven by a windmill. In spite of the usefulness of the invention of artificial ventilation it failed its purpose in this case, for it did not affect the lice which, as we know now, were really responsible for the typhus.

Hales's measurement of the blood pressure was carried

out, not on a human being, but on his horse. He fastened a large glass tube directly to an artery. The blood rose in the tube to a height of six feet or more and pulsated with each beat of the heart. This was the first real advance in the

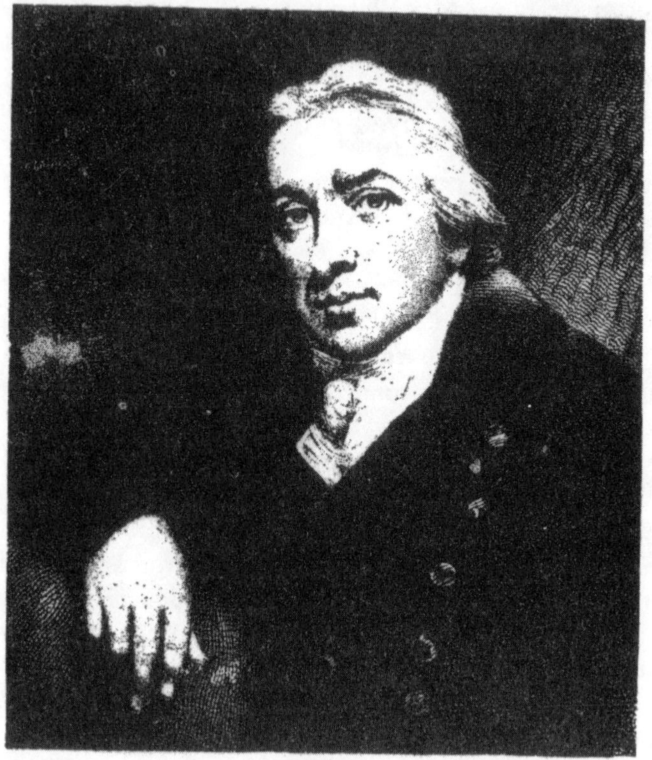

Edward Jenner.

physiology of the circulation of the blood since the days of Harvey, more than a century before. The physician of today finds in the measurement of the blood pressure one of his most useful methods of diagnosis, but needless to say he does not measure it on his patients as Hales did, but by a much simpler method, and a painless one. He finds out how tightly the arm must be squeezed by a rubber cuff into which air is blown from a bulb, to shut off momentarily the flow of blood. The pressure needed is the same as the pressure of the blood in the arteries.

So far in our account of eighteenth-century medicine, we have not dealt kindly with the doctors of Europe; physiology we have seen in the hands of the chemists and of a preacher; the doctors were more interested in fashions and systems and theories than in discovering facts. These were defects of the period. But in any time strong and earnest men may overcome such handicaps. And there were strong men of medicine in the eighteenth century. Although they were not scientists in the sense that the chemist Lavoisier was, although they were not seeking the fundamental facts of physiology as he and Harvey did, they nevertheless made practical contributions of vast importance to the progress of medicine. Three such men were Giovanni Morgagni, John Hunter, and Edward Jenner.

Morgagni takes us again to the famous University of Padua where Vesalius had carried out his dissections, where Sanctorious had taught, and where Harvey had studied. Morgagni held the position of professor of anatomy, the same post that Vesalius had held two hundred years before. Vesalius had studied the normal structure of the body and from his work we gained the first true understanding of human anatomy. Morgagni's attention was held by the abnormal structures of the body, those that were caused by disease, and he gave us our first knowledge of what is called pathology.

Many physicians before Morgagni had noticed that changes in the normal structure had occurred in the bodies of men who had died from disease. They had seen strange growths; they had found stones in the gall bladder; they had seen lungs red and firm like the liver instead of soft and pink as is the normal lung. These for Morgagni were clues to his discoveries; and just as Lavoisier had disclosed the secret of why men breathe, so Morgagni disclosed the reason why diseases give rise to symptoms.

Whenever he had the opportunity he dissected the bodies

AN

INQUIRY

INTO

THE CAUSES AND EFFECTS

OF

THE VARIOLÆ VACCINÆ,

A DISEASE

DISCOVERED IN SOME OF THE WESTERN COUNTIES OF ENGLAND,

PARTICULARLY

GLOUCESTERSHIRE,

AND KNOWN BY THE NAME OF

THE COW POX.

BY EDWARD JENNER, M.D. F.R.S. &c.

——QUID NOBIS CERTIUS IPSIS
SENSIBUS ESSE POTEST, QUO VERA AC FALSA NOTEMUS.

LUCRETIUS.

London:

PRINTED, FOR THE AUTHOR.

BY SAMPSON LOW, N°. 7, BERWICK STREET, SOHO:

AND SOLD BY LAW, AVE-MARIA LANE; AND MURRAY AND HIGHLEY, FLEET STREET

1798.

Title-page of Jenner's announcement of vaccination.

of those who had died of disease. He found, as other men had, changes in the organs. But he went further; he studied these changes in relation to the disease from which the man had died and to the symptoms which his illness had shown.

As he gradually accumulated his observations concerning one disease after another, he wrote of them in letters to his numerous friends in medicine. They in turn studied and confirmed his findings. Finally, in 1761, when Morgagni was seventy-nine years old, he published his life's work in a book—the first book of pathology. Thus only one hundred and thirty-nine years before the beginning of the twentieth century, physicians for the first time learned something of the changes in the body caused by diseases and of the symptoms that arose from them. With the aid of this knowledge the physician, by merely studying the symptoms, could determine the changes in the body caused by the disease. In the progress of medicine Morgagni takes his place with the great leaders: Hippocrates described the symptoms of disease, Sydenham the nature of diseases, and Morgagni the changes caused by diseases.

Morgagni's work was only the beginning of the great study of pathology which year by year since his time has brought us nearer the answer to the problem of what disease is. He did not use a microscope in his study; his descriptions were only of the changes that appeared to the naked eye. It was past the middle of the nineteenth century that the great Prussian scientist, Rudolf Virchow, carried Morgagni's work forward another stride and showed the nature of the changes produced by disease in the cells that make up the tissues.

The first field of medicine to profit from the study of pathology was surgery. Surgery, as we know it now, aims to correct by operation disease states within the body. Without a knowledge of pathology, surgery is a mere skilled trade of amputating limbs, treating wounds, and correcting those disturbances that can be seen or felt from the surface. Surgery before the work of John Hunter was little more than that. In the opening years of the eighteenth century it was much as Ambroise Paré had left it in the sixteenth. The physician still looked upon the surgeon as a man of inferior rank. But that social barrier was being broken down. In America, by force of necessity, the physician performed surgical operations. In France, in the early years of the eighteenth century, the surgeons publicly revolted against the physicians, refusing to open the doors of their meeting room to the procession of doctors clad in full regalia with ermine-trimmed robes. Left standing in the street in a snowstorm the ridiculous appearance of the doctors amused the spectators. The

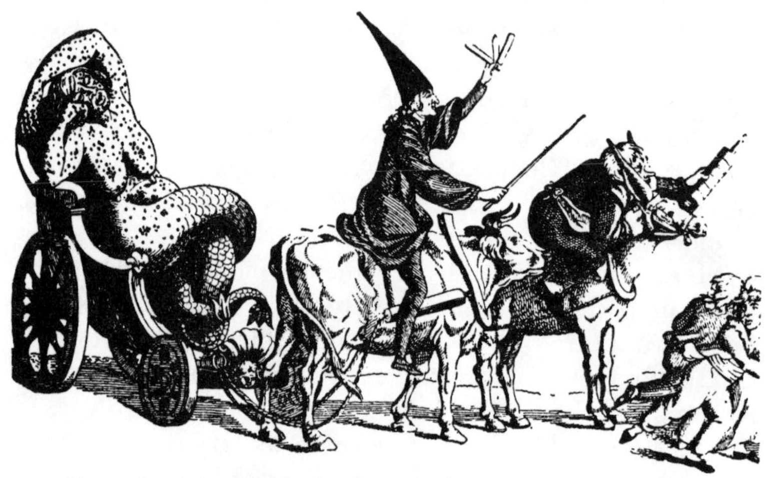

An anti-vaccination caricature published in 1800 intended to discourage the use of vaccination.

people sided with the surgeons and finally the fashionable physicians admitted the surgeons to an equal standing with them. In England a similar change was brought about in a way vastly more important to the progress of surgery.

John Hunter based surgery upon pathology and physiology. At his hands it acquired the aims of modern surgery. It was no longer sufficient for the surgeon to know merely anatomy and the tricks of his trade. Instead he must study physiology, pathology, diagnosis—in short, study all of medicine—and learn the operations of surgery in addition.

Under the influence of John Hunter surgery became a profession.

But even with this change there was still a vast difference between surgery then and now. Two of the greatest discoveries were to come in the nineteenth century—the use of antiseptics to prevent infections, and of anæsthetics to abolish pain. Until the middle of the nineteenth century, people under operation bore their pain as best they could, and were held down in their struggles by powerful men. The almost universal infection that followed prevented surgeons from performing operations within the abdomen; infection there was more deadly in its effect than anywhere else in the body.

John Hunter, like Sydenham in the previous century, had only snatches of education. He refused flatly to learn Latin. As a young man failing to do well in various occupations, he was sent from his Scottish home to London to assist his brother William, a prominent surgeon and teacher. In the dissecting room John found his place. He worked indefatigably; he dissected not only men but every variety of animal he could find in order to compare the structures of their bodies. He collected an enormous museum of specimens which is preserved today in the Royal College of Surgeons. There you will find his two greatest curiosities: the skeleton of a Sicilian dwarf, a girl of ten who was only one foot, eight inches high, and the skeleton of the famous Irish giant who was seven feet, six and a half inches. And what a time he had getting that enormous skeleton of O'Brien! When the giant became ill, Hunter watched over him with such solicitude that the poor man suspected the surgeon's ulterior motives. He made his friends promise faithfully that when he died they would never lose sight of his body until they had sealed it in a lead casket and sunk it in the sea. Nevertheless the skeleton stands today in the Hunterian Collection.

John Hunter leads us directly to the last of our medical heroes of the eighteenth century—Edward Jenner. Jenner was a pupil of Hunter, but, leaving him, he became a country practitioner in Gloucestershire. He was a man of pleasing appearance and kindly, gentle ways. He was also one of the greatest medical discoverers of all times. He gave us vaccination against smallpox.

A tradition among the dairy folks of the countryside led him to make his discovery. Now and again Jenner was called to inoculate against smallpox the members of some farmer's family. And often he could not succeed in giving the smallpox in this way to people who handled cows. "They've had the cowpox," said the farmers. That was the tradition. Those who had the disease called cowpox would never afterwards take the smallpox.

Cowpox appeared in the dairy cattle as small pus-filled sores on the skin. Men and girls handling the cattle sometimes acquired similar sores. Beyond the local effect which lasted only a short time, they were not ill. And yet tradition insisted that those who had had the cowpox never took the smallpox.

Here to Jenner was a thrilling possibility—something safe and simple to take the place of inoculation. But he had learned from John Hunter the principles of science. He could not jump at conclusions; he must obtain proof by experiment.

In 1796 cowpox broke out on a farm in Gloucestershire; a dairy maid named Sarah Nelmes contracted the disease. Jenner took from her sores a tiny drop of pus and put it in a scratch on the arm of an eight-year-old boy named James Phipps. Soon a small sore appeared on the boy's arm; he had the mark of cowpox only in that one place; it healed and left a tiny scar. Jenner waited. A month went by and then he again made a small scratch on the boy's arm; this time he rubbed over it the pus from the sores of a man with smallpox—he inoculated the boy. James did not become ill. Again a few months later Jenner inoculated him and still he did not take the smallpox. The tradition was true; cowpox protected against smallpox. Jenner wrote an account of his experiment and sent it to the Royal Society for publication in the *Transactions*. His letter was returned unpublished. The observation, the members of the Society thought, was

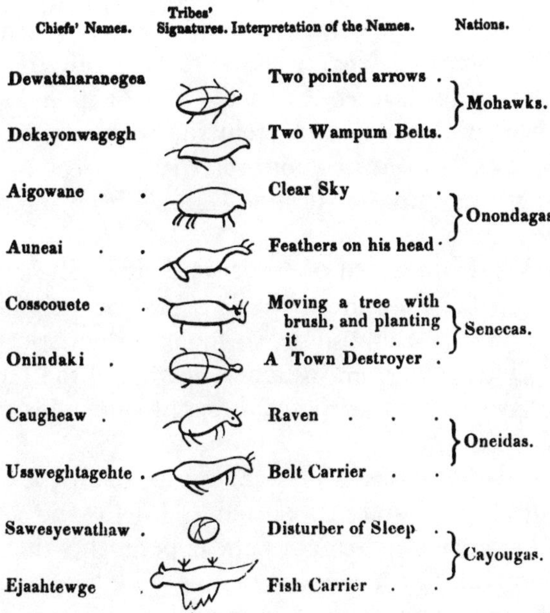

Chiefs' Names.	Tribes' Signatures.	Interpretation of the Names.	Nations.
Dewataharanegea		Two pointed arrows	Mohawks.
Dekayonwagegh		Two Wampum Belts.	
Aigowane		Clear Sky	Onondagas.
Auneai		Feathers on his head	
Cosscouete		Moving a tree with brush, and planting it	Senecas.
Onindaki		A Town Destroyer	
Caugheaw		Raven	Oneidas.
Ussweghtagehte		Belt Carrier	
Sawesyewathaw		Disturber of Sleep	Cayougas.
Ejaahtewge		Fish Carrier	

Signatures of Indian chiefs on the tribute to Jenner.

too amazing to be true. It was a mere chance that James had not taken the smallpox.

Encouraged by John Hunter, Jenner repeated his experiment on other subjects. He got the same result: cowpox protected against smallpox.

The evidence was beyond question, and so in 1798 Jenner published a book called *An Inquiry into the Causes and Effects of the Variolæ Vaccinæ*. It is only seventy-five pages long, but it is one of the great masterpieces in medical literature. It is literally because of that book that you and I have not had smallpox either from infection or by inoculation, which vaccination replaced.

Even Edward Jenner, in those closing years of the eighteenth century, could not in his writing wholly escape the affectation of his time. But fortunately he used most of it in the opening paragraphs of his book, which read:

"The deviation of Man from the state in which he was originally placed by Nature seems to have proved to him a prolific source of diseases. From the love of splendour, from indulgences of luxury, and from his fondness for amusement, he has familiarised himself with a great number of animals, which may not originally have been intended for his associates.

"The Wolf, disarmed of ferocity, is now pillowed in the lady's lap. The Cat, the little Tyger of our island, whose natural home is the forest, is equally domesticated and caressed. The Cow, the Hog, the Sheep, and the Horse, are all, for a variety of purposes, brought under his care and domination."

After this florid preamble leading up to cowpox, he discarded his fine style and reported as briefly and as clearly as would any scientist of today the experiments that demonstrated the validity of vaccination.

In the early days of the practice of vaccination, the procedure followed was in one respect vastly different from that of today. In Jenner's time no one knew anything about bacterial infection. The virus of the cowpox was taken from human subjects and passed from arm to arm. Infection sometimes followed, for bacteria were thus spread from one person to another. Today the virus is obtained only from calves kept in stables almost as clean as is the operating room of a hospital. The modern vaccine virus is a vastly purer product than the cleanest milk we drink.

In spite of crude methods, men of Jenner's time, faced constantly with the horrors of smallpox and the dangers of inoculation, could appreciate the blessing of vaccination.

From all over the world people paid tribute to Jenner. The American Indians sent a deputation to thank him personally and to bring him gifts. The Dowager Empress of Russia sent him a ring and gave the name Vaccinoff to the first child vaccinated in Russia. Napoleon ordered all the men of his great army vaccinated, just a little more than a quarter of a century after George Washington had ordered the men of the Continental Army inoculated.

The pathetic eagerness with which vaccination was welcomed by men who had seen their families ravaged with smallpox and the primitive way in which vaccination was given in the early years of the nineteenth century, led to one of the strangest of all voyages. In 1805, seven years after Jenner's announcement of his method for safely preventing smallpox, a ship set sail from Spain to the Spanish possessions in the New World. Its cargo was children. Each week two of the children were vaccinated from the sores on the arms of the two who had been vaccinated the week before. These children were the living bearers of vaccine virus to the lands where, nearly three hundred years before, the Spanish explorers had introduced the smallpox from Europe. Millions of people in the New World had died of the disease; millions of them are saved each year by the medical contribution of the eighteenth-century country doctor—Edward Jenner.

Florence Nightingale

Part Nine

MEDICINE AT THE BEDSIDE

IN THE OPERATING ROOM

IN BARRACKS AND PRISONS

CHAPTER XXV

Medicine at the Bedside

IN the year 1782 there was a vacancy in the staff of the Necker Hospital in Paris. A young physician named Jean Nicolas Corvisart presented himself before the board of governors and applied for the post. His medical qualifications were excellent, his recommendations the best. But he was refused the position. He was rejected because he wore no powdered wig!

But eighteenth-century emphasis on such matters was near its end. The Reign of Terror began in 1793. Fashionable heads, stripped of their wigs, fell under the knife of Dr. Guillotin's invention. These were days of chaos. All corporations aided or controlled by the state were abolished. There was no longer any regulation of medical practice; anyone could call himself a doctor and treat the sick. There was indeed no place where anyone could be trained in medicine; the medical schools were closed.

But doctors and especially surgeons were greatly needed. France was at war with Austria; she was at war with herself. The wounded must be cared for by trained men. New schools must be established. The old ones had taught the traditions of medicine from ancient texts long out of date. This was an era of a new democracy and a new progress. Men with aristocratic ways and old-fashioned ideas must yield to the new.

Medical education was a century—yes, three centuries—behind the times. The learned doctors still quibbled over the "authorities"; they ignored Paracelsus; they ignored Sydenham and Harvey and Sanctorius and Morgagni. Men were needed who would look not backward, but forward, who would seize and use everything that the new sciences offered for treating and preventing disease.

Medical education in the general form in which we know

it now grew out of the French Revolution. In the new schools of Paris there were laboratories for scientific study; students were taught at the bedside in the hospital, as Sydenham would have taught them. And it was Corvisart—he

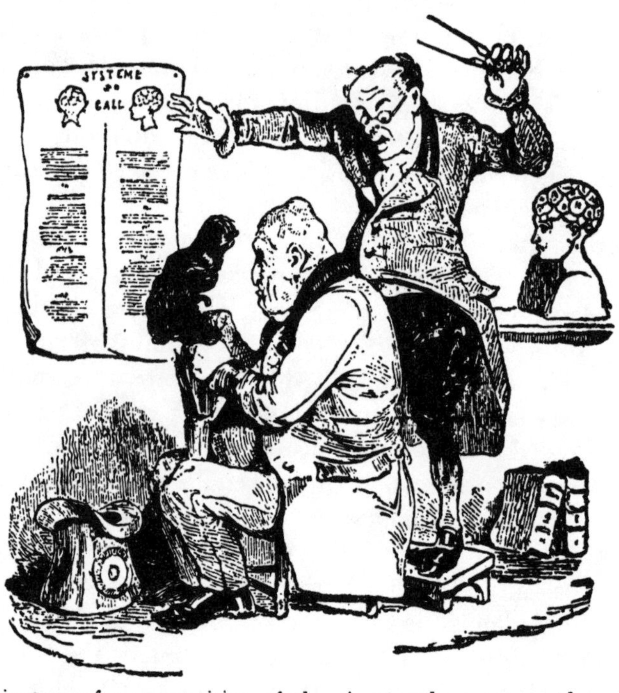

A caricature of a superstition of the nineteenth century—phrenology.

who wore no wig—who did the teaching, for under the new *régime*, he had become the leading professor of medicine.

Observe—train the senses to perceive the symptoms of disease—that was his watchword. He collected accurate observations in order to learn the natural history of diseases. And when possible he followed the example of Morgagni and noted from dissection, from autopsy, the changes in the body that caused the symptoms of disease.

This was in spirit modern medical education, but in those opening years of the nineteenth century few of the modern aids of diagnosis were available to Corvisart. Like Hippocrates, like Sydenham, he used only his bare hands and his keen senses in studying disease. True, more fortunate than Sanctorius, he had a watch and could easily count the pulse. But he was eager for other methods to aid in the elusive study of diseases.

He discovered that in 1761—the same year that Morgagni's book appeared—a Viennese doctor named Leopold Auenbrugger had published a book on what is called percussion. It was a small book, only ninety-five pages. It had failed to impress physicians and had been nearly forgotten. But Corvisart saw in it the possibility of a greatly needed means of diagnosis. He translated the book and amplified it from his own observations until it grew to more than four hundred pages. Corvisart gave full credit for the discovery to Auenbrugger.

In the preface of his little book, *Inventum novum ex percussione thoracis humani*, Auenbrugger had written: "I here present the reader with a new sign which I have discovered for detecting diseases of the chest. This consists in the percussion of the human thorax, whereby according to the character of the particular sounds elicited, an opinion is formed of the internal state. . . . In making public my discoveries . . . I have not been unconscious of the dangers I must encounter, since it has always been the fate of those who have illustrated or improved the arts and sciences by their discoveries to be beset by envy, malice, hatred, destruction and calumny."

But Auenbrugger was wrong in his prediction. His discovery was first received with indifference and then actually revised with praise by Corvisart.

Percussion is today a commonplace of medicine, something with which everyone is familiar who has been examined by a doctor. The physician taps with his finger on the chest and listens to detect the slight differences in the sounds as he percusses one place after another.

Over the lungs, since they are filled with air, the gentle tap on the chest elicits a reverberation like that of a muffled drum. Over the heart and liver the sound is dull. When there are diseased areas in the lungs they, too, may give out a dull note or one that sounds to the doctor's ear quite different from the reverberation of the normal chest. The percussion discovered by Auenbrugger and popularized by Corvisart, is one of the indispensable means of diagnosing disease in the lungs.

In 1807 Corvisart became the personal physician of Napoleon Bonaparte; he died in 1821. But the principles he taught were used by his pupils. And soon one of them discovered an instrument to aid in finding the symptoms of disease—the stethoscope—to be used in what is called auscultation, an art as indispensable to the modern physician as is that of percussion.

In auscultation the physician listens to the sounds that come from the lungs and from the heart. The gentle "swish" of air as it passes through the tiny bronchial tubes may be altered in disease, and harsh crackling or bubbling sounds appear; the regular "lub-dub" of the normal heart beat may be blurred with murmurs. These sounds allow the physician, with his trained ear, to "see" into the chest and find the seat of disease and learn its nature.

Long before the nineteenth-century physicians had occasionally practiced auscultation, but their observations had little meaning until the pathology of Morgagni showed the way of finding out the disease state from which the abnormal sounds arose. Even then, auscultation did not come into wide use; it was difficult indeed with the bare ear pressed to the chest to hear the faint sounds that denoted disease.

René Laënnec, physician-in-chief to the Necker Hospital —from which his teacher Corvisart had been turned away because he wore no wig—saw great possibilities in auscultation. He also found great difficulties in it. The patients in the hospital of those days, for all the seeming modernity of medicine, were often unwashed and infested with vermin.

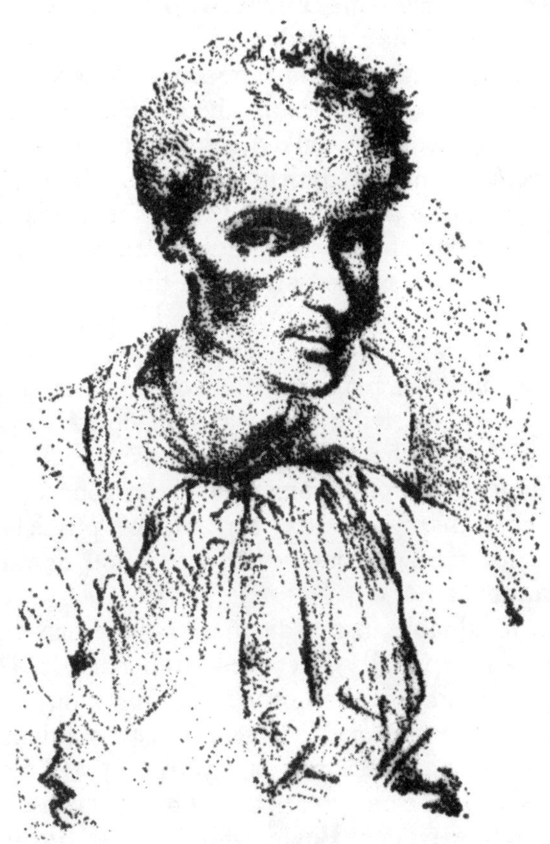

René Laënnec.

Putting the ear to a dirty chest was far from pleasant for a fastidious physician such as Laënnec. And there were even greater difficulties. Some patients were so fat that the faint sounds from the chest were deadened and lost.

It was in fact this very difficulty that led Laënnec to the

invention of the stethoscope. He had as a patient a fat girl suffering from heart disease; not a sound could he get from her well-insulated chest. One day on his way to the hospital, Laënnec chanced to walk through the gardens of the Louvre. He paused to watch some children at play on a pile of lumber. One child put his ear to the end of a long beam; another went to the opposite end and tapped on the wood. The signal traveled through the beam. There Laënnec saw the answer to his problem. He walked quickly to the hospital and in the room of his fat patient he seized a paper-covered book, rolled it into a cylinder and to the amazement of the onlookers put one end of this crude instrument against the patient's chest and applied his ear to the other. To his joy he heard the heart sounds clearly and those of breathing louder than he had ever heard them before.

Soon Laënnec was making little wooden "trumpets" on a turning lathe. The stethoscope was well on its way toward its modern form—the one with which we are all familiar: a tiny funnel to be put against the chest, connected to the rubber tubes that go to the ears of the physician. And equally important, Laënnec each day found new uses for his invention.

It was invaluable in the diagnosis of the one disease in which he was especially interested—tuberculosis. Half the patients who came to the hospitals of those days had this disease, so the stethoscope disclosed. After more than a thousand autopsies, Laënnec knew nearly all that we know today of this disease, save one great fact—how it is caused. It was he, and a fellow-student Boyle, who showed that the disease could appear in any part of the body as small lumps which they called tubercles—hence tuberculosis. Nearly a half century was to pass before the German doctor, Robert Koch, showed that these lumps are caused by a certain kind of bacteria.

In 1819 Laënnec published his famous book, *Traité de l'auscultation médiate*. In 1826 he died of tuberculosis.

Percussion and auscultation, the physician's two great methods of examination, were first used in the opening years of the nineteenth century; a third—the most amazing of all methods—was discovered in the closing years of the same century: the X-ray. This time the discoverer was not a physician, but a physicist. In the intervening years the progress of medicine had become inseparably connected with the progress of physics and chemistry and, indeed, all branches of science. No sooner was a discovery made in science than the doctor seized upon it, searching to find in it some valuable use in the diagnosis, the treatment, or prevention of disease. Medicine had lost its old-fashioned ways, it had fallen into step with science. In the seventeenth century the thermometer and the pulse pendulum of Sanctorius lay neglected; in the closing years of the nineteenth century Wilhelm Konrad Roentgen's discovery of the X-ray was seized upon and used in medicine within a month after he had announced it.

Roentgen was a professor in the Department of Physics at the University of Würzburg in Germany. He experimented with electrical discharges from an induction coil through a bulb called a Crookes tube. When the electrical discharge was passed the bulb glowed with a yellowish, greenish light. If a piece of paper coated with certain metallic salts was held in the light the coating glowed with a curious phosphorescence.

On November 18, 1895, Roentgen, working in his darkened laboratory, chanced to cover the Crookes tube with black paper to exclude all light. Then, with the tube darkened, he turned on the electrical discharge. No visible light appeared, but the coated paper lying on the table suddenly glowed with a mysterious ghostly light. It shone as brightly as it had before he put the black paper over the tube. Roentgen picked up the paper and turned its coated surface away from the tube. It continued to glow. An invisible ray was shining through the paper. He held a piece of metal before the paper; a shadow was cast; he held his hand before it and saw what no one had ever seen before—the shadow of the bones of his hand. The invisible ray that lighted up the paper passed through human flesh. And what is more, these same rays affected photographic film. It was possible to take

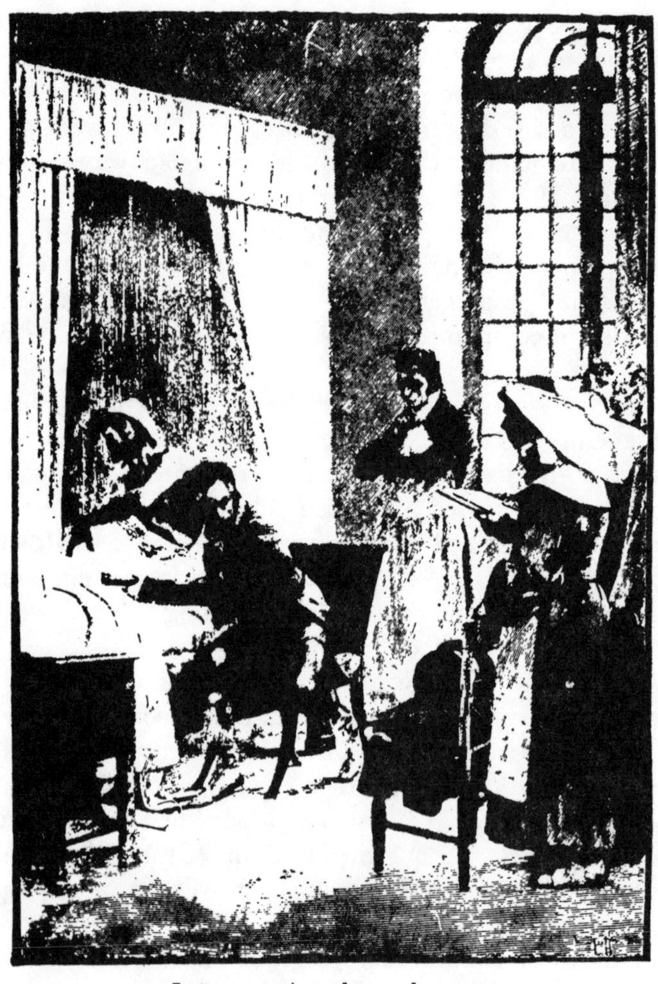

Laënnec using the stethoscope.

pictures of bone and structures beneath the surface of the skin.

Early in January, 1896, Professor Roentgen told a group of scientists at Würzburg of his discovery of what he called the X-ray. But even before that his secret had leaked out. Accounts appeared in the newspapers of all countries; but they were not accurate, and from them the reader got odd notions indeed of the new ray. It was believed that it could be used anywhere at any time. An English merchant promptly advertised X-ray proof clothes for modest ladies. A bill was introduced into the legislature of New Jersey prohibiting the use of X-rays in opera glasses at the theater and a professor in a New York university talked of using X-rays to penetrate the thick skulls of dull students and project knowledge directly into their brains. The doctors, however, were quick to sense the true possibilities of the X-ray.

In the four decades that have passed since Roentgen announced his discovery, the X-ray has become one of the most valuable methods of diagnosis—a method that allows the physician to actually see within the body and detect the changes which Morgagni first showed as foci of diseases.

By the time the X-ray had been discovered, medical education had been through nearly a century of progress since the days of Corvisart. Great schools had grown up throughout the world. Medical progress had become international. For a time, at the hands of some great teacher, one school or another grew supreme and became the Mecca for doctors—as England had been for the doctors of colonial America.

Following France, the schools of Vienna and Berlin led for a time in medical progress. In Berlin the pathology of Morgagni was carried a long step forward, as we have already said, by Dr. Rudolf Virchow. Virchow was born in 1821—the same year that Corvisart died; he graduated from medical school in 1843, and that year began his teaching as an assistant in the school in Berlin.

A great scientific discovery was in those years attracting the attention of physicians with its possibilities for a nearer approach to the nature of disease. Physicians recognized that organs, and even tissues of the body, might become disordered and appear abnormal; that the symptoms of disease might arise from these changes. But there was still the age-long question of what is disease? Why and how do the changes appear in the flesh? There was only a vague theory for answer. In these years so near our own, the theory of Hippocrates and Galen—of the disordered humors—was still advanced to explain the cause of disease.

In the seventeenth century when the microscope was a scientific novelty, men had seen that some plant substances seemed to be made up of tiny blocks or cells. Gradually, with the perfection of the microscope, details were seen in the structure of these units. And finally, in the nineteenth century, the microscope disclosed the fact that human flesh was likewise made up of cells. The cell was the smallest unit of living tissue. The tissues of the body were aggregations of cells; one tissue differed from another because of the differences in the cells of which they were constructed. When flesh grew, the increase in size was due to the multiplication of cells. When it was diseased—and this was Virchow's discovery—it was the cells that were changed and disordered. Their disorder in turn affected the appearance of the tissue to the naked eye—causing the changes which Morgagni had described.

With that knowledge, the microscope became another of the indispensable instruments for the study of disease. To-day the modern physician turns to his microscope to study the blood: to count the red cells, for if they are lacking anæmia exists; to count the white cells in order to judge from their number the possibility of a patient's having an infection; to examine tissues suspected of harboring that anarchy of cell growth that we call cancer. The microscope serves a thousand purposes in the study of disease.

Rudolf Virchow, who gave us the modern cellular theory of disease, lived until 1902.

Structure is only one aspect of tissues and organs; function is another. Physiology as well as pathology must make its contribution to medical progress. And one of the earliest

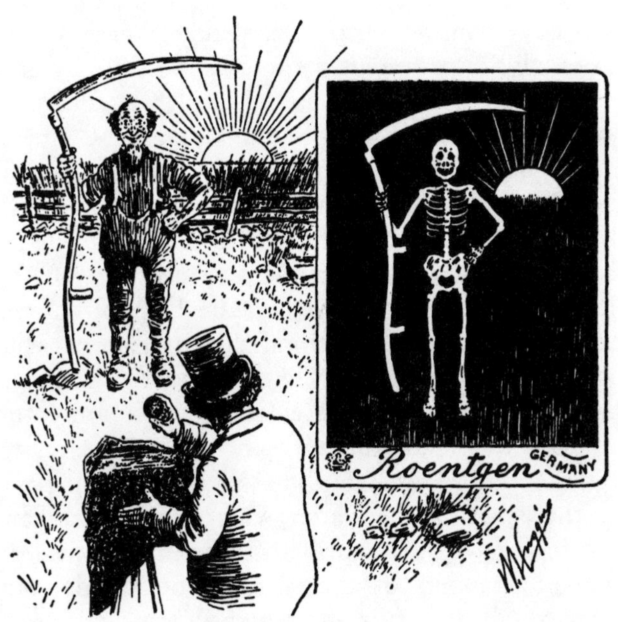

An early cartoon of Roentgen's discovery of the X-ray published in Life.

and most important of its advances takes us from the learned professors of the cities of Europe to a simple army surgeon in the backwoods of America. It was William Beaumont, stationed in the early years of the nineteenth century at the frontier post, Fort Mackinac, who gave us the first clear account of what happens in the stomach during the digestion of food.

There had been many theories to explain digestion. Some

men had thought that the food was ground up in the stomach; others that it "cooked" or simmered there; still others —and they had performed experiments on birds and dogs and even on themselves—were certain that the food underwent some sort of fermentation. But no one was certain. The stomach was looked upon as a mill, a fermenting vat, or a stewpan.

It was Beaumont who proved that digestion was a chemical process; his experiments were made possible by an accident.

Beaumont was born in 1785 at Lebanon, Connecticut. Leaving home in 1806 with all of his possessions—a horse and sled, a barrel of cider, and one hundred dollars—he set out to make his way alone in the world. For a time he taught school and then, becoming interested in medicine, he decided to be a doctor. He did not go to a medical school—American medical education was far behind that of Europe—but instead took an apprenticeship with a practicing physician. After two years of study, he enlisted in the army for the War of 1812 as an assistant surgeon.

After the war he was stationed at the trading post and fort on the island in the waters where Lake Michigan and Lake Huron unite. In the spring of the year, the traders and hunters and trappers of the surrounding woods came to Mackinac to sell their furs and replenish their stock of food. In the spring of 1822 a gun was discharged by accident into the midst of the crowd that filled the store. A French Canadian named Alexis St. Martin received the full charge in the abdomen. Surgeon Beaumont was called from the fort to treat him. It seemed impossible at first to save his life; a great gaping wound had been opened into his stomach. For three years Beaumont nursed him. Finally there came a day when Alexis, thin and pale, could walk about. But the wound had not healed completely, nor would it ever heal; a small flap of flesh covered an opening that led into the stomach; when the flap was pushed aside the interior of the stomach could be seen. Beaumont realized the possibilities that existed for actually watching digestion and the movements of the stomach. He employed Alexis and day by day he carried on his investigations. He studied the rate at which various kinds of food were digested; he collected the secretion formed; he noted the effect of alcohol and of indigestible food. For two months the studies went on and then Alexis deserted Beaumont. He returned to Canada, married and had two children; there, after four years of search, Beaumont finally found him. Again the experiments were undertaken and carried on for two years. In 1833 Beaumont published his work: *Experiments and Observations on the Gastric Juice and the Physiology of Digestion*—the first medical contribution to experimental science to come from America and one that established the basis of our present knowledge of digestion in the stomach.

Beaumont died at the age of 68; his patient Alexis lived to be 83.

Chance alone gave Beaumont the opportunity to make his contribution to physiology. The study of that subject was carried on by the great French physiologist, Claude Bernard, who really founded what is called experimental medicine. But even his discoveries were often as much due to accident as was that of Beaumont. Thus it was by chance that he found that the liver stores, for future use, sugar brought to it from the digestion of food in the intestines. The studies that followed from that observation laid the groundwork for a great discovery of the twentieth century—a means for controlling the disease diabetes, in which the body fails to burn sugar. Discovery after discovery came from his investigations; knowledge of digestion in the intestines, the way the blood vessels are controlled in size, the first facts concerning what are called internal secretions (chemical substances that control the functions of the body), the action of certain poisons, and many, many more. But perhaps most important of all was the fact that it was he who made physicians see for the first time that the organs of the body do not act independently but are linked together and work together and must be studied together. The liver, the heart, the lungs, were to be looked upon only in their relation to the man as a whole. This was a step that had a profound influence on the development of modern physiology.

In this chapter we have seen medical progress taking new

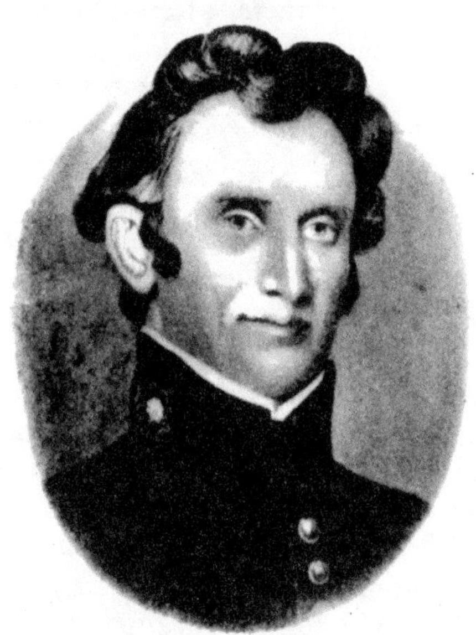

William Beaumont.

shape as the result of great discoveries and new conceptions and medical education well launched toward its modern form. The doctor of today was being shaped in the years that gave us Corvisart, Virchow, Beaumont, and Bernard. But medical education in the early part of the century was sometimes faced with a peculiar difficulty; it was one that led to a morbid chapter in medical history. There was intensive opposition to anatomical dissection and it was only after the anatomy riots and the notorious murders of Burke and Hare, that the modern anatomy laws were passed. Under these laws the unclaimed bodies of paupers are turned over to medical schools for the dissection so essential to medical education.

In the eighteenth and early nineteenth centuries there were no laws of this kind in England or America. Bodies were sometimes obtained by robbing graves. And suspicion of grave robbery was often turned against those who taught anatomy. Dr. William Shippen, Jr., of Philadelphia, the surgeon-general in the American Revolution, was once shot at by a mob angered by rumors of grave robbery. In 1788 in New York City a mob stormed a hospital where dissections were performed and burned the anatomical collection. The doctors took refuge in jail and the militia was called out. Seven rioters were killed and several severely wounded. The following year the state legislature authorized the dissection of the bodies of men executed for burglary, arson, and murder.

In 1831 Massachusetts passed the first law in this country making available for dissection "deceased persons, required to be buried at publick expence." That law and those to come after it in most of the other states, were the aftermath of a great medical scandal that occurred in Edinburgh, Scotland, then a prominent center of anatomical instruction.

Men called "Resurrectionists" often supplied the schools by robbing graves. In 1827, William Hare and William Burke in partnership undertook a less laborious way of obtaining bodies—they used the simple expedient of murder. Sixteen bodies were obtained in this way and sold before they were detected. They were careful to attack only those whose disappearance would attract little attention. Suspicion was finally aroused when they murdered a good-natured but feeble-minded man, a character on the streets of Edinburgh, known as "Daft Jamie." They were arrested. Hare turned state's evidence; Burke was hanged in 1829 before a gathering of thirty thousand people—among them it is said was Sir Walter Scott. This sensational and disreputable episode led to the passage of laws to provide for the dissection necessary in medical schools.

CHAPTER XXVI

In the Operating Room

THERE are men living today who were born before the time when means were found for relieving the pain of surgical operation. There are many people who can remember from their own experience when there was no way of preventing the infection that almost invariably followed any operation, or indeed, any wound. In those days, less than a lifetime removed from our own, surgical operation was the last resort of necessity, to be tried only when all other forms of treatment had failed.

Today most of us at some time in our lives are treated by surgery, but a vastly different surgery from what our grandfathers knew. We no longer need view an operation with horror, but rather with some calm and a genuine thankfulness that we live in a time when the discoveries of the nineteenth century have given us the oblivion of anæsthesia that does away with pain and the safety of antisepsis and asepsis that removes the danger of infection. These medical discoveries have kept from our lives many of the cruelest hardships our ancestors suffered.

From earliest time men had tried to overcome the pain of operation. Drugs and alcohol, numbing of flesh with cold or pressure, and hypnotism were all tried and none was successful. Pain was apparently inevitable, an ordeal not only for the patient, but for the surgeon. In compassion the surgeon attempted to shorten the agony by working with the greatest speed; and when an operation had to be completed in a few seconds, it could not be the careful and precise procedure that the best surgery requires.

It is strange how often discoveries lie already made before our eyes without our really seeing them. In 1800 the English chemist Sir Humphrey Davy recorded the fact that inhalation of the gas nitrous oxide produced unconsciousness; he wrote: "It may probably be used with advantage in surgical operations." But no one used it for nearly half a century.

Surgical anæsthesia was an American discovery that was discovered twice within a few years. The first physician to use an anæsthetic for an operation was Crawford Long of Georgia. He used ether. This substance had been known for many years; some doctors even were aware of the fact that if its vapors were inhaled, drunkenness and unconsciousness might follow. Dr. Long was the first to put this chance observation to practical use.

In March, 1842, he removed a small tumor from the neck of a patient; during the operation the man inhaled the fumes of ether. He suffered no pain. Unfortunately, Dr. Long did not publish a report of his success; indeed his discovery remained unknown until the effects of ether had been rediscovered and anæsthesia had become an accepted part of surgery.

Strange to say, before ether again came into use the anæsthetic effects of nitrous oxide were again discovered, and this time by a dentist of Hartford, Connecticut, named Horace Wells.

In the forties, lectures were a popular form of entertainment. And in 1844 a man named Colton gave a series of lectures in Hartford on the new discoveries of chemistry. He demonstrated in his lectures the effects of nitrous oxide. His advertisement in the newspapers announced that he would allow members of the audience to inhale the gas which would make them laugh and talk and sing. He promised to have twelve strong men in the front row to protect the spectators against harm from the exuberant antics of those who became drunk from the gas.

Horace Wells and a friend attended the lecture. The friend volunteered as one of the subjects. Dazed from the gas, he became pugnacious and, so the story says, jumped from the stage to grapple with one of the "strong men" in the front row. The guardian of safety fled and after him went Wells's friend. To cut short the chase, he jumped over the back of a bench. He caught his leg and fell to the floor. Sobered by the blow he made his way shamefacedly back to his seat beside Wells. The lecture continued; and then suddenly the man with Wells noticed that his leg was bleeding.

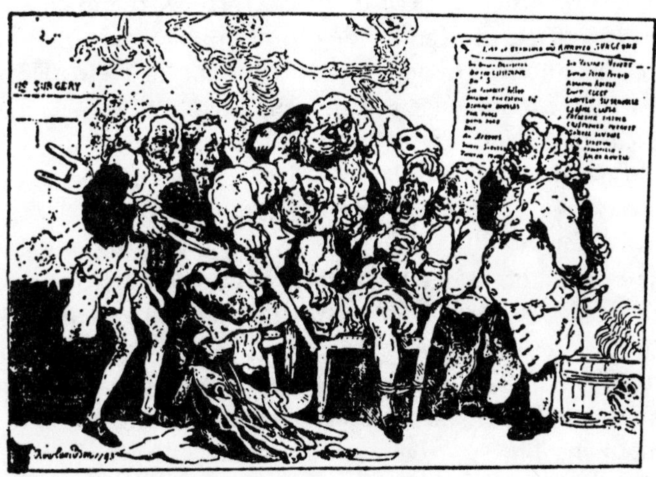

A caricature of eighteenth-century surgery.

He pulled up his trousers to expose a ragged gash that he had received when he struck against the bench. He was surprised at the sight of the wound, for he had felt no pain. Wells questioned him closely; still he insisted that he had not felt the blow.

The next day Horace Wells prepared a bag of nitrous oxide; he had a tooth pulled as he inhaled the "laughing gas," and he felt nothing. Convinced that he had arrived at a long sought goal, he went to Boston to the Massachusetts General Hospital and offered to exhibit the properties of nitrous oxide. But there his efforts failed. Without special apparatus nitrous oxide is difficult to administer; the patient whose tooth he extracted revived from the gas before the operation was over and screamed his pain. Wells went home discouraged.

But another dentist named William Morton, who knew Wells, continued where he left off. Morton was a student in the Harvard School of Medicine, as well as a dentist. One of his professors, a chemist named Jackson, suggested to him that he try ether instead of gas. Morton experimented on himself and on the family dog, and finally used ether with success as an anæsthetic for the extraction of teeth. He was ready then for his great venture, the use of ether for a major surgical operation. He asked Dr. Warren, chief surgeon of the Massachusetts General Hospital, for permission to make the test. The request was granted; the day was set for October 16. This was in 1846.

The story of that demonstration has become one of the classics of medicine. Rumor spread that some medical student had presumed to offer a method for abolishing the pain of operation. The gallery of the operating amphitheater was crowded with incredulous spectators. The patient was brought in. The surgeon waited, dressed in formal morning clothes—in those days surgeons did not wear white gowns, nor did they wash their hands before operating, but only afterward, for Lister had not yet shown that infection might come from dirty hands. At the appointed time the surgeon, the patient, the strong men to hold him down in his struggles, the spectators, were all ready, but Morton was not present. A quarter of an hour passed, and then Dr. Warren, taking his knife in hand, turned to the spectators and said, "As Dr. Morton has not arrived, I presume he is otherwise engaged." The audience smiled—they had been skeptical all along. Dr. Warren touched his knife to the skin of the shrinking patient. At that moment—so the story goes—the door opened and in came Morton. He had been delayed in completing an apparatus to administer the ether. Dr. Warren stepped back, pointed to the man strapped to the operating table, and said, "Well, sir, your patient is ready." Amid the silence of the spectators, surrounded by unsympathetic faces, Morton administered the ether. In a few minutes he looked up and said, "Dr. Warren, *your* patient is ready." The incredulous audience watched in silence as the operation was begun. The patient gave no sign of pain; he was obviously alive—everyone could see his breathing; he slept. With the completion of the operation, Dr. Warren turned to the spectators, and said, "Gentlemen, this is no humbug."

Anæsthesia for surgical operation was a demonstrated reality. But the men in that operating room did not call it anæsthesia; the phenomenon was new and there was no term in the language to describe it. Oliver Wendell Holmes later coined the words anæsthesia, anæsthetic, and anæsthetist.

The operating room at the Massachusetts General Hospital where the demonstration was made has stood unchanged ever since that day in 1846, a memorial to the first public demonstration of the blessing of anæsthesia. If by chance you visit it, you will realize that its very appearance also commemorates a second great discovery in surgery. It is an ordinary room of the period, with wooden floors, carpet strips and drab painted walls. It has no white tiles or shining metal, and none of the scrupulous cleanliness of the modern operating room. The story of the change with all that it embodies in freedom from infection takes us from America to Scotland.

In 1854 a young surgeon, an English Quaker named Joseph Lister, went to Edinburgh. Six years later he had risen to the position of professor of surgery in the University of Glasgow and embarked on the career that made him the greatest surgeon of all times. The problem that held his attention was infection in wounds. The formation of pus, the development of fever, were believed to be due to the state of the weather, and to evil smells in the air, or else were considered inevitable in all wounds resulting from violence and indeed, as we have seen, a regular part of healing. Infection, whatever its cause, made surgery a discouraging task. Lister operated skilfully and cared for his patients carefully; they did well for a day or two, and then the infection set in. Half or more died of what we should call blood poisoning. A surgical operation in Lister's hospital or in any other at the time was nearly as dangerous as bubonic plague. What made matters worse was that it seemed to make little difference whether the operation was grave or slight. In either case the infection came and the blood poisoning followed.

Lister, studying the problem, observed a curious fact which gave him the clue to his discovery. There were men in the wards with broken legs and broken arms. They were wounded, but the wound was under the skin. Such wounds did not become infected. The air did not reach them. Something from the air, reasoned Lister, poisoned the wound and caused infection.

The next clue came from the work of a French chemist, Louis Pasteur. He had been employed by the wine industry of France to study the diseases of wines. Wines sometimes became "sick," lost their pleasant odor and spoiled. Pasteur found that the sickness was due to the growth of bacteria that got into the wine from the air. To prevent the growth of these "germs," he had developed a process of treating the wine by heat. The process has ever since been known by his name, "Pasteurization."

Lister, reading of Pasteur's discovery, saw a similarity between the putrefaction of wine and the infection of wounds. The something from the air that caused the "putrefaction" in open wounds might well be bacteria. If that should prove true, then he had to prevent the bacteria from getting in the wound or, if that were impossible, kill them before they had multiplied and spread.

He decided to start his experiments with a wound that was already infected. But first he must find something with

A **GRAND EXHIBITION** of the effects produced by inhaling NITROUS OXIDE, EXHILARATING or LAUGHING GAS! will be given at *UNION HALL, THIS (Tuesday) EVENING, Dec.* 10th, 1844.

FORTY GALLONS OF GAS will be prepared and administered to all in the audience who desire to inhale it.

TWELVE YOUNG MEN have volunteered to inhale the Gas, to commence the entertainment.

EIGHT STRONG MEN are engaged to occupy the front seats, to protect those under the influence of the Gas from injuring themselves or others. This course is adopted that no apprehension of danger may be entertained. Probably no one will attempt to fight.

THE EFFECT of the GAS is to make those who inhale it either Laugh, Sing, Dance, Speak or Fight, &c., &c., according to the leading trait of their character. They seem to retain consciousness enough to not say or do that which they would have occasion to regret.

N. B. The Gas will be administered only to gentlemen of the first respectability. The object is to make the entertainment in every respect a genteel affair.

MR. COLTON, who offers this entertainment, gave two of the same character last Spring, in the Broadway Tabernacle, New York which were attended by over four thousand ladies and gentlemen, a full account of which may be found in the New Mirror of April 6th, by N P. Willis. Being on a visit to Hartford, he offers this entertainment at the earnest solicitation of friends. It is his wish and intention to *deserve* and receive the patronage of the first class. He believes he can make them laugh more than they have for six months previous. The entertainment is *scientific* to those who *make* it scientific.

Those who inhale the Gas once, are always anxious to inhale it the second time. There is not an exception to this rule.

No language can describe the delightful sensation produced. Robert Southey, (poet) once said that "the atmosphere of the highest of all possible heavens must be composed of this Gas."

For a full account of the effect produced upon some of the most distinguished men of Europe, see Hooper's Medical Dictionary, under the head of Nitrogen.

Mr. COLTON will be the first to inhale the Gas.

The History and properties of the Gas will be explained at the commencement of the entertainment.

The entertainment will close with a few of the most surprising CHEMICAL EXPERIMENTS.

Mr. COLTON will give a private entertainment to those Ladies who desire to inhale the Gas, TUESDAY, between 12 and 1 o'clock, FREE. None but Ladies will be admitted. This is *intended* for those who desire to inhale the Gas although others will be admitted.

Entertainment to commence at 7 o'clock. Tickets 25 cents—for sale at the principal Bookstores and at the Door.

dec 10 1d

Colton's announcement in the Hartford Courant, *December 10, 1844.*

which to kill the bacteria; obviously he could not Pasteurize a man. He turned to chemical substances in the hope of finding one that would kill bacteria. Strangely enough, at this time his attention was called to the use of carbolic acid in treating sewage to prevent unpleasant odors. He decided to try it.

His preparations were now made, but he waited ten months for the arrival of a case in which he could feel justified in trying the experiment. Finally a man suffering from a compound fracture was brought to the hospital. A compound fracture is one in which the ends of the broken bone are forced through the flesh and skin, making an open wound. Simple fractures, those in which there is no opening to the air, healed in Lister's wards, as we have said, without infection. Compound fractures were always infected, and in Lister's time, for lack of a way to control the spread of infection, it was usually necessary to amputate the limb. Even then the result was often fatal.

Lister applied carbolic acid to the wound of the fracture and built a small tent over it to exclude the air. In spite of all these precautions, infection developed, blood poisoning followed, and the patient died. But Lister persisted. For later cases he washed his instruments in carbolic acid; he dipped his hands in the antiseptic, and sprayed a mist of it in the air about the room; he took every precaution to clean the wound and to keep bacteria from entering it. This time he succeeded; pus did not form or blood poisoning occur. The infection was controlled.

Soon he was using the spray of carbolic acid in the operating room and carrying out in all operations the procedure that had succeeded with the compound fracture. Infection and fever disappeared; the clean wounds healed quickly and safely. Vastly fewer deaths occurred.

In those early days Lister was convinced that the germs causing infection came from the air. In fact, so strongly did he insist upon the unpleasant spray of carbolic acid in the air of the operating room that other surgeons thought he was trying to introduce a new medicine; their attention was distracted from the fundamental principle he was advocating —the principle of preventing the spread of infection by the use of antiseptics. Lister went his way calmly, indifferent to opposition, performing safely operations which other surgeons feared to do and saving the lives of the patients in his wards.

Reports of Lister's work spread to the continent and soon foreign surgeons came to visit him and learn his methods. The Franco-Prussian War broke out and antiseptics were used on the wounded with great success.

Gradually as experience grew, the belief that the germs of infection came from the air gave way to the knowledge that they came from filth ground into wounds, from the unclean hands and instruments of the surgeons, and from dirty bandages. So cleanliness—surgical cleanliness or asepsis—became the dominant idea of surgery. The modern operating room, the scrupulously clean hospital, the white-gowned surgeon, all are the result of Lister's discovery that infection in wounds is due to the presence of bacteria.

With the new safe surgery, freed from the fear of ever-present infection, surgeons for the first time could operate successfully on parts of the body where few had ever dared to operate—especially the abdomen and joints. Before Lister's time, men and women and children had appendicitis just as they do today. But the surgeon, even if he had fully understood the condition, could not have saved their lives by operation. The dangers of infection were far too great. A whole new field of surgery was opened up by Lister's discovery. And what is equally important, for the first time in all history, medicine had given a reason for cleanliness, in the home and office and factory as well as in the hospital and operating room. But cleanliness did not wholly replace the use of antiseptics even in the operating room. Instruments could be sterilized with heat, but not the surgeon's hands or the patient's skin. For these antiseptics must be used. And besides, there were still wounds from accidents in which bacteria were present. Knowledge of the need of antiseptics spread, until now everyone knows of their necessity in the first aid treatment of even slight injuries. Fortunately we today have better and safer antiseptics than the carbolic acid that was first used.

Lister died in 1912—two years too soon to see the greatest vindication of his principles of antisepsis made in the World War, on the germ-ridden battlefields of France and Belgium. Thousands upon thousands of veterans who live today owe their lives to Lister, just as do hundreds of thousands of other men and women and children wounded in peacetime accidents or in operations.

CHAPTER XXVII

In Barracks and Prisons

AGAIN we return to the time of the French Revolution, to the events that gave Corvisart his opportunity for reorganizing medical education and that cost Lavoisier his head. Great national changes were underway: the States-General had assembled, the Bastille had been stormed, the Rights of Man proclaimed, the palace invaded, the king beheaded, and France was a republic. The Commune ruled. Out of fanaticism and patriotism and oratory, the members of that body shaped the policies of a nation and defined the Rights of Man. The extreme radicals were gaining power rapidly and the Reign of Terror was about to burst on France.

But an event perhaps more important to the future of the civilized world than those of politics and bloodshed was brought to pass amid the turmoil by a frail and timid doctor named Philippe Pinel. He had nerved himself to appear before the Commune and asked to be allowed to plead for the rights of his patients. He was repulsed. Again and again he came, and finally the burly Couthon, the firebrand of the Commune, condescended to listen to his plea.

Pinel told Couthon that if all men had equal rights then his poor insane patients in the prison of Bicêtre should share in them. They were chained in filthy dungeons; their fate was far more unjust than had been that of the common man at the hands of the aristocrat before the Revolution; they should be sheltered in kindness and given reasonable liberty.

Couthon, although he regarded Pinel as a wild visionary, was touched on a sensitive spot—his treasured reputation for equality. He consented to go with Pinel to the prison. Long used though he was to deal with the savage element of society, he flinched before the scene at the Bicêtre. In the damp corridors of an underground prison he was greeted by the shouts and execrations of three hundred lunatics, by the creaking of chains, the pounding of manacles against iron bars. Couthon exclaimed to Pinel, *"Ah, ça! citoyen, es-tu fou toi-même de vouloir déchainer de pareils animaux?"* (Citizen, are you crazy yourself to want to unchain such beasts?). Pinel insisted. Retreating from the filthy cells,

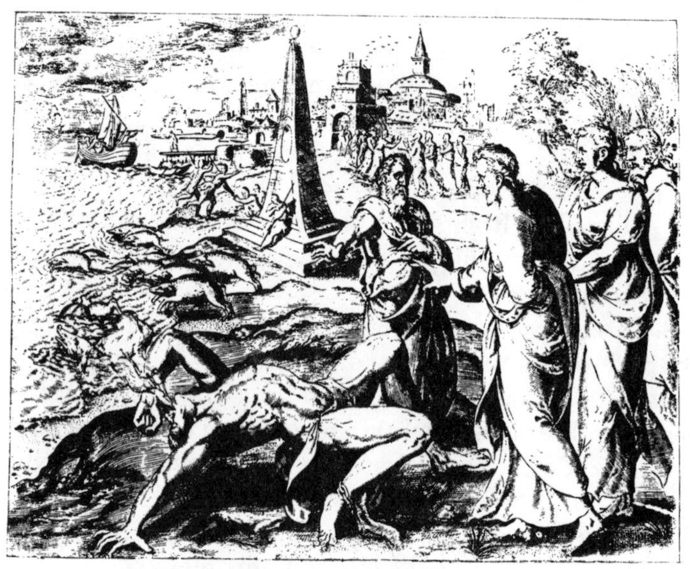

Casting the demons into the swine.

Couthon said, "Do as you will; but your own life will be sacrificed to this false mercy." Couthon left; Pinel began his great experiment in the humane care of the mentally ill.

He commenced with an English captain who had been in chains for forty years. The man had killed an attendant with a blow from his manacles; the keepers approached him cautiously watching his every move. But Pinel walked ahead and entered his cell unattended. He talked to the man quietly and offered him the freedom of the prison yard if he would promise to behave "like a gentleman." The promise was given and the chains cut off. The poor man, for want of exercise, could not walk at first. Finally he managed to creep to the door. And he wept in ecstasy at the sight of the trees and sky.

Within a few days Pinel released from their chains more than fifty men who had been violently insane. The removal of restraint, the kindliness they received, wrought a change in them. They were still insane, still needed careful watching and help, but the violence of their mania, aggravated by chains and brutality, yielded to gentleness. They were no longer rebellious and disorderly.

Pinel's experiment, as we shall see, was destined to spread and grow into a great humanitarian movement which has completely altered not only the care of the insane, but also our attitude toward mental illness.

Pinel and Corvisart were the same age; they were friends, but two men could hardly have been more different in appearance and personality. Corvisart was stocky, round, vigorous, hail-fellow-well-met, and above all, practical. Pinel was slender, frail, retiring, meticulous in manner, visionary in his ideas. Corvisart set a useful, practical example in medical education and in diagnosis; Pinel originated a fundamental ethical change in civilization.

Pinel started his career as a student by entering a school of divinity, but he became interested in philosophy and then in natural history; it was only at the age of thirty that he finally decided that medicine should be his career. For a time he followed the fashions of the day and developed a classification of diseases. But again his interest shifted; one of his friends became insane and according to custom, was locked up and treated like a vicious animal. He escaped and hid in the woods; a few days later his skeleton was found; he had been devoured by wolves. The event made a horrible impression on Pinel; in the hope of benefiting men like his friend, he turned his medical interest to the study of insanity.

Under his influence the prison asylums of Paris, the Bicêtre and the Salpêtrière, became hospitals.

The brutality manifested toward the insane in the closing years of the eighteenth century was dictated by the belief that they were consciously unruly and destructive; that they

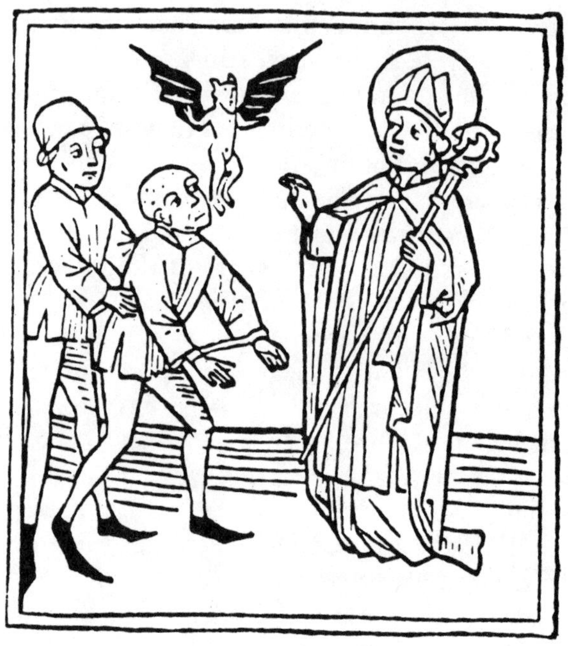

Driving out a demon.

were intentionally malicious. The insane were looked upon not at all as human beings; but literally as wild beasts to be brought to reason with chains and torture. There was no sympathy for them. The men of the early nineteenth century were compassionate to physical suffering and kind to animals; but they had not yet learned to sympathize with the mentally ill. There was no true understanding of the nature of mental disease.

In all ages the attitude toward the insane had been determined by the prevailing view concerning the cause of insanity. Among primitive peoples the insane were often held in high respect as being nearer to the spirits or gods than ordinary men. The insane man in his hallucinations heard voices—spirit voices—that no one else could hear; he talked to unseen creatures. He was superior to ordinary men. Even today in some Oriental countries the insane and feebleminded are tolerated in kindness in the belief that their wits are already in Heaven.

But there was another belief regarding the insane which was to have unpleasant consequences. A spirit might enter a man's body and take possession of his faculties; he would then speak with the man's voice and hear with his ears. The man "possessed" could be brought back to normal only by driving out the spirit with medicine or magic ritual. The idea of possession dominated the attitude toward insanity for thousands of years.

The belief persisted after the appearance of the Christian religion, but views concerning spirits changed. Good spirits could no longer possess men, only evil ones, demons. The good spirits had taken the shape of angels, and although they could guide and advise men, they could not possess them.

Consequently, if the insane man's behavior took on a religious character, if he prayed and mortified the flesh, if he spoke with many holy words, he was not considered possessed; indeed he might be regarded as one deserving to be a saint. But if he were blasphemous, violent, or unruly, then indeed he was possessed of a demon. Exorcism with prayer and ritual was the treatment; if this failed, he might be beaten for his stubbornness in refusing to relinquish the demon.

At a still later date, another belief flourished that brought even less sympathy to the insane. It was the idea that witches made a voluntary bargain with the devil. As we have said in earlier chapters, many of the witches burned were unfortunate insane people.

Gradually belief in "possession" and in witchcraft began

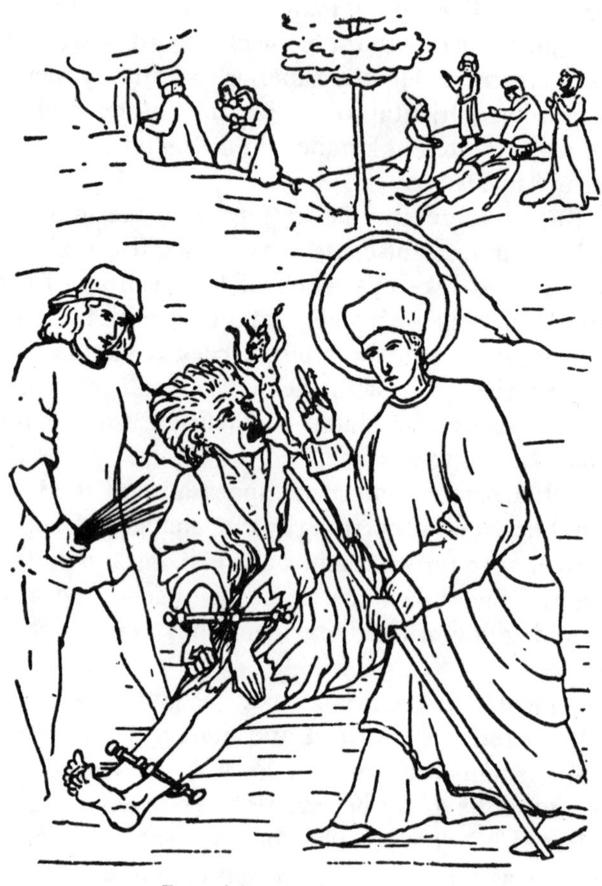

Exorcising an insane man.

to die out. But the lot of the insane was no better; indeed, if possible, it was worse. No longer were demons or the devil responsible for their victims; the victims themselves were to blame. They were like wild beasts: their irrational ways were due to inherent maliciousness. And like beasts, they were to be brought under control by force.

Such was the state of affairs when Pinel asked permission from the French Commune to try the experiment of treating the insane as sick men.

His experiment, as we have seen, was a success. Under kindly care, violence and disorder diminished. It was still necessary to have institutions for the mentally ill, as it was to have hospitals for the physically ill. But these new institutions were to be truly hospitals for care and help, and not prisons.

Pinel's theory that insanity was a mental illness, deserving the same study and sympathy as physical sickness, spread slowly among physicians; here and there an institution was opened for the new treatment of the insane. But the idea did not reach the general population; their attitude remained unchanged; to them the insane were still not human beings.

It was in America that the great reform was extended to give the public the understanding that insanity was a form of sickness. At the beginning of the nineteenth century the United States had one asylum; it was located in Virginia; the hospital of Philadelphia had, as we have said, cells where the insane could be locked up. Forty years later there were eight institutions in America where the mentally ill could receive care, but few of them were hospitals supported by state funds. Most of the mentally ill, if violent, were still locked in barns and sheds, or jails, or county poor farms. If they were harmless, they were sometimes auctioned off to the bidder who would take the smallest sum for their care, or else turned loose on country roads to become tramps.

That was the situation when a seemingly insignificant event occurred, but one that was destined to spread the reform that Pinel had started throughout the world. On Sunday, March 28, 1841, a school teacher of Boston, Miss Dorothea Lynde Dix, was asked to give Sunday School instruction to the inmates of the East Cambridge House of Correction. Here for the first time she was brought in contact with the frightful conditions in the jails of that time. She found twenty women crowded together into one very dirty room. No provision was made for heat, for among them were several who were insane, and because of their violence, a stove was dangerous. Miss Dix was shocked. She decided to do what she could to remedy the condition.

In the forties of the last century aggressive women were

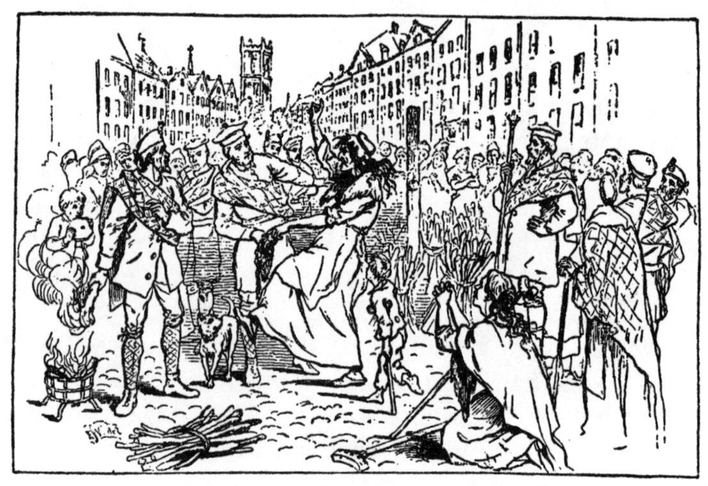

Burning a witch.

not looked upon with favor—a woman's place was in the home, not in public affairs. Accordingly Miss Dix asked a Dr. Howe of Boston to protest in his own name in the newspaper against the brutalities she had seen. His letter had no effect. Miss Dix set out quietly to visit every prison and poorhouse in the state of Massachusetts. It took her two years to do it. Then she wrote a memorial to the State Legislature. It began with these words: "About two years since . . . duty prompted me to visit the prisons and almshouses in the vicinity of this metropolis. . . . Every investigation has given depth to the conviction that it is only by decided, prompt and vigorous legislation that the evils to which I refer, and which I shall proceed more fully to illustrate, can be remedied. I shall be obliged to speak with great plainness, and to reveal many things revolting to the taste, from which

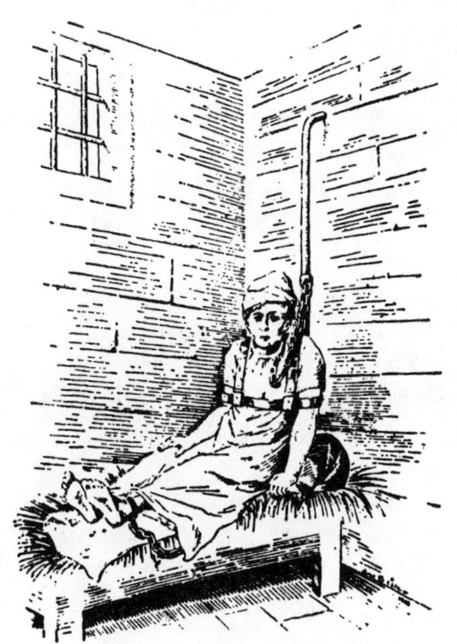

Insane girl in prison.

my woman's nature shrinks with peculiar sensitiveness. But truth is the highest consideration. I shall tell what I have seen."

Her memorial goes on to describe specifically the revolting scenes in the jails and poor farms where the insane were chained in dungeons and often starved and frozen. It was a gruesome document, a veritable indictment of civilization. In response to it, action was prompt; the Massachusetts Legislature unanimously voted to appropriate funds to establish state-supported hospitals and provide humane care for all the mentally ill of the state.

Miss Dix, however, realized that the abuses she had helped to correct in one state still existed in the others. Her work had barely begun. In the next forty years she visited every state in the Union, and England and Scotland as well. Her procedure was always the same—an investigation and a memorial. The response was always the same—the appropriation of funds and the erection of a hospital. In this country thirty-two new state institutions were started as a result of her work, and, what is equally important, under her disclosures the sentiment of the public changed. The people of this country—indeed of the whole civilized world—were made conscious of a grave abuse, and given a new ideal—sympathy for the mentally ill.

In spite of her great work, Dorothea Lynde Dix is little known today. The name of another medical humanitarian of the nineteenth century is much more familiar—a woman whom Longfellow has described in Santa Filomena:

On England's annals, through the long
Hereafter of her speech and song,
That light its rays shall cast
From portals of the past.

A Lady with a Lamp shall stand
In the great history of the land,
A noble type of good
Heroic womanhood.

The "Lady with the Lamp" was Florence Nightingale. In 1915, during the World War, a statuary group was unveiled in London in memory of an earlier conflict, the Crimean War. One of the figures in that group was Florence Nightingale. Except for members of royalty it was the first statue in honor of a woman to be erected in London.

During the Crimean War Florence Nightingale founded

modern trained nursing. She did not found nursing but she made it a respected profession. Women in all centuries had given their services to aid the sick and injured; but they were rarely trained to this calling. The Sisters of Charity of the Catholic Church had from early days devoted their lives to nursing, but in the nineteenth century they were of

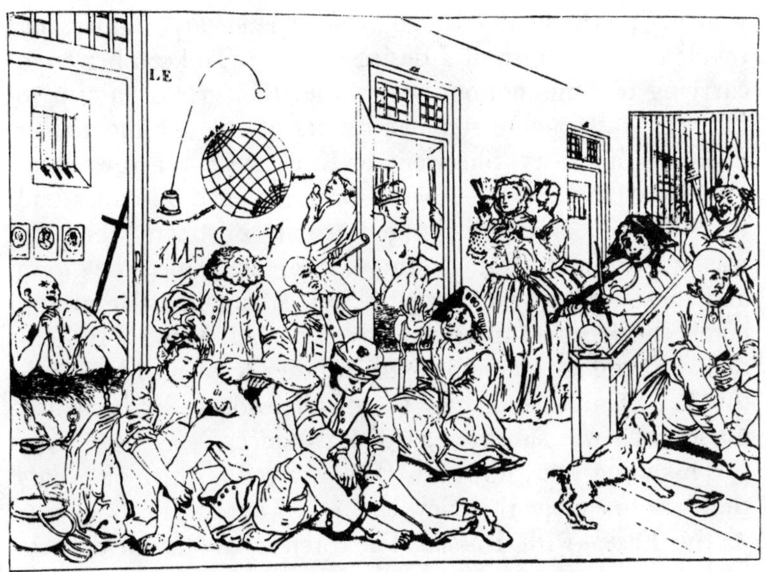

Hogarth's picture of Bedlam.

little practical use in the hospitals of England and America. An absurd prudery had grown up. In consequence a series of restrictions were imposed even upon the Sisters of Charity. They could watch the sick, maintain discipline in the hospitals, but the actual care of the sick was carried out by women who were too low in social caste or intelligence to be ashamed of their degraded occupation of professional nursing. These were the days before Lister's discovery; the hospitals in the hands of slovenly drunken nurses were indescribably filthy. No one went to a hospital when ill who could possibly avoid it; people stayed at home, even for surgical operations.

Florence Nightingale was a well-bred English girl of the nineteenth century, but she revolted against the idea that young women should live at home, without any means of earning their living, and wait to be married. One of her great interests in life was establishing the independence of women. To the utter outrage of her friends and family, her revolt took the form of a desire to nurse. To keep her from carrying out this notion, her mother took her on a trip to visit the fashionable summer resorts of the continent. But Florence ran away. She went to Kaiserswerth, a town near Düsseldorf, where a Lutheran pastor named Fliedner had started a school for discharged female prisoners whom he was attempting to train as nurses. Florence joined the group and there learned the first principles of nursing. Returning home, she became superintendent of a small hospital in London. But though she hoped for it, other women did not follow her example and show their independence by becoming nurses. She was simply regarded as "queer."

This same year, however, there started a series of events that was to change this view entirely. There was talk of war in the East—with Russia. The French and English fleets had steamed to a position at the mouth of the Dardanelles. A year later the western forces had joined with Turkey and the Crimean War began. Today we may turn to Tennyson's "Charge of the Light Brigade" for the story of the war; but in 1854, news of a far less romantic cast came to London from a newspaper correspondent named Russell. Before his reports were censored, he told some unpleasant facts about the conditions of the war hospitals. Among other things he said that there were no nurses whatever to take care of sick and wounded English soldiers.

The public was aroused. A call was issued for volunteers. Women responded; but none, save Florence Nightingale, knew anything of organized nursing. Put in full charge of the entire nursing service of the English Army she managed to collect thirty-eight women, ten of whom were nuns, who knew something of practical nursing. This little band was to care for all the sick and wounded of the British Army.

On November 4, 1854, they landed at Scutari, a suburb of Constantinople. The hospital there was a deserted bar-

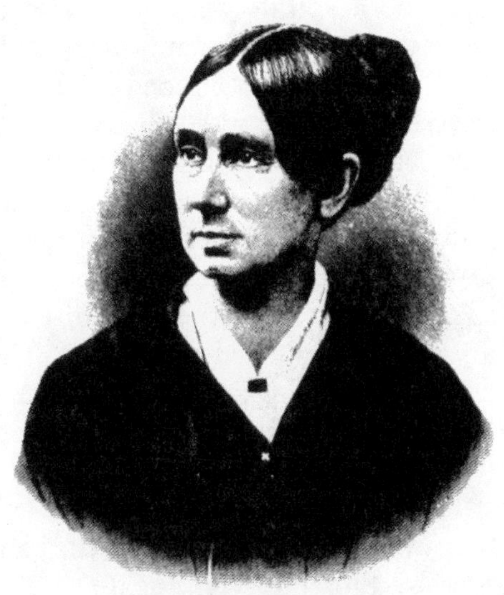

Dorothea Lynde Dix.

racks intended to accommodate a thousand men. Four thousand sick and wounded soldiers were crowded into it. Four miles of beds—and thirty-eight nurses! The beds were bare boards on trestles; there was no other equipment in the hospital. Army regulations required each soldier to bring his own clothing to the hospital; none was issued even to men carried from the battlefield in rags. The windows of the barracks were tightly closed. The floor was rotten and unswept. There was no laundry. The doors were shut at night and opened only in the morning to pass out the dead. There was no one at all to care for the sick during the night.

Florence Nightingale undertook to remedy the situation. She was at once confronted by official red tape. The regulations must be obeyed. But Miss Nightingale, as we have implied, was a strong-minded lady. Her temper was as short as the colonel's; her sarcasm matched his. She took orders from no one; she gave them instead. Supplies were issued; the windows of the hospitals were opened; a laundry was built. To the army officer in command she must have seemed a raging demon, but to the wounded soldiers she was an angel of mercy. No sacrifice was too great in her work of "helping the patient to live." At night she walked through the long wards of the barracks, lamp in hand, ministering to the soldiers. The lamp became her emblem.

In 1856 the war ended. The troopers returned home. Thousands of men carried back the story of the "Lady with the Lamp" to whom they owed their lives. They were the advocates of trained nursing; before their appeal prudery crumbled. Soon funds were raised and schools opened where young women could be trained as nurses.

No practical advance ever made in medicine has brought greater comfort and greater help to the sick than the trained nursing founded by Florence Nightingale.

But her inspiration was destined to lead to an even greater humanitarian reform. In 1859, a Swiss named Henri Dunant stood on a hillside overlooking the battle of Magenta and Solferino. His mind, tortured by the scene before him, turned to Florence Nightingale's work of relief. Could it be extended to relieve the suffering on the battlefield? He conceived there the idea that grew to be the great humanitarian principle for which the Red Cross stands today.

On that June day, Dunant saw the allied armies of France and Italy under Napoleon III engaged in battle with the army of Austria. Forty thousand men were killed or wounded. There was no treaty to protect the doctors of the armies; they, of necessity, followed the troops as the allies drove the Austrians from the field. The wounded lay unattended, deserted except by the people of the neighboring villages. The peasants came with carts; the wounded who had lain on the ground perhaps for days were loaded into them and carried over rough roads to the towns. There were no doctors or nurses to care for them; the women of the town ministered as best they could—but only to their own compatriots. From sheer neglect thousands of men died who could readily have been saved if provision had been made for their care.

Dunant went among the wounded, giving such help as he could. On the altar steps of a church he found an Austrian chasseur, horribly wounded, who had had nothing to eat for three days. He bathed his wounds and gave him bouillon to drink; the man lifted his benefactor's hand to his lips. Dunant, weeping, turned to the women of the town, and urged them to make no distinction in the care of the wounded, telling them that all wounded men were their brothers, no matter in what cause they had fought.

This was indeed a new ideal of humanity—a universal brotherhood with the ill and needy. In the past there had been a few attempts to put military hospitals under a flag of truce, but usually the wounded had been neglected or actually killed. The Knights Hospitalers of the Crusades and the Sisters of Charity had given their services without distinction to race or creed or nation. But Dunant was suggesting something greater—an international alliance which would raise the wounded above all ties of race or nation and make them brothers of every man. To that end he wanted not only the wounded, but the doctor, the nurse, and the hospital as well, to be fully protected by truce of war.

He wrote a book called *Un souvenir de Solferino;* in it he described the scenes he had witnessed, and set forth his ideas for an international alliance. He worked enthusiastically to bring the plan before the rulers of the European countries.

In 1863, four years after Solferino, his efforts were rewarded. A meeting was held at Geneva; fourteen countries were represented. Each agreed to follow Dunant's suggestion. These nations banded together in an international alliance to aid the wounded and to provide succor in time of disaster. They agreed that the injured man, the physician, and the nurse were thereafter to be considered neutrals, and the hospital a sanctuary.

An international army of a new kind—one that was dedicated to the interests of humanity—was founded. That army, too, was to have an emblem, a flag to rally under, a distinguishing mark that would be respected by all men in time of war and peace. In tribute to Dunant, the emblem chosen was the Swiss flag with colors reversed—the red cross on the white background.

HBoerhaave

Part Ten

THE LABORATORY

THE FRONTIERS OF DISEASE

THE GOAL

CHAPTER XXVIII

The Laboratory

IN the nineteenth century a search that had been going on for more than one hundred and fifty centuries ended. The spirits which primitive man had thought responsible for pestilential disease were finally seen and identified as bacteria. When spread out on a thin slip of glass and viewed through a microscope, there was nothing supernatural about these creatures. Quite the contrary; they appeared harmless—merely tiny rods or minute spheres like infinitesimal berries, or slender filaments coiled into corkscrew forms.

Leeuwenhoek, in the seventeenth century, had seen these minute plants through his crude microscope. They were then merely scientific curiosities. Until late in the nineteenth century no one dreamed that they played a part in human affairs. It was the work of Pasteur, Lister, and Koch that brought bacteria into prominence and into disrepute. Since those days we have become painfully conscious of an invisible population of the world—a ruthless murderous population.

But this attitude is totally unfair to the great family of bacteria. By far the greater portion of them spend their humble lives toiling, as Pliny with his teleology would have said, in the interest of mankind. The fact is that without bacteria the human race could not exist. Nothing would decay; fallen plants, dead animals would not disintegrate into soil and so nourish other growths that nourish man. Most bacteria are the harmless benefactors of all visible living things. Most of them cannot thrive on living flesh; put into a wound they would die. It is the unfortunate ability of a few to grow on living human flesh that makes them disease bacteria. The insignificant presence of a few thousand or even a million bacteria in the flesh, does not make them harmful; but rather their ability to grow there, to become billions and trillions until their overwhelming numbers force the body to recognize their presence. The body defends itself; the defence gives rise to the symptoms of disease.

The rogue bacteria, which through the centuries have learned to prey on human flesh, have each their special habits. Some are harmless except in open wounds; and there one kind may produce pus, another blood poisoning. Others cannot live in wounds, and find conditions suited to their growth only in the throat or perhaps the intestines. Different symptoms of disease result from these habits of growth of the various kinds of disease bacteria, giving rise to what are called specific infectious diseases. One kind and only one produces typhoid fever; a quite distinct variety gives rise to diphtheria; while still another produces scarlet fever.

It was Pasteur who taught us the life history of bacteria; Lister who found that they produced infection in wounds; and Koch who showed that they were the cause of the specific infectious diseases.

Louis Pasteur was not a physician; he was a chemist. Born at Dôle, France, in 1822, the son of a tanner, he went as a young man to Paris to the École Normale. There he showed such talent for science that he became an assistant to one of his teachers. Soon Pasteur made an important discovery: tartaric acid from wine existed in several forms; each was composed of exactly the same chemical elements in exactly the same amounts, but when a beam of light from a quartz prism was passed through the crystals of the acid, some turned the beam to the right, others to the left, and still others affected it not at all. This difference, as Pasteur was the first to demonstrate, was due to a difference in the arrangement of the elements that made up the acid.

Thus at the very beginning of his career, he founded a whole new branch of chemistry, one known as stereochemistry—based on the position of the atom in the molecule. His reputation was made, and he was offered teaching positions in other schools. For a time he taught at Dijon and then Strasbourg; but soon he was called to become dean of the

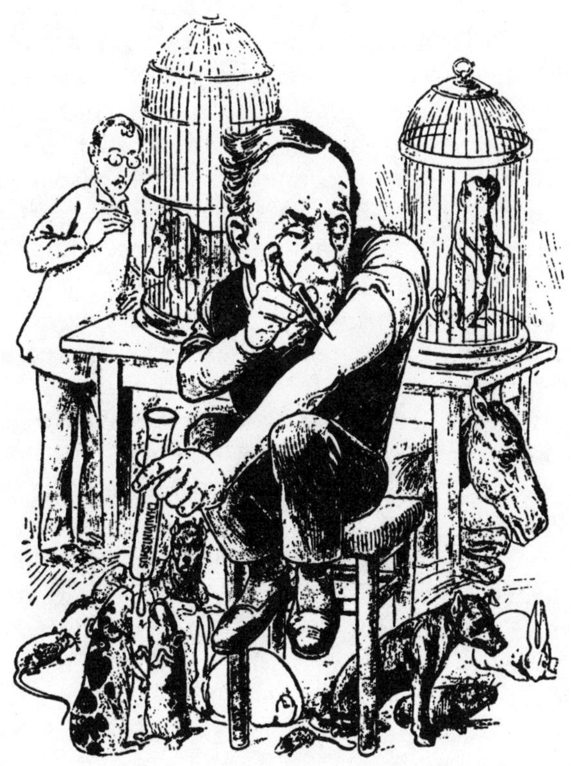

A caricature of Pasteur.

faculty of natural science at Lille. This city was the center for the manufacture of alcohol, and Pasteur turned his attention to the problem of fermentation.

It was known that sugar was converted into alcohol by the action of a microscopic plant called yeast. The living yeast used the sugar for food, and alcohol was formed as a waste product. But there were other changes besides that of fermentation; wine soured, and so did milk; butter became rancid and meat putrefied. Were these alterations likewise due to living things?

Pasteur's microscope disclosed in all souring and spoiling food substances the presence of bacteria. But then came the question: were bacteria the cause of the change or the result; did they produce putrefaction or were they a product of it? Here again was the old problem of spontaneous generation of life. In the seventeenth century Redi had shown that maggots did not arise spontaneously in spoiled meat but came from the eggs of flies. In the nineteenth century Pasteur repeated the experiments using bacteria. Fluids such as wine or bouillon, that had been heated to kill any bacteria already present, did not sour or putrefy as long as air was excluded. But if air containing bacteria was allowed to come in contact with them, putrefaction began as soon as the bacteria multiplied in the fluid. Pasteur proved conclusively that bacteria come only from other bacteria.

The "sickness" of wine was caused by bacteria; it could be prevented by heating—"Pasteurization"—which killed the bacteria. That was a discovery of enormous value to the wine industry; it was the one, as we have seen, that guided Lister in his discovery of the cause of wound infection.

The bacterial population of the world, which up to this time had been ignored, now suddenly came into startling prominence. Did bacteria cause disease in men and animals? That was the question.

Pasteur first applied his discoveries not to human beings but to silk worms. Silk growing, like the manufacture of wines, was one of the great industries of France. A disease had broken out; the caterpillars were dying. Pasteur found out that certain bacteria were affecting the worms and showed the silk growers how to breed healthy stock.

Five years were taken up in the investigation that saved the silk industry of France and, even more important, showed that bacteria could produce disease. By this time other men were becoming interested in bacteria, and particularly a German country physician named Robert Koch. He was twenty-one years younger than Pasteur and when Pasteur was showing that the disease of silk worms was caused by bacteria, he was just beginning his practice in the district of Wollstein. Koch had a hobby; he was a botanist of a kind, but the plants he studied were bacteria. His young wife had made him a present of a microscope; his office soon became a crude laboratory. Between calls on his patients he cultivated his collection of bacteria with all the enthusiasm that an amateur gardener spends on flowers or vegetables. Koch was learning the habits of bacteria, finding out how to raise them; he was establishing the principles of modern bacteriology.

In the countryside where Koch practiced there was prevalent a disease of sheep and cattle called splenic fever or anthrax. It sometimes spread as a fatal malady to the men who handled the animals or their hides. As early as 1849 a veterinary surgeon, examining animals which had died of anthrax had, through his microscope, seen in their blood large rod-shaped bacteria. In 1863 a physician had put some of the blood containing these bacteria into a sheep; the sheep developed anthrax and died. The experiment seemed to show conclusively that the disease was caused by the bacteria; it would have been proved except for one fact. The blood of the sick animals caused the disease even when no bacteria could be found in it. There again was the question that had confronted Pasteur—were the bacteria the cause or the result of the disease?

This problem Koch undertook to solve. In his laboratory he grew the bacteria from the blood of diseased animals; they appeared as long delicate threads in the nutrient fluids which he used for their cultivation. But if a drop of the fluid was put on a piece of glass and allowed to dry, a change took place in the filaments. Dot-like areas appeared on them.

The large bacteria shriveled and died but the minute dots persisted. When these were put in broth they grew like seeds and produced the large bacteria. These in turn multiplied so that from a few of the "spores," as the dots are called, a great number of bacteria could be produced.

Here then was a possible answer to the question why blood from sick animals that showed no bacteria could still produce disease. Only the minute spores were present. Experiments proved that. Anthrax was due to a specific bacterium, but one that had the peculiar property, shared by a few disease bacteria, of existing in two forms. The spores were far more resistant to drying, to heat, to antiseptics, than were the long rod-shaped forms that came with active growth. The spores clinging to the wool of sheep, or to the grass of pastures, could persist for many months. If they were eaten, or if they entered wounds, they developed into the tender rod-shaped form and multiplied. Anthrax resulted.

Koch made his discoveries known. He described the life history of the anthrax bacterium and proved it to be the cause of a specific infectious disease.

In time Koch became the director of the Institute for Infectious Diseases at Berlin, and it was there in 1882 that he made one of his greatest discoveries. He found the cause of tuberculosis. He showed that tuberculosis was not due, as men had supposed, to "bad" heredity or to weakened constitutions; it was caused by a bacterium, the tubercle bacillus. The swellings called tubercles that René Laënnec had found in the flesh of men sick with the disease were the result of the growth of these bacteria. Tuberculosis was an infection. Koch's discovery made possible for the first time the development of means to prevent consumption which until our time has killed more men than perhaps any other disease. Today it has lost its place as "captain of the men of Death"; each year it yields more and more to the efforts which point now to its eventual eradication—efforts to prevent the spread of the bacteria which Koch discovered to be its cause.

After Koch had set the example the bacteria responsible for most of the infectious diseases were discovered in rapid succession—those of cholera, typhoid, bubonic plague, dysentery, and diphtheria, and many others.

At last a means of preventing infectious diseases—by controlling the spread of disease bacteria—had been found. Modern sanitation and modern public health grew out of the discoveries in bacteriology made late in the nineteenth century.

But the discoveries led into other channels as well—treatment and personal prevention. It was Pasteur who by chance observation discovered the possibilities of vaccines. He had isolated a bacterium that caused cholera in chickens and he was growing the organism in tubes of broth in his laboratory. Every few days he would take a drop from a tube and add it to fresh broth in another tube. Left too long, the bacteria by their prodigious multiplication would overcrowd the broth; they would apparently become weakened and, left long enough, would actually exterminate themselves.

A drop or two of the broth containing the actively growing bacteria, given to a chicken, caused it to sicken with cholera and die. But one day in his experiments Pasteur chanced to use an old culture, one in which the bacteria had lived for several weeks. This time the chickens, although they seemed sick for a day or two, did not die. Obviously the bacteria had been weakened by their own overcrowding and had lost their deadly properties. They could no longer multiply in the flesh of the chicken. That was a fact readily explained. But here was something else. Pasteur again gave these same chickens cholera germs, this time fresh and vigorous ones that killed quickly and certainly—but they did not kill these particular chickens. These chickens could not be given cholera; they could eat the bacteria with impunity. Why? The dose of weakened cholera germs had rendered them immune to the disease. Their bodies had been able to cope with the weakened bacteria and had developed protection against a second attack. This was an immunity similar to that observed in nearly all infectious diseases: after we

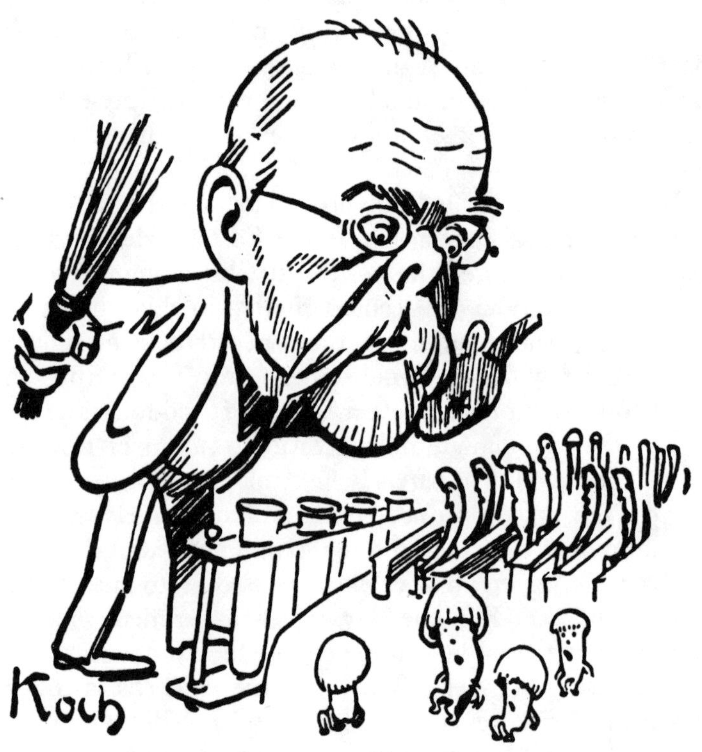

Caricature of Dr. Koch "culturing" bacteria.

have once had a disease we are not likely to acquire it again. Weakened or even dead bacteria then might be used to produce immunity safely, produce it without the dangers of the disease itself.

Pasteur applied his discovery of what he called vaccines to the prevention of anthrax. He prepared a culture of the anthrax bacilli and then made it harmless; that is, he killed the bacteria. His vaccine was a sort of soup of the vegetable called the anthrax bacillus. He injected some of the vaccine into half the cattle in a herd. After a few days he repeated the injection. And then into all the cattle he injected living and virulent anthrax bacteria. The untreated cattle sickened and died; those given the vaccine were not affected. The dead bacteria had rendered them immune.

Next came the question: what change did the vaccine produce in the body—what was the nature of immunity? That problem has not even now been answered fully, but in studying it, one of Koch's pupils, named Emil von Behring, made a great practical discovery. He found that some bacteria, as they grew on the flesh, formed poisons which were absorbed and carried into the blood, injuring the nerves or other delicate tissues of the body. In immunity there was something in the blood that neutralized this poison. It was an antidote or antitoxin. Thus blood of a man who had had diphtheria, because of the antitoxin it held, neutralized the poison given off by the diphtheria bacteria. This antitoxin could be produced in animals by injecting small and non-fatal amounts of the bacterial poison. The fluid of the blood, the serum, held the antitoxin. Here again was a new weapon in fighting disease. In diphtheria—then a prevalent and fatal disease—the child infected with the bacteria was making his own antitoxin, but often not as fast as the bacteria were producing the toxin. Help could be given by supplying antitoxin. Soon antitoxin was used by physicians in all civilized countries; the results were amazingly successful. Diphtheria ceased to be the dreaded disease it once was.

The principle applied to diphtheria yielded equally beneficent results with another and even more deadly disease—tetanus or lockjaw. Infection from this bacterium comes from filth and dirt ground into wounds or carried deep into the flesh in slender puncture wounds such as those made by nails or the prongs of rakes. The disease is so severe and can so readily be prevented by antitoxin that this treatment is now a regular part of the medical care of accidental injuries.

One of the few diseases that rank with tetanus in its extremely deadly nature is hydrophobia, or rabies. And this disease, in time, was conquered by Pasteur.

In 1881 he reported to the French Academy of Science that the virus of rabies is found in the saliva of animals which have the disease. Year by year the progress of his work can be followed in the pages of the papers of the Academy. He told how he found the virus in nerves; how it traveled to the brain and there, acting on the nerve cells, caused madness.

It took weeks or months for the virus to travel from the bite to the brain. But Pasteur could produce rabies in animals quickly by putting the virus directly into the brain; or he could weaken the virus by passing it from one animal to another. And then by taking out and drying the nervous tissues that held it he made a vaccine. He injected dogs with the weakened virus. Then he put with them an equal number of dogs unprotected by vaccination, and turned a frantically mad dog loose among the group. All were bitten. The unprotected dogs developed rabies; those vaccinated did not. Here was a method that might eradicate rabies. Pasteur suggested that all the dogs in France be vaccinated. But there were obstacles; there were stray dogs that could not be captured and there were wolves that harbored rabies. It seemed that, after all, the treatment which offered so much hope might fail of practical use. Pasteur had not then thought of applying the vaccine to men already bitten.

It was the affair of a boy named Joseph Meister that gave Pasteur the idea of using the vaccine to stop the spread of the virus within the body. Joseph and his mother came from Alsace to Pasteur's laboratory. The nine-year-old boy had been bitten in fourteen places by a rabid dog. His death was almost certain. Pasteur was not a physician; he was a chemist. Doctors called in consultation recommended the experiment of giving the vaccine, for the boy was doomed otherwise. On the evening of July 6, 1885, Pasteur made the first injection. He gave ten more. Joseph did not develop rabies.

Soon there was another patient, a shepherd boy named Jean Jupille who, seeing a mad dog throw itself upon a group of six young children, had taken his whip and rushed to their aid. The dog had seized his hand, but the boy threw the animal to the ground, forced open its mouth to release the mangled hand, and although bitten many times, held the dog until he could tie its mouth shut with the whip cord and beat it to death with his wooden shoe.

Jean was treated by Pasteur. He too survived. And today in the courtyard of the Pasteur Institute in Paris there is a statue showing this shepherd boy struggling with the mad dog. But the true memorials to Pasteur, Koch, and Von Behring are not in stone but in human beings who have been freed of suffering—who are alive even—because of their work.

CHAPTER XXIX

The Frontiers of Disease

THERE is a legend of a ghost ship called *The Flying Dutchman.* In southern waters on moonlight nights the sailors saw her, so they said, as, with sails filled, she glided by them without crew or helmsman. *The Flying Dutchman* was an evil omen; her legend was the sailors' picturesque way of expressing their dread of the "yellow jack"—that mysterious disease of the tropics. And there really were ships that became Flying Dutchmen of a kind. Yellow jack—the yellow fever—broke out on board; the crew perished to a man; the ship became a derelict carried before the winds, drifting with the currents.

Yellow fever, so it seemed, struck only at the white man. The negroes on the coast of Africa and in the West Indies never took the disease; only the sailors, soldiers, travelers, merchants who came to those places, died of it. When, just before the opening of the eighteenth century, the king's ship *Tiger* lay at the Barbados, her captain buried six hundred men in two years, although his full crew was only two hundred and twenty. He "pressed" sailors out of every merchant ship that came to the Islands to keep his own crew manned.

Yellow fever, carried in the merchant ships, reached the Atlantic coast of America in the eighteenth century; the inhabitants of Boston, New Haven, and Philadelphia more than once suffered from the disease. In the summer of 1793, nearly ten per cent of the population of Philadelphia died of the "American plague," as it was called. The city resembled London in the days of the bubonic plague. People fled, hoping to escape. New York and other cities posted armed guards to prevent the entrance of anyone from Philadelphia. Burial of the dead was carried out by negroes; they were exempt from the disease; it was only the white man who suffered—or so it was believed.

In reality we know now that the exemption was not natural, but acquired. In the native home of the negroes, yellow fever was a nearly universal disease. Among children, as compared to adults, it was a mild malady. The native children all had it and obtained life-long immunity. But when the adult white man came to Africa, to the West Indies, or to parts of South America, or when the disease spread to northern cities and attacked adults, it assumed its severest form, and the mortality was high.

Yellow fever serves to illustrate what may be called a biological balance between bacteria and man; it also illustrates the penalties of disturbing the balances that nature imposes. What is true of yellow fever is true also of most of the infectious diseases.

Looked at in a wholly impersonal way, there is an element of fair play in the matter of infectious disease. Only a few such maladies are almost invariably fatal, like hydrophobia and tetanus; most are comparatively mild in children; and nearly all confer immunity with one attack.

These are the elements that enter into the natural biological balance that existed when disease was universally present and completely uncontrolled.

A baby at birth carries from its mother a temporary immunity against the diseases to which she is immune. That once meant all the common infectious diseases. For a few months the baby is protected against disease; then gradually the immunity diminishes. One after another in the past the disease bacteria gained a foothold, and specific infectious diseases appeared—measles, scarlet fever, smallpox, whooping cough, typhoid fever, typhus perhaps, cholera, and bubonic plague; and in the tropical regions, yellow fever, and, even in the temperate zone, malaria and nearly always tuberculosis. In all the diseases except malaria and tuberculosis, immunity resulted in those who did not die and even for these two a tolerance of a sort developed. After the baptism of disease the child had little need of sanitation, little benefit from modern preventive medicine. He had paid his tribute to the bacterial world and thereafter he could live immune to it.

But there was one great drawback to satisfying this biological balance which gave safety to the adult. For all their comparative mildness in diseases of childhood, the bacteria often killed. Formerly more young people died than survived to obtain their immunities. Nature took heavy toll of life.

Modern prevention of infection began with the first sketchy attempts at quarantine; progressed with the efforts in the early nineteenth century to clean the towns and cover up the sewers; and bounded forward with tremendous impetus following the discoveries of Pasteur, Lister, and Koch. In consequence the lives of many boys and girls who in earlier generations would have died from infectious diseases were saved. During the nineteenth century the average length of life was doubled.

Save for vaccination against smallpox, the efforts of preventive medicine have been mainly to keep disease bacteria from reaching men and infecting them. In consequence there have grown up generations which, though they have escaped the penalties of disease and lived to adult years, have also lost the benefits—immunity to infection. Our ancestors, with their immunity to the diseases common in their time, were like the natives of the tropics in respect to yellow fever—we today are like the travelers, the sailors, the soldiers, and the merchants who went unprotected to the West Indies and to the coast of Africa.

In fact, this situation is exactly duplicated by the infections that we now call tropical diseases. There are in reality few diseases that are limited to any part of the world. Those that are, are mainly limited because they depend on some tropical insect for their transmission. The tsetse fly, which causes the African sleeping sickness, is still peculiar to Africa, although its haunts have spread. Yellow fever appeared in Philadelphia but could not survive the winter there, for the mosquito that carried it died with the frost. The hookworm of the tropics and of our southern states, likewise is killed in the soil by freezing weather. But diseases that we now often consider wholly tropical—the malarias, the choleras, the plagues, the dysenteries—were all diseases that our ancestors knew well in their northern homes. They have been driven out of the temperate zone by an active civilization and intensive sanitation. But they have not been eliminated; they retreated to strongholds in less progressive regions—the tropics—and there in warmth and filth they flourish.

When the trader of the nineteenth or twentieth century went to tropical regions, he was moving backwards in sanitary history. There he met, not bizarre diseases, but those known to his own ancestors a hundred or two hundred years ago. He found the natives of the tropics living in the natural biological balance with disease, just as the inhabitants of Europe and of North America had lived—but the trader, reared in civilization, had sacrificed his immunity.

True he could shun the tropics and live only in those regions made safe for him by sanitation. But modern progress did not take that path.

Medicine, for its advance, had drawn on the natural sciences; it had developed preventive medicine. Engineering and invention, drawing on these same sources, had achieved the miracles of transportation and communication. The steamboat, the canal and the railroad, the telegraph and the cable, made the once enormous world grow smaller—not in miles but in hours. The journey from England to America changed from months to days; the once distant tropical wilderness moved closer to the northern regions. The frontiers of civilization expanded rapidly and extended beyond the shelter of medical protection. Planters and merchants and travelers now went to regions once known only to explorers and soldiers. The white men met in the tropics the diseases of their own past. The conquest of the tropics meant a struggle, not against men, but against disease.

The tropical fevers bred in swamps were mostly malarias. And malaria was a disease known well to the ancient Romans, widely prevalent in France in the time of Louis XIV, and in England in the days of Charles II. It was the ague, the chills and fever, of the colonists of North America. The first step toward controlling it was taken in the tropics. About 1630 the Countess of Chinchon, visiting Lima where her husband was a viceroy of the Spanish possessions, sickened with malaria. In spite of all treatment she burned with the fever and shivered with chills of the disease. One day an Indian brought her the bark of a tree, the native remedy for the disease. There was a legend that years before a tribesman, nearly dead of fever, had fallen beside a pool of water in which lay a broken tree. Tortured with thirst, he dragged himself to the water and drank. The fluid was bitter with the taste of bark. But something in the bitter water drove away the fever; the man recovered. The bark of that kind of tree became the native remedy for fever. The countess took the bark, and her fever went away. Two years later the remedy was carried to Europe by the Jesuit priests; it was called Jesuit powder, or, in honor of the countess, chinchona bark. Its use was popularized in medical practice by Sydenham. We call its active element quinine.

For the milder forms of malarial fever quinine is a specific cure; it is also a preventive against the disease. Due to the use of quinine and the development of sanitation, the malaria of Europe and North America began to disappear; with the drug, the traveler, the missionary, and the soldier could go with far greater safety into the fever-infested regions of the tropics. But malaria in its severest form still existed there.

The knowledge that will lead to the eventual eradication

of the disease came in 1880. That year Alphonse Laveran, an army surgeon in Algeria, discovered in the blood of victims of malaria a microscopic animal parasite. It was not a bacterium but a single-celled form of animal life. In 1897 Ronald Ross of the Indian medical service discovered this same parasite in the stomach of Anopheles mosquitoes that had sucked the blood of men with malaria. The next year he showed that the parasites were in the saliva of the insect and were deposited in the blood of other men by the bite of the mosquito. Malaria did not spread from man to man by contact as did smallpox and diphtheria—an intermediary was required. This intermediary was that particular breed of mosquito called the Anopheles. The mosquito, considered formerly only a pest, now appeared in a new guise as the carrier of a deadly disease.

The attitude toward the louse and flea and even the common fly was to change just as the attitude toward the mosquito had. As carriers of disease these insects assumed a new importance in the scheme of life.

The discovery of the part that the mosquito played in infecting men with malaria made possible the control of the disease. Eradicate the mosquito; drain swamps; get rid of stagnant water or oil its surface so that mosquitoes could not breed in it—those were the essentials for controlling malaria.

Centuries ago the disease got its name, as we have said, from the Italian words meaning "bad air," for men had long known that the chills and fever came to those who lived near swamps and stagnant water. To avoid the mists and miasma, men had moved to healthier regions. In the closing years of the nineteenth century they learned to avoid the mosquito instead of the mist. The spade and the drainage ditch became the instruments of preventive medicine. The conquest of the tropics began. Typhoid and cholera also yielded before supplies of clean drinking water and the sewer.

There still remained the less widely spread but far more deadly yellow fever. Against it, quinine offered no relief. It remained a constant menace to the traveler in the West Indies and South America; and even in the early years of the twentieth century it reached our southern states in epidemics.

Expanding trade and commerce focused attention on a jungle region of South America. Speed could be gained, miles of journey saved, if a canal could be cut across the isthmus that tied the continents together. Late in the nineteenth century the great French engineer, De Lesseps, who had built the Suez Canal, undertook to separate the Americas. He failed. His engineering skill was adequate to the task, the means were available, but disease drove the workmen from the zone. Yellow fever made Panama "the white man's grave." The tropical jungle spread over the deserted machinery of the French; the railroad they had built rusted and crumbled away. It was said without exaggeration that under each crosstie lay the body of a workman, a sacrifice to the diseases which then had their stronghold in the tropics.

In 1904 the United States undertook to build the canal across the same region. It succeeded. Today the Panama Zone is one of the healthiest regions in the world. It is made healthy and kept healthy by the unremitting efforts of preventive medicine.

Most of the discoveries that have given us means for control of the diseases prevalent in the tropics have been made by physicians in the army medical service. It was an army commission headed by Major Walter Reed that in the year 1900 discovered how to control yellow fever.

The disease was present in Cuba during the Spanish-American War. Many soldiers lost their lives from it. At the close of the war a commission was appointed to investigate it and found that yellow fever was not caused by visible bacteria, or even a microscopic animal parasite. But there was present in the blood of men who had been infected for twelve or fifteen days something that would produce the disease but that could not be seen even under the most powerful microscope and would pass through a filter of porcelain far too fine to allow the passage of the smallest known bacteria. The infectious substance was one called a virus—a filterable virus.

The most important question was: how was the virus transmitted? Dr. Carlos Finlay of Havana had suggested years before that mosquitoes might play a part. Walter Reed and his commission investigated the possibility. They experimented on men who volunteered to expose themselves to the bite of infected mosquitoes or to have the virus injected into their bodies. One member of the commission, Lezear, died of the fever contracted from an accidental mosquito bite in the yellow fever ward of the hospital.

The experiments proved conclusively that a certain species of mosquito, the *Aëdes ægypti*, was responsible for the spread of yellow fever. Its bite carried the virus from the sick to the well man.

This particular mosquito has habits different from the Anopheles that transmits malaria. *Aëdes ægypti* is far more domestic; it lives in water barrels about houses, in the water in discarded tin cans, in sagging drain pipes. It cannot survive the freezing weather of the north, and for that reason the outbreaks of yellow fever in the temperate zone had occurred only in the summer time. The yellow fever mosquito does not fly over long distances; those that had caused the northern outbreaks had been carried by ships from South America or the West Indies.

In 1901 Major William Gorgas put to use the knowledge supplied by Walter Reed and his commission to free Havana of yellow fever. He surrounded everyone who had the disease with screens to keep away mosquitoes, he drained the breeding places, cleaned up the city, screened water barrels, killed mosquitoes. Three months later, for the first time in one hundred and fifty years there was not one case of yellow fever in Havana.

It was William Gorgas, now a general, who carried the same measures of sanitation to Panama and made "the white man's grave" a healthy place to live. But so long as infectious diseases still exist—and they do exist in the jungles on both sides of the zone of Panama—sanitation must continue unremittingly. If the medical measures that keep the Canal Zone healthy today were dropped, in a decade Panama would again be as fever ridden as it was at the opening of the twentieth century. We should not be able to use the Canal for fear of disease.

Today the visitors to Panama see in stone and steel and concrete a memorial to the engineering progress of the century. The medical triumph is not visible, or obvious. The greatest victories of medicine are negative—the absence of disease. Yet without these negative victories—so easily accepted and forgotten—the engineering miracle of steel and speed could not exist.

CHAPTER XXX

The Goal

IN the nineteenth century Darwin formulated the theory of evolution. Man, as well as everything else in the world, was changing, evolving. Human egotism and human hope interpreted change as progress. With scant evidence to support it, the belief was accepted and firmly held that the human race is moving generation by generation toward some desirable goal, improving its condition, growing better, and at the same time making the world a better place to live in.

Progress inevitably involves a goal toward which the progress is made. The mere fact, however, that there may be grave doubts concerning the goals we are seeking, strange to say, does not seem to affect belief in the inherent goodness of progress. Yet in matters pertaining to government, economics, and sociology there are today widely different views as to the desirable goal. It has even been questioned by some people whether invention with its multitude of amazing engineering achievements, pointed to and exclaimed over as the very acme of modern progress, has led us toward happier ways of living. And without a definite goal, progress is purposeless.

Medicine is in sharp contrast to these things. Its goal has never been uncertain. It is the control of disease, prevention of suffering and prolongation of life. That has been its aim since primitive man was first confronted with disease.

We have traced through our chapters the devious course that men have followed in striving for the goal of health. Today, more secure against disease than any previous generation of the race, we can look back in sympathy and pity to the centuries when men sought blindly for the goal that seems now almost within our grasp. Yet it is entirely possible that with the scientific revelations yet to come, future generations will in turn look back to our day with the same sympathy, the same pity.

But whatever happens, the opening of the twentieth century will continue to mark an epoch—the completion of a great cycle in the history of medicine. In these years in the midst of a rapid succession of discoveries, medicine suddenly went backwards. Instead of evolving a new form it assumed one long discarded—that in which the medicine of primitive people had appeared. Medicine, after the lapse of thousands of years, again took up its social leadership.

In the days before civilization medicine had been the preeminent social force. The medicine man led his tribe in its struggle against misfortune. He not only treated the individual patient in illness and injury, but in public ceremony he dispersed the spirits that threatened all his people with disease and pestilence.

Under the influence of civilization medicine shrank in importance. In earlier chapters we have traced the steps in the change. We have seen belief in spirits as the cause of disease discarded; we have seen religion separated from medicine. In that parting, religion assumed the social leadership; to medicine were left merely the maladies of the individual man. The priest in public ceremony guided the welfare of his people; he shaped their beliefs, their customs, their behavior. The physician on the contrary had nothing to offer to the general welfare. His place was in the seclusion of the sickroom. In times of pestilence men did not turn to the physician for protection; they turned in hope to the priest.

It was the great discoveries of the nineteenth century that brought the doctor from the bedside to take his place in social leadership. This time he was not to wage a futile war against the spirits, but armed with knowledge he was to fight successfully to preserve the health of nations—of all mankind.

In the few years of its new leadership medicine has profoundly altered the manners and customs of men, their beliefs, and their ideals.

We have seen the ethical concepts of civilization alter before the humanitarian innovations of Pinel and Dix and Nightingale and Dunant. But the greatest contribution of medicine to public welfare was intelligent cleanliness as a means of preventing the spread of infection. Modern sanitation had its origin in the discoveries of Pasteur, Lister, and Koch. Led by the physician, the civilized world began to clean up, and as it became cleaner the mortality from disease declined and the average length of life increased.

Sanitation extended into every phase of civilized life. The modern sewage system, the inspection of food, the pasteurization of milk, the purification of water, the disposal of refuse, the use of fly screens, refrigeration, the new doctrines of personal cleanliness, antiseptics to prevent wound infection, the individual drinking cup, and the individual towel—things commonplace to all of us—mark the influence of sanitation. Changing laws and changing customs indicate its progress; its successes are proved by the fact that the average length of life has tripled since the eighteenth century; they are felt in a sense of security against disease never before experienced by mankind.

There can be little question that the discovery of the bacterial causes of infection—made so near to our own day—ranks in importance with those fundamental discoveries made countless years ago that are the very basis of civilization—the use of fire, the principle of the wheel, the domestication of animals, the raising of crops, the invention of writing. Indeed, measured by its effects on the conditions of life, the bacterial cause of infection is the only discovery made during recorded history that takes its place among those fundamentals of civilization.

Sanitation has become a basic necessity of human existence. Today when disaster comes upon men, when lands are desolated by fire, earthquake or volcano, the first call is for food; the second is for physicians to institute the measures which control the spread of pestilential disease.

The prevention of communicable disease by the sanitation arising from the discovery of the bacterial cause of infection has yielded such striking results that it has tended to obscure another and equally important social aspect of medicine—health promotion. Health is something more than the mere absence of disease. Health and vigor and growth to the utmost of the individual's capacity come only from satisfying the needs of the body. It has become the duty of the physician to define these requirements and to educate the public. This is his social obligation.

Modern knowledge of food values due to medical education has changed the dietary habits of civilized man. The result of one of these discoveries now greets nearly all babies soon after their arrival—the nursing bottle full of prepared milk. Only a little more than a hundred years ago bottle feeding was almost the equivalent of a death warrant. Even under the best conditions, sixty to seventy per cent of the babies deprived of mothers' milk died. Today, with the knowledge gained of diet, a baby suffers no serious handicap in being raised on a bottle and most of them are at least partially fed that way.

The modern knowledge of dietary requirements came from the same source as the discovery of the bacterial cause of infection—the application of the natural sciences to medical problems. Such terms as calories, proteins, carbohydrates, roughage, mineral needs, and vitamin requirements were only a few years ago the technical words of the research laboratory. Now they are household terms. The public has followed with eager interest the discovery of one vitamin after another; it has seen scurvy, the disease that killed the crews on the sailing vessels of the great explorers, yield to fruit juice—the same fruit juice that for the same reason a mother now feeds to her young baby. Disappearing rapidly, too, is that disease in which the bones became deformed—rickets—for medicine has shown that this once mysterious disturbance yields to a vitamin. This vitamin is a peculiar one—the only one that can be formed in the human body; the ultra-violet light of sunshine produces it. Today the baby has his sun bath, or failing that, he drinks his sunshine from his bottle as vitamin D. Growth-promoting vitamin A has brought green vegetables and butter and milk to the table. And with these foods comes vitamin B, which prevents the disease beriberi and makes the muscle of the intestines more vigorous in its action.

Of the minerals the body needs, iron and calcium and iodine are the ones that medicine has shown to be most often lacking. In consequence, spinach, molasses, and milk have been given a new virtue in the home; and iodine has become a matter of legislation. In some sections of our country the tiny trace of iodine found in most drinking water is lacking; a swelling of the neck, a certain kind of goiter, may develop unless the deficiency is supplied. In consequence iodine is added to the table salt.

Almost as mysterious in action as the vitamins are those peculiar chemical substances described three quarters of a century ago by Claude Bernard—the internal secretions found in minute amounts within the body and poured into the blood to exert, as we know now, a profound influence on growth and health. Through lack of secretion from a gland of the neck, the thyroid, a child will fail to grow in stature and in mind, and will become a stunted imbecile. The dwarf and the giant of the side show suffer from a disturbance of a gland in the skull, the pituitary, the dwarf from too little secretion, the giant from too much. Medical discovery day by day is finding more of these secretions, isolating the chemical forces that control the human body. At least two secretions have already become valuable remedial substances. The child stunted by lack of secretion from the thyroid gland can be made to grow and become normal if fed precisely the right amount of the thyroid gland of a sheep. But few of the internal secretions that have been discovered can be taken by mouth; they are destroyed by digestion. That is the case with the second of the commonly used secretions which is called for in the treatment of diabetes. In diabetes, the pancreas gland, which forms a digestive fluid for the intestines, is diseased. The digestive fluid is formed, but an internal secretion also made in the gland is lacking. The man so affected can digest sugar and starches but cannot use them in his body for fuel—and he sickens. In bygone days diabetes was often fatal. But now it need not be, for medical research has shown that this internal secretion of the pancreas can be used as a medicament and given with a hypodermic needle. It is called insulin.

The doctor of today, for all his successes in the field of social leadership, for all his conquests in the laboratory, still wrestles with diseases at the bedside of the individual patient just as did Hippocrates and Sydenham and all those generations of men who devoted their lives to ease the suffering of their fellow men. His problems still lie before him, complex and mysterious, some of them, as the problem of life itself, but the doctor confronts them today with an experience in art and science that has accumulated in the two hundred centuries our story has covered.

INDEX